Relational Perspectives on the Body

T0386503

RELATIONAL PERSPECTIVES BOOK SERIES

STEPHEN A. MITCHELL AND LEWIS ARON
SERIES EDITORS

In Preparation

Emmanuel Ghent
Process and Paradox

Karen J. Maroda
Surrender and Transformation: Mutuality in Relational Analysis

Relational Perspectives on the Body

edited by
LEWIS ARON
and
FRANCES SOMMER ANDERSON

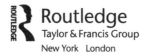

Routledge
Taylor & Francis Group
New York   London

First published by Lawrence Erlbaum Associates, Inc. Publishers
10 Industrial Avenue
Mahwah, New Jersey 07430

Reprinted 2009 by Routledge

Routledge

270 Madison Avenue
New York, NY 10016

2 Park Square, Milton Park
Abingdon, Oxon OX14 4RN, UK

First paperback edition 2000

LIBRARY OF CONGRESS CATALOGING-IN-PUBLICATION DATA

Relational perspectives on the body / edited by Lewis Aron and Frances
Sommer Anderson
    p. cm
  Includes bibliographical references and index.
  ISBN 0-88163-343-7
  1. Body schema. 2. Psychoanalysis. 3. Mind and body.
4. Body, Human—Symbolic aspects. 5. Interpersonal
relations—physiological aspects. I. Aron, Lewis. II.
Anderson, Frances Sommer, 1948-.
 616.89-dc21   1998

                        98-19363
                        CIP

10 9 8 7 6 5 4 3 2

With love,
For my mother,
Gertrude Aron
L.A.

With gratitude to my mother,
Julia Mae Thompson
In memory of my father,
Donald Anderson
F.S.A.

CONTENTS

IV. THE PLACE OF BODILY EXPERIENCE IN THE PSYCHOANALYTIC PROCESS

CONTRIBUTORS

FRANCES SOMMER ANDERSON, PH.D. (EDITOR)
Clinical Assistant Professor of Psychiatry, New York University School of Medicine; Psychologist, Bellevue Hospital; Adjunct Clinical Supervisor, Clinical Psychology Doctoral Program, The City University of New York.

LEWIS ARON, PH.D., ABPP (EDITOR)
Director, New York University Postdoctoral Program in Psychotherapy and Psychoanalysis; President, Division of Psychoanalysis, (39), American Psychological Association; author of *A Meeting of Minds* (TAP, 1991) and an Associate Editor of *Psychoanalytic Dialogues*.

RON BALAMUTH, PH.D.
Clinical Assistant Professor of Psychology, Doctoral Psychology Program, New York University; Adjunct Assistant Professor, Teacher's College, Columbia University; Faculty, National Institute for the Psychotherapies, New York City.

MURIEL DIMEN, PH.D.
Clinical Professor of Psychology, New York University Postdoctoral Program in Psychotherapy and Psychoanalysis; Fellow, New York Institute for the Humanities, New York University; author of *Surviving Sexual Contradictions* and many essays on gender, psychoanalysis, and social theory, and Associate Editor, *Studies in Gender and Sexuality.*

BARBARA K. EISOLD, PH.D., ABPP
Clinical Supervisor, New York University Medical College, New York University School of Applied Psychology, and Ferkauf Graduate School; Consultant for "I Have a Dream Foundation."

LINDA GUNSBERG, PH.D.
Chair, Family Forensic Psychology Training Program, Washington Square Institute, New York City; Supervisor, Child Therapy Practicum, Ph.D. Program in Clinical Psychology, City College of The City University of New York.

ADRIENNE HARRIS, PH.D.
Faculty and Supervisor, New York University Postdoctoral Program in Psychotherapy and Psychoanalysis.

KAREN HOPENWASSER, M.D.
Clinical Assistant Professor of Psychiatry, Cornell University Medical Center; private practice, New York City.

KERSTIN KUPFERMANN, M.A.
Faculty, New York School for Psychoanalytic Psychotherapy and Psychoanalysis, New York City; Clinical Assistant Professor, Department of Psychiatry and Behavioral Science, State University of New York, Stony Brook.

TAMSIN LOOKER, PH.D.
Faculty and Supervisor, National Institute for the Psychotherapies; private practice, New York City.

BARBARA PIZER, ED.D., ABPP
Faculty and Supervising Analyst, Massachusetts Institute for Psychoanalysis; Instructor in Psychology, Department of Psychiatry, Harvard Medical School.

ISAAC TYLIM, PSY.D.
Fellow and Faculty, Institute for Psychoanalytic Training and Research, New York City; Training Analyst, International Psychoanalytic Association; Supervisor, New York University Postdoctoral Program in Psychotherapy and Psychoanalysis; Coordinator, Inpatient Psychology, Maimonides Medical Center, Brooklyn, New York.

HARRIET KIMBLE WRYE, PH.D., ABPP
Training and Supervising Analyst, Los Angeles Institute and Society for Psychoanalytic Studies (LAISPS) and the International Psycho-Analytical Association (IPA). Coauthor, with Judith Welles, *Narration of Desire* (TAP, 1994).

ACKNOWLEDGMENTS

We are both members of the "Postdoc Community"—a group constituted by those affiliated with the New York University Postdoctoral
Program in Psychotherapy and Psychoanalysis. We would each like
to express our appreciation to all the candidates, graduates, and faculty of this remarkably stimulating and supportive community, so
many of whom have had a part in helping us work on this project. We
are grateful to Elaine Martin, a graduate of the Postdoc, for accepting
our invitation to photograph an image for our bookjacket.

At The Analytic Press, our thanks to Paul Stepansky, Ph.D., who
believed in our project and provided enthusiastic support throughout. Eleanor Starke Kobrin (Lenni) has been a pleasure to work with,
especially when she helped us confront all those red marks she provided as an excellent copyeditor. Thanks to Joan Riegel and all the
other staff who have worked to make our undertaking a success.

We have been lucky to work with an exceptional group of contributors, each of whom is making unique, cutting edge contributions
to contemporary psychoanalytic theory and practice. They have
enthusiastically provided high quality chapters, making our job as
editors easier and most rewarding.

LA and FSA

Among the many rewards and pleasures of teaching at the New York
University Postdoctoral Program in Psychotherapy and Psychoanalysis, perhaps the most wonderful is being exposed to many students
who are themselves experienced, seasoned, and creative psychologists who have a great deal to teach in return. I met Frances Sommer
Anderson when she was in a course I was co-instructing at the Postdoc.
Later she took my theory and clinical courses. Students on this advanced level are also colleagues, and Fran was as sophisticated a
clinician as I have encountered. With her rich and varied clinical

experience, her keen interest in the relational dimension of psychoanalytic theory and practice, and her expertise in the intensive treatment of psychosomatic disorders, I found a collaborator and invited
her to join me in this project. It was only as we worked together solic-
iting, collecting, and editing manuscripts over the past years that I
learned how energetic, disciplined, responsible, scholarly, and innovative Fran can be. I thank her for being so consistently supportive
and good humored as she carried on this project during stretches
when I had taken on too much.

Stephen Mitchell, with whom I coedit the Relational Perspectives
Book Series, explicitly suggested that the body was in need of theorization by relational psychoanalysts. Steve has been a good friend,
mentor, editor, and source of continuous support, stimulation, and
intellectual excitement.

My love and gratitude to my wife, Janie, and to my children, Benjamin, Raphi, and Kirya, who are the joy of my life.

LA

I am grateful to Lewis Aron for the opportunity to collaborate on this
book. His infinite patience, flexibility, boundless energy, sense of
humor, and ability to remain focused despite the press of multiple
responsibilities made learning the intricacies of publishing easier than
I dared hope.

My contribution to this project has been enhanced by teachers,
colleagues, and friends. Among many, Jean Hendricks introduced me
to the "mind-body problem" in my first psychology course and, offering enthusiasm and encouragement, reappeared in my life when I
started to work on this book; Arlene Feinblatt, Ph.D. and John Sarno,
M.D. at Rusk Institute-New York University Medical Center, and Eric
Sherman, Psy.D., an NYU Postdoc colleague have been stimulating
collaborators in treating people with musculoskeletal pain for the last
18 years; Joyce McDougall has given unflagging support throughout.
Marcia Lesser and Meeta L'Huillier have taught me much about the
body in the last 20 years. Florence Wilson and Joan McDermott were
ready to help when I needed them. Judith Langis and Desirée Ledet
provided excellent body care that increased my stamina when I needed
to work long hours.

Herzog, Fog, and the late Yitzak, my feline affect regulators, spent weekends beside me as I revised my manuscript and edited the book. Thea Sommer, my stepdaughter, continues to hearten me as she courageously tackles the most difficult obstacles to open communication and personal growth.

To my husband, William Sommer: Your love, your belief in me, and your patience have helped me reach personal and professional milestones I never envisioned. Your integrity, intellectual rigor, sense of humor, and good heart will always inspire me.

FSA

PREFACE

In this collection of contemporary psychoanalytic perspectives, the analysts will be instructive, illuminating, and provocative to the reader who seeks knowledge of ways that the body and bodily experience both construct and are constructed in the relational matrix. Our book is a response to Stephen Mitchell's (1996) call for relational theorists to attend to the place of the body and somatic experience in their models. For an overview of the history and development of the Relational tradition in psychoanalysis, we refer the reader to Aron (1996) and Mitchell and Aron (in press).

When we planned the structure of the book, we invited analysts strongly interested in the place of the body in contemporary psychoanalysis to free associate to our title, *Relational Perspectives on the Body*. In organizing the contents of the book, we created sections to direct the reader to a pattern that we saw in the manuscripts. We emphasize that this is only one of many ways the chapters could be arranged, and we invite the reader to find additional themes.

Lewis Aron introduces the book with a discussion of the body in drive and relational theoretical models. Following this orientation, in Section I, "Relational Constructions of the Body," three relational analysts, Lewis Aron, Adrienne Harris, and Muriel Dimen, synthesize contemporary, sometimes divergent, multiple theoretical trends and influences to provide innovative relational models of psyche-soma integration.

Aron brings together two areas of interest in the psychoanalytic process—the role of the body and the development and use of reflexive self-awareness. He argues for an intersubjective, "two-body" psychology. Integrating the contributions of leading contemporary psychoanalytic theorists and researchers—for example, Bach, Auerbach and Blatt, Fonagy and Target, Bromberg, Davies, Krystal, McDougall, van der Kolk, Taylor, and Young-Eisendrath—Aron delineates the role of the body in mentalization and relates the clinical body to the reflexive mind.

Harris and Dimen have studied feminism and the body for many years. Harris, focusing on "bodies in relationship," describes a relational body that is interpersonal and fluid. She contends that the body is a "complex imaginary construction" rather than the substrate of mind or a parallel to mental life. Harris integrates contemporary relational theory (Mitchell, Bromberg, and Aron), feminist relational theory (Dimen, Goldner, and Benjamin), French psychoanalytic and psychosomatic theory (Green, Anzieu, and Houzel), and feminist philosophies of the body (Brennan, Grosz, and Gates). Dimen finds "flies in the postmodern ointment." She advocates for the experienced and experiencing body, revealed in a two-person matrix, and for a breathing rather than a hungry body in our relational theory-building and practice. She critiques, among others, determinism, Lacan, and Foucault and alerts us to the danger that lies in any theory that throws out nature and overvalues culture.

In Section II, "Linking Mind and Body," the authors grapple with a legacy of determinism—the dichotomization of mind and body. Harriet Kimble Wrye, striving to relink the "entire" body and mind— that is, the body before and after words—elaborates a way to access primitive bodily states of mind in the psychoanalytic process through the maternal erotic transference and the maternal erotic countertransference. This approach requires the analyst to overcome intellectual prejudices toward the body and to attend to kinesthetic and sensory cues in the relational matrix. Linda Gunsberg and Isaac Tylim take up the topic of "ownership" of the body and mind through naming. Addressing the "pregender" body and the preoedipal mother's powerful hold on her child's internal world, the authors review the contributions of Fain, McDougall, and Krystal. Gunsberg and Tylim contribute the concept of "ownership of the body–mind," which cannot be accomplished without bringing the analyst's body and mind into the psychoanalytic process.

In Section III, "The Material Body in the Relational Matrix," we refer to the way the physical body can become a focus in the psychoanalytic process. Kerstin Kupfermann provides the first report, to our knowledge, of psychoanalytic treatment of Munchausen Syndrome, or Factitious Disorder. In the report of her creative, courageous work with a young woman with a history of extreme childhood sexual and physical abuse by her parents and their friends, Kupfermann delineates the techniques she used to facilitate a process of corrective symbiosis by way of symbolic realization. When her analysand developed "colon cancer," a factitious disorder, Kupfermann used a multidimensional therapeutic approach to treat and help resolve this complex symptom presentation. Her contribution will be provocative and instructive for all analysts, especially for those who treat trauma survivors.

Barbara Eisold discusses her work with a young woman with a sex-linked, genetic anomaly that resulted in stunted growth. The woman experienced this and other physical and environmental attributes as shameful humiliations and created an alternative self-state for relief and recreation. In delineating the treatment process, Eisold describes the way her experience of the patient's stature, skin color, and expectations of the world were shaped by socioeconomic difference.

Barbara Pizer addresses another topic that is rarely dealt with in the psychoanalytic treatment process—breast cancer. She openly and vividly shares her experience of having a life-threatening, body-altering illness and reflects on the way that body awareness contributes to the development of the analytic self and the self of the analytic partner. Addressing taboos on discourse about the body, sensuality, and death, she advocates that the analyst address concrete body experiences of change, loss, and felt betrayal. Pizer describes cancer as an "unavoidable blight on dialogue." Her contribution begins to fill an enormous void in our analytic discourse.

The final section, "The Place of Bodily Experience in the Psychoanalytic Process," extends and enhances a theme that runs throughout the preceding sections—the importance of the analyst's and the analysand's somatic experience in the relational matrix. Karen Hopenwasser discusses dissociation, memory, and somatic symptoms in the context of current neurobiological theory and the shift to what she calls "post-Cartesian neurophilosophy." In her clinical vignettes, she stresses the importance of respecting somatic memories in the treatment process.

The last three papers in Section IV grew out of the Body Study Group of Frances Sommer Anderson, Ron Balamuth, Tamsin Looker, and Zeborah Schachtel, colleagues at the NYU Postdoc. Looker, using her experience with parents and their young children, takes the position that "psychosomatic disharmony" is rooted in the child's relationship to the mother's body and, thereby, to the mother's own psychosomatic dissociation. She illustrates the special role of "constructive aggression" in healing this split. She argues that the analyst must surrender to body-based experience and bodily imagery, both aggressive and loving, before abstracting and verbalizing. Balamuth draws our attention to "absence of aliveness" in the psychoanalytic process and traces it to traumatic experience that "dis-members" the body from memory and "lived body experience." He discusses the importance of enactments as a source of lived body experiences that the analyst can use in the treatment process and encourages the analyst to free associate to her/his own body. In the final chapter, Anderson discusses her approach to psychoanalytic treatment of musculoskeletal back pain, illustrating how dissociated affect can lead to back pain and other physical symptoms and documenting the mutative impact of the analyst's affective participation in the psychoanalytic process, for example, through visceral sensations and bodily imagery. She demonstrates the power of the psychoanalytic process to relieve physical pain of long duration without the use of medical, that is, "physical," interventions.

We hope that these relational perspectives will engage you, enliven you, and help you embody new approaches to the age-old mind-body problem.

REFERENCES

Aron, L. (1996), *A Meeting of Minds*. Hillsdale, NJ: The Analytic Press.
Mitchell, S. (1996), Editorial statement. *Psychoanal. Dial.,* 6:1–3.
———— & Aron (in press), *The Relational Tradition in Psychoanalysis*. Hillsdale, NJ: The Analytic Press.

INTRODUCTION

The Body in Drive and Relational Models

Lewis Aron

Commenting on some hypothetical future time when scientific research would narrow "the age-old gap between mind and body," Winnicott (1949) wrote, "I venture to predict that then the antithesis which has baffled all the philosophers will be found to be based on an illusion" (p. 243). Ultimately, for Winnicott, the mind did not really exist as an entity; rather, the psyche referred to "the imaginative elaboration of somatic parts, feelings, and functions, that is, of physical aliveness (p. 244). Winnicott may be seen as elaborating here on an idea that was first articulated by Freud.

In what has become a well-known adage, Freud (1923) declared that "the ego is first and foremost a bodily ego" (p. 26), by which he meant, as he went on to elaborate, that "the ego is ultimately derived from bodily sensations, chiefly from those springing from the surface of the body" (pp. 26–27). As Freud so often used the term ego to refer to one's self, this maxim has been taken to mean that one's self or one's self-representation is first and foremost a bodily self. One's image of oneself or one's self-representation originates in one's bodily sensations and is a reflection of one's body image. For Freud (1915), "the somatic process which occurs in an organ or part of the body" (p. 123) was "the source," not only of instinctual drives, but of one's very sense of self. For Freud the body was central to psychology for two distinct reasons. Our bodies, our sensations, particularly the sensations of our skin surfaces (our "feelings and touchings") are critical in shaping our images of ourselves. This line of thinking leads to a theoretical focus on our bodies and our feelings, or affects, as central in the construction of the self. It is clear that in infancy our bodily sensations are greatly affected by the qualities of the "holding" and "handling" that we receive from caregivers, and so it is not much of an extension to suggest that our self is first and foremost a body-as-experienced-being-handled-and-held-by-other-self, in other words, our self is an intersubjective-bodily-self.

For Freud (1915), the body was also important, however, in that our drives act as a "demand made upon the mind for work in conse-quence of its connection with the body" (p. 122). For Freud, it was the body that drives the mind, and at least in this passage, Freud's acceptance of Cartesian dualism is apparent, although, like the rest of us, Freud seems to have struggled with these ideas about how to conceptualize body and mind. It is important to emphasize that Freud was making two distinct and independent points in this regard: the first has to do with the body's role in the construction of the self-concept and in the experience of agency; the second point has to do with the role of bodily based motivations or drives. Whether or not contemporary psychoanalysis accepts Freud's dual-drive theory, and whatever our philosophical view on the mind–body issue, we may nevertheless make use of the equally Freudian notion that what is fundamental to the construction of the self is the body and its affects. One obvious difference between these two theoretical strategies is that it is easier to conceptualize the impact of other people on the body and on affective experience than it is to see how drives are con-structed by the interpersonal environment, although some theorists have argued for just such an understanding of drives, thus altering the meaning of drives as endogenous motivations (Greenberg and Mitchell, 1983; see also Peskin, 1997).

Very often in psychoanalytic writing these two conceptual-izations about the body and the place of instinct are not sufficiently differentiated. This very blurring of the meaning of instinctual drive and of bodily life and experience may be traced back to Freud's writ-ings. Consider, for example, the following eloquent passage by Loewald (1980). Loewald was discussing Freud's notion of instinct, *Triebe*. Loewald was trying to establish that, for Freud, "instinct and the life of the body . . . are one and the same. They become separate only when we begin to distinguish between soma and psyche" (p. 126). For Loewald, included in Freud's notion of *Triebe* was

> the life of the body, of bodily needs and habits and func-
> tions, kisses and excrements and intercourse, tastes and

smells and sights, body noises and sensations, caresses
and punishments, tics and gait and movements, facial expression, the penis and the vagina and the tongue and arms
and hands and feet and legs and hair, pain and pleasure,
physical excitement and lassitude, violence and bliss—all
this is the body in the context of human life [p. 125].

Jay Greenberg (1991), in what I believe is the most articulate
and lucid discussion of the place of the body in psychoanalytic
metapsychology, suggests that, for Freud, drives were largely conceptualized as bodily phenomena. Greenberg cites Schur (1966) as
pointing out that there was no psychological interpretation of the
drives until long after Freud had discussed them biologically.
Greenberg goes on to argue that the Freudian (1915) idea that drives
were "on the frontier between the mental and the somatic" (p. 122)
was a rather late addition to Freud's thinking and that, even here,
Freud insisted on the somatic origins of the drives. Indeed, in the
famous passage from "Instincts and Their Vicissitudes" from which I
have been quoting, Freud explicitly stated that he was considering
"mental life from a *biological* point of view" (p. 121). Freud and, following his lead, all the early psychoanalysts adopted what Greenberg
termed a "somatic strategy" (p. 100) in building psychoanalytic theory.
In the somatic strategy, all psychological needs are ultimately reduc-
ible to the body and bodily needs. When we have traced the origins
of a psychological need back to its somatic source, then we have
reached motivational bedrock and it cannot be further analyzed. The
body is the very foundation of psychoanalysis. Greenberg makes what
seems to me a compelling case for adopting alternative theoretical
strategies so that drives may be conceptualized as psychological
motivations rather than as fundamentally somatic phenomena (a point
of view recently supported by Peskin, 1997, writing from the point of
view of evolutionary biology).
     If we keep in mind the distinction that I have made between an
emphasis on the body as the source of the drives and an emphasis on
the child's experience of the body as the foundation for the self, then
we may judge these two somatic strategies quite distinctly and independently. Consider Greenberg's rejection of Fred Pine's (1985) assertion that one of the defining features of psychoanalysis is that
"bodily based experiences of drive and gratification" are central components of intrapsychic life. What Greenberg objects to in Pine's definition is the assumption that drives are bodily based phenomena. If
we modify Pine's statement somewhat, however, it takes on a different meaning, one that would be more acceptable even to Greenberg.

Would we not all agree that experiences of the body (rather than bodily based experiences) are central components of psychological life? My point is that, whether or not we subscribe to Freud's bodily based drive theory, we are still left with the psychological experience of the body as fundamental to psychoanalysis. For the sake of clarity, I should also specify that no one, not even the most radical of relational theorists, denies that bodily urges matter in human life. What has been a matter of dispute among theoreticians is whether or not a comprehensive psychoanalytic theory should place drives at the center of its theoretical structure and how best to conceptualize how many drives to posit, which particular motivations are most explanatory, and the relation of these motivations to the body and to biology.

In his final work, *Psychoanalysis in Transition*, Merton Gill (1994) devoted a chapter to "The Body in Psychoanalysis." Relying on the distinction between "the body as such" and "the body in terms of its meanings" (p. 139), he described the former subject as the realm of the natural sciences and the latter as the domain of the hermeneutic point of view. Gill correctly pointed out that Freudian theory, more than other systems of psychology and psychoanalysis, accords sexuality a basic and overriding importance. I want to highlight that whether or to what extent the experience of the body and bodily functions, including sexuality, are given a central place in our theory must be considered independently from the status of drive theory. One may reject Freudian dual-drive theory as the ultimate basis of human motivation and nevertheless maintain that the body, sensorimotor experience, and human (including infantile) sexuality are central to psychological life. Roy Schafer (1983) has elaborated just such a position. While criticizing the classical drive metapsychology, he nonetheless adheres to a Freudian narrative, which he defines as including an emphasis on "bodily zones, modes, and substances, particularly the mouth, anus, and genitalia; and in conjunction with these zones, the modes of swallowing and spitting out, retaining and expelling, intruding and enclosing, and the concrete conceptions of words, feelings, ideas, and events as food, feces, urine, semen, babies, and so on" (p. 224). Thus one may place bodily events, including sexuality, as central to the theory and practice of psychoanalysis without necessarily endorsing Freud's bodily based dual-drive metapsychology.

Gill (1994) made the point, however, that we need to distinguish between bodily zones, with their modes and substances, and metaphoric expression of the ideas of these zones, with their modes and substances. Freudian narratives, according to Gill, are, too often, re-

ductive to the body as concrete and miss the opportunity to interpret conceptions about the body as metaphoric. To illustrate, Gill
suggested that the withholding of feces might be a metaphoric expression of the personality trait of stinginess, but that stinginess, on
the other hand, might be expressed by the withholding of ideas, with
the mind depicted as a bowel and ideas rendered as feces. According
to Gill, "in classical analysis, if stinginess and anal withholding occur
together, the stinginess is likely to be seen as a metaphor for anal
withholding rather than the anal withholding as a metaphor for stinginess" (p. 141). Castration anxiety and penis envy are concepts that
may be used to illustrate this same problem, for each may have both
material and metaphorical meanings. The classical bias is to reduce
the metaphoric to the concrete bodily part or function and to miss
the opportunity to interpret conceptions about the body as metaphors as well.

I remember that when I was in analytic training I would frequently
hear (or tell) a joke along these lines: Students would say that, if you
told a Freudian supervisor about a case organized around problems
related to intimacy, then you would be told about the meaning of this
in terms of the patient's conflicted sexuality. If, on the other hand,
you told an interpersonal supervisor about a case in which the
patient's sexuality played a central role, then you would likely be told
to look at the underlying difficulties in the patient's capacity for intimacy. There was, I believe, much truth to this joke. Both groups used
theoretical structures, metapsychologies, to guide their analytic listening; and, whereas the Freudians tended to highlight bodily phenomena, particularly sexuality, as at the core, the interpersonalists
tended to put interpersonal events at the center and to view sexuality as derivative of such interpersonal experience as intimacy. What
was surface for one analyst was depth for the other.

The interpersonal attitude regarding the relation between such
bodily phenomena as sexuality and interpersonal and cultural meanings was best described by Singer (1965), who explicated and further
developed the interpersonal tradition of Fromm, Sullivan, and Fromm-
Reichman. At one fascinating point in his text, Singer self-reflectively
questioned how it is that, after rejecting libido theory and refusing to
place sexuality at the center of all considerations, his clinical illustra-
tions so frequently dealt with sexual disturbances and sexual sym-
bolizations? He answered as follows:

> The apparent contradiction is reduced if it is clear that the
> rejection of libido theory does not entail a disregard for or

even a diminution of the importance of sexual impulse and
behavior. Sexual disturbances and problems [are con-
ceived] as pointed reflections of wider and more general
difficulties in living, reflections of the person's outlook and
orientation vis-a-vis himself as a physically independent
unit and his concomitant outlook upon others. *A person's
sexual behavior is then seen as a manifestation of his orientation rather than its cause.* . . . . [S]exuality lends itself more
readily than any other behavior to symbolic expression of
attitudes toward oneself, others, and life itself [p. 96, italics added].

Singer illustrated this position by discussing the mythological symbol of the "winged phallus." According to Singer, Freud had suggested
that the connection between flying and male sexuality is a consequence of both flying and penile erections defying the laws of gravity.
Singer argued, by way of contrast, that from an interpersonal perspective there are any number of affective tones associated with flying, such as the defiance of restrictive ties as in the Icarus myth or
the exhilaration of conquering space. Rather than reducing the symbol of flying to phallic sexuality, Singer suggested that flying may be
associated with any number of sexual or nonsexual issues.

   I want to extend Singer's point, since he did not spell out all the
implications of this approach. I see this analysis as leading in two
directions. First, it opens up the realm of symbolic meanings such
that the symbol of flying is not necessarily reduced to phallic sexuality but may take its meaning from any affect stirred up within a given
interpersonal/cultural context. Second, and this is the point that Singer
did not explicate, even if one chooses to connect the symbol of flying
to penile erections, Singer's interpersonal approach does not stop
the analysis at this point; the chain of signification does not end with
our coming to the happy thought of the erect penis. Rather, the erection itself is subject to analysis in terms of the affects and immediate
interpersonal situation that it may symbolize.

   My elaboration of Singer's interpersonal position may be usefully compared to Benjamin's (1991, 1992, 1995) approach to recon-
sidering the place of penis envy in contemporary psychoanalysis.
Benjamin argues that bodily symbols should be understood metaphorically to represent certain relationships (such as certain identifications). One may see the striking similarity to Singer's (1965)
interpersonal position when Benjamin (1991) suggests that penis envy
may symbolize aspects of the ideal love of the father such as "the
embodiment of ideal, but sacrificed, aspects of self, particularly as-

pects of autonomy, excitement, and activity in the world" (p. 418). The similarity between Benjamin's approach and Singer's may be best explained historically by the fact that Benjamin draws on the early criticism of Freud's theory of sexuality by Karen Horney (1967), who insisted that penis envy was not the explanation but rather something that itself needed to be explained. Horney's cultural approach also made its mark on the interpersonalists with whom she was associated.

In what has become, for good reason, a much-cited passage, Mitchell (1988a) has offered several explanations for the centrality of bodily, and specifically sexual, experience as an expression of interactive and relational meanings rather than as a result of the internal pressure of biological drives. He suggests four reasons why sexuality is a central organizer of childhood experience. First, because bodily sensations, processes, and events dominate a child's early experience, bodily events are drawn on and elaborated imaginatively so that the child can construct and represent a view of the world and of the important people in it. Second, since sexuality involves both an interpenetration of bodies and desires and contact with the bodies' boundaries and openings, it is ideally suited to represent longings, conflicts, and negotiations in the relations between self and others. Third, bodily, and especially sexual, experience entails powerful surges that are used to express the dynamics of conflict and interpersonally generated affect.

> Fourth, the very privacy, secrecy, and exclusion in one's experience of one's parent's sexuality make it perfectly designed to take on meanings concerning a division of interpersonal realms, the accessible vs. the inaccessible, the visible vs. the shadowy, surface vs. depth. Sexuality takes on all the intensity of passionate struggles to make contact, to engage, to overcome isolation and exlusion [p. 103].

Interestingly, although Mitchell's background and training are in interpersonal psychoanalysis and while he has championed the contributions of the interpersonal school in many other areas, he (like Benjamin) does not highlight the continuity of his analysis of sexuality and bodily phenomena with that of the interpersonal tradition. In my view, this neglect of the interpersonal tradition in discussions of the body and bodily metaphors in psychoanalysis reflects the fact that, by contesting the fundamental place of the drives in psychoanalysis, and of sexuality in particular, interpersonalists gave up too much and seemingly lost sight of the body. By attempting to differentiate themselves from the Freudians, the interpersonalists may have created an atmosphere in which for analysts to acknowledge sexuality and the body as an area of focus in their clinical work was to risk being viewed as "too Freudian."

A personal story may illustrate the nature of the problem. After graduating from a classical analytic training program, I began supervision with Mitchell in an attempt to broaden my thinking. Soon after beginning, Steve and I noticed that we often came at the material from different angles, and we set out to discuss how we each had arrived at our respective viewpoints. I told him that in my training I had been taught to "think body." I remembered one woman supervisor from whom I had learned a great deal, who told me repeatedly as we would listen together to a patient's free associations to "think body, think sex, think dirty." I still consider this to have been excellent clinical advice. (I might add that it was also useful for me personally to have a woman in authority tell me that not only was it all right, but it was expected and useful, for me to think sexy and dirty. The impact of this advice was heightened by my having a male analyst at the time who helped me to work through the significance of this event. Hence, in my personally elaborated psychic experience, I found a new parental couple providing me with a fresh message about the body and sexuality.) But to return to the story of my supervision with Steve: he responded to me by saying that he felt that in his own training, he had been taught to "think parental character" (see Mitchell, 1988b). The interpersonal position

> stresses the formative impact of parental character. . . . the emotional life of the child is filled with and shaped by the contours of parental character and is constructed out of actual interactions. The parents' issues become the child's issues; the kinds of interaction they make possible determine the metaphors that ultimately are utilized by the child to constitute the intrapsychic [p. 490].

Arriving at this understanding was helpful to both Steve and me, for we could each see how our analytic traditions had shaped us to view the same material from a different perspective. It should be clear that there is no contradiction between the positions; there is no reason why a clinician cannot hear material while listening for both the body and parental character. Nevertheless, our theories and listening perspectives are important because they assuredly guide what we attend to and how we understand what we hear. If classical analysts tend to listen for the bodily, they do so at least partially because of the historical impact of the centrality of drive theory. If interpersonal analysts have tended to neglect the body to some extent, it may well be that, in reacting against drive theory, they unnecessarily neglected bodily metaphors. Whatever we (contemporary psychoanalysts of any theoretical orientation) may ultimately decide about the heuristic value of Freud's dual-drive theory, we may still profit from the momentous legacy bequeathed us in Freud's recognition that a person's very self is constructed out of bodily experience. We may benefit, too, from the therapeutic corollary of this principle that in clinical psychoanalysis the analyst needs to attend to all sorts of direct and symbolic expressions of the patient's experience of the body.

Mitchell (1996) outlined those areas of psychoanalysis that most urgently need to be addressed by relational analysts. He wrote, "In terms of theory, there is a need for rational authors to address more directly those domains of experience with which classical Freudian theory was most centrally concerned: sexuality, aggression, the body, constitution" (p. 2). This book, *Relational Perspectives on the Body,* emerged out of this call for renewed attention to the place of the body and somatic experience within a relational paradigm.

Psychoanalysis (across all of its various schools) has increasingly moved in a relational direction. Simultaneously with this shift from a drive-centered to a relational theory, the profession of psychoanalysis has undergone a demedicalization, which may have further shifted the attention of psychoanalysis away from the body. Nonmedically trained analysts may well have felt less sure of themselves in attending to and studying bodily based and psychosomatic phenomena. It is the intention of this book to bring the focus of psychoanalysis back to the body, to the bodily rooted self, to bodily based communication, to bodily and affective experience, and to somatic and psychosomatic phenomena, now all viewed in a relational context.

REFERENCES

Benjamin, J. (1991), Father and daughter: Identification with difference—A contribution to gender heterodoxy. *Psychoanal. Dial.,* 1:277–299.
———— (1992), Reply to Schwartz. *Pschoanal. Dial.,* 2:417–424.
———— (1995), *Like Subjects, Love Objects.* New Haven, CT: Yale University Press.
Freud, S. (1915), Instincts and their vicissitudes. *Standard Edition,* 14:117–140. London: Hogarth Press, 1957.

—— (1923), The ego and the id. *Standard Edition,* 19:3–68. London: Hogarth Press, 1961.

Gill, M. M. (1994), *Psychoanalysis in Transition.* Hillsdale, NJ: The Analytic Press.

Greenberg, J. (1991), *Oedipus and Beyond.* Cambridge, MA: Harvard University Press.

—— & Mitchell, S. (1983), *Object Relations in Psychoanalytic Theory.* Cambridge, MA: Harvard University Press.

Horney, K. (1967), *Feminine Psychology.* New York: Norton.

Loewald, H. W. (1980), *Papers on Psychoanalysis.* New Haven, CT: Yale University Press.

Mitchell, S. (1996), Editorial statement. *Psychoanal. Dial.,* 6:1–3.

—— (1988a), *Relational Concepts in Psychoanalysis.* Cambridge, MA: Harvard University Press.

—— (1988b), The intrapsychic and the interpersonal: Different theories, different domains, or historical artifacts? *Psychoanal. Inq.,* 8:472–496.

Peskin, M. M. (1997), Drive theory revisited. *Psychoanal. Quart.,* 66:377–402.

Pine, F. (1985), *Developmental Theory and Clinical Process.* New Haven, CT: Yale University Press.

Schafer, R. (1983), *The Analytic Attitude.* New York: Basic Books.

Schur, M. (1966), *The Id and the Regulatory Principles of Mental Functioning.* New York: International Universities Press.

Singer, E. (1965), *Key Concepts in Psychotherapy.* New York: Basic Books, 1970.

Winnicott, D. W. (1949), Mind and its relation to the psyche-soma. In: *Through Paediatrics to Psycho-Analysis.* New York: Basic Books, 1975, pp. 243–254.

PART I

*Relational Constructions
of the Body*

1

THE CLINICAL BODY
AND THE REFLEXIVE MIND

Lewis Aron

The body, bodily sensations, bodily experience, bodily metaphor, and bodily imagery play a central role in the psychoanalytic process. The psychoanalytic process, however, is often thought to be quintessentially an exercise in the use, development, and enhancement of reflexive self-awareness or psychological mindedness. In this chapter, I bring together these two broad areas of study: the role of the body in the psychoanalytic enterprise and the self-reflexive function of the mind: the clinical body and the reflexive mind. I focus our attention on the place of the body in the mind's self-reflexive functioning, and the effects on the body when self-reflexive functioning is impaired. Extending this to the realm of the intersubjective, I will consider the mutual impact of the mind and the body on each other as the psychoanalytic situation entails two individuals jointly processing, experiencing, and reflecting on psychosomatic phenomena. Hence, whereas I have previously elaborated on a meeting of minds (Aron, 1996), here I describe the mutual interplay of body–mind and mind–body (Grotstein, 1997), a sort of return from a *two-person psychology* to Rickman's original idea of a two-body psychology (cited in Balint, 1950, p. 123).

Self-reflexivity (the capacity to experience, observe, and reflect on oneself as both a subject and an object) is at the very heart of the

My thanks to Fran Sommer Anderson, John S. Auerbach, Stephen A. Mitchell, and J. Christopher Muran who made valuable contributions to this chapter.

clinical psychoanalytic process, and in this chapter I explore the body's role in self-reflexive functioning as well as the body's involvement when self-reflexive functioning fails. The construction of a bodily self requires self-reflexivity, and self-reflexivity emerges through intersubjectivity. On the other hand, under normal conditions, intersubjectivity (and for that matter any subjectivity) is always embodied. Trauma is responsible for disruptions in the development of self-reflexivity, intersubjectivity, and embodiment. I believe that research into and clinical study of self-reflexivity (and especially the relationship among self-reflexivity, intersubjectivity, embodiment, and trauma) is among the most promising areas of psychological research and psychoanalytic investigation taking place today.

SELF-REFLEXIVE FUNCTIONING, MENTALIZATION, AND PSYCHOLOGICAL MINDEDNESS: AN OVERVIEW

To begin with, my technical use of the term self-reflexivity needs to be carefully distinguished from the more usual understanding of self-reflection. Self-reflection ordinarily connotes a cognitive process in which one thinks about oneself as if from the outside, that is, as if examining oneself as an object of thought. The way I am using self-reflexivity here, by contrast, includes the dialectical process of experiencing oneself as a subject as well as of reflecting on oneself as an object. It is not, therefore, exclusively an intellectual observational function, but an experiential and affective function as well.

My understanding of self-reflexivity has been decisively shaped by the writings of Sheldon Bach (1985, 1994), although, in recent years, the topic of self-reflexivity has emerged at the cutting edge of psychoanalytic thought and has been taken up by numerous theorists from divergent points of view. I am particularly indebted to the work of John Auerbach and Sidney Blatt (Auerbach, 1993; Auerbach and Blatt, 1996) which, like mine, was heavily influenced by the earlier work of Bach. But I also believe that there is a convergence of interest taking shape in this area as seen in Peter Fonagy and Mary Target's (Fonagy and Target, 1995, 1996, 1998; Target and Fonagy, 1996) fascinating studies of reflective mental functioning, or what they call the person's capacity for "mentalization," as well as with a good deal of what we have been learning about the impact of trauma on thinking, states of consciousness, self-regulation, and dissociation (Bromberg, 1996; Davies, 1996; Krystal, 1988; van der Kolk, 1996); on related developments in the study of psychosomatics and alexithymia (Nemiah and Sifneos, 1970; Taylor, 1992a, b); and on understanding the ways in which people benefit from psychoanalysis itself, especially in clarifying what is meant by what we commonly refer to as "psychological mindedness" (McCallum and Piper, 1997).

Self-reflexive functioning is the basis on which participation in the psychoanalytic process rests for both the patient and the analyst. Self-reflexive functioning is also a critical psychological capacity that is impaired in different ways across the various psychopathological forms as a result of psychological conflict, deficit, and trauma. In this chapter, I discuss the role of the body in mentalization and relate the clinical body to the reflexive mind.

SELF-REFLEXIVE FUNCTIONING

I am using the technical term self-reflexivity in a very specific way to refer to the mental capacity to move back and forth, and to maintain the tension, between a view of the self as a subject and a view of the self as an object. The distinction between these two perspectives on the self can be traced back very clearly at least to William James's (1890) distinction between the I and the me.[1] James described the "me" aspects of self as the actual qualities that define the self-as-known. These include, for James, material (body, possessions), social (roles and relations), and spiritual characteristics (consciousness and psychological mechanisms). The "me" in James's theory of the self refers to the person's self-concept, all that a person can know about oneself through one's own observations or through feedback from others. In this sense, the "me" has been referred to as the more objective aspect of the self. Interestingly, in regard to my focus in this essay, James believed that the body and the "bodily me" lie at the bottom of the hierarchy formed by these constituents of the "me" and provide the structural basis to the "me." In this respect, James's ideas about the self anticipated those of Freud as I will describe later.[2]

For James, the "I" refers to the self-as-knower in that the essence of the "I" is its subjectivity.[3] The "me" is often referred to as the objective self and the "I" referred to as the subjective self. I think that this terminology is misleading because it does not make clear how we might think of the self-concept as objective. I suggest that it is much clearer and closer to James's meaning to refer to James's "me" as the sense of the "self-as-object," and to the "I" as the "self-as-subject." James's theory of the self, then, is a comprehensive one that includes a) the sense of the self-as-subject, the "I," as an integrated experience of agency, continuity, distinctness, and reflection constituting the self that initiates, organizes and interprets experience, and b) the self-as-object, the "me," the self as observed by a subject, which forms the basis of the self-concept.[4]

Bach (1985) distinguishes between "subjective awareness" and "objective self-awareness." According to Bach, in certain states of consciousness, which he refers to as subjective awareness, we are totally immersed in our own thoughts and actions; in these states, we are aware of ourselves as agents or the subjects of thought and action. In contrast, there are other states of consciousness, referred to as objective self-awareness, in which we take our selves as the objects of our thoughts or actions.

> Thus, one might say that the child is confronted with the double or complementary task of establishing a sense of self as a center for action and thought and of viewing this self in the context of other selves as a thing among other things. What is required is both a subjectification and an objectification, two different perspectives on the same self [p. 53].

Bach (1985, 1994) suggests that a good deal of narcissistic and borderline pathology, including such structurally related conditions as perversions, addictions, eating disorders, and psychosomatic disorders, may be best understood in terms of the patient's inability to maintain appropriate tension between these two perspectives on the self. When immersed in a state of consciousness of subjective awareness, the self is experienced as the agent, in Kohut's (1977) words, as "a center of initiative and a recipient of impressions" (p. 99). At the extreme, this may lead a patient to experience grandiosity and a sense of entitlement and be unable to experience the self as an object among other objects or a self among other selves. When immersed in the state of consciousness of objective self-awareness, the patient can view himself or herself only as an object among other objects and cannot experience the sense of agency or vitality that comes with being a subject, a distinct center of thoughts, feelings, and actions. Although some patients (with certain forms of pathology) are more apt to maintain one side of this polarity over another (for example, overinflated narcissists tend to maintain states of subjective awareness, whereas depressives tend to maintain states of objective self-awareness), nevertheless, according to Bach, the real problem with all of these patients is that they have persistent difficulties moving back and forth between the two perspectives on the self and integrating them into their representational world.

Bach (1994) proposes that it is an important developmental achievement for a person "to integrate his sense of wholeness and aliveness (subjective awareness) with his parent's and his own developing perspective on himself as one person among many others (objective self-awareness)" (p. 46). Accordingly, psychopathology is understood as a person's inability to tolerate ambiguity and paradox, to deal with metaphor, or to maintain multiple points of view, especially about the self.[5] Instead, in psychopathology, we find polarization, splitting, either-or thinking, manic and depressive mood swings, and sadomasochistic role reversals.[6]

Auerbach and Blatt (Auerbach, 1993; Auerbach and Blatt, 1996) have drawn on Bach's and others' work to elaborate what they refer to as self-reflexivity. Reflexive self-awareness, or self-reflexivity, is the capacity to move easily between subjective and objective perspectives on the self, or to put this in the terms that I prefer, self-reflexivity refers to the capacity to maintain the dynamic tension between experiencing oneself as a subject and as an object. Auerbach (1993) suggests that these two experiences of the self are fundamentally incompatible:

> Because one cannot simultaneously regard oneself as an object and immerse oneself in one's own subjectivity, except perhaps during mystical experiences or states of ecstasy, and because these two modalities for self-knowledge can result in highly discrepant self-images, the capacity for reflexive self-awareness necessarily produces psychological tension and conflict, especially about one's conception of oneself [p. 77].

Auerbach, following Bach, goes on to elaborate narcissism as an attempt to escape the conflicts that result from self-reflexivity. He writes, "Kernberg's narcissists, in their shameless grandiosity and entitlement, overemphasize subjective self-awareness; Kohut's narcissists, in their shame ridden hypersensitivity, vulnerability, and submissiveness, overemphasize objective self-awareness" (p. 83). Once again, to put this into somewhat different terms, those narcissists who overemphasize subjective awareness tend to view themselves only as a subject, and not as one object among other objects or one subject among other subjects, for to view oneself as a subject among other subjects is to objectify oneself. Because they do not see themselves as one among many, they appear to be grandiose and to have a sense of entitlement. Those narcissists who emphasize objective self-awareness tend to view themselves predominantly as one object among many, without experiencing themselves as a subject, agent, or center of initiative. Therefore, they seem to be vulnerable and fragile, with little sense of control over their lives, an inability to will.

The Auerbach and Blatt (1996) study is extremely rich and has many implications regarding the body's role in the establishment of the self-representation and in self-reflexivity. I cannot review the study in detail here, but, before moving on, I do want to highlight two issues that have particular relevance to the body. First, Auerbach and Blatt make the interesting distinction between two different dynamic explanations for bodily self-mutilation. They suggest that, because people with schizophrenia lack a sense of embodiment, attacks on the body are not experienced as attacks on the self, although the schizophrenic may be attempting to establish some sense of existence in attacking his or her body.[7] Borderlines, in contrast, who do have a core sense of self, are often attempting to overcome the depersonalization or dissociation that excessive self-focus can elicit. Borderline persons have an impaired ability to regulate their self-reflexive function, and they attempt to augment this self-regulation through a concrete enactment that restores some sense of themselves as feeling subjects.

Another area that is dealt with in a most interesting way by Auerbach and Blatt concerns the impact of bodily changes during adolescence on self-reflexive functioning, which itself undergoes dramatic transformation during adolescence because of the advent of new cognitive abilities at that time. To summarize very briefly, genital maturity tends to coincide with the emergence of a systematic mode of self-reflection under the influence of formal operational thought. Adolescents must then integrate bodily experiences and urges into their body image and self-representation. Doing so requires integrating subjective awareness and objective self-awareness. It is a particular challenge to those schizoid adolescents who have not established a core sense of themselves prior to adolescence and who, under the influence of newly formed cognitive operations, desperately look inward in search of vitality, agency, and selfhood, but who find instead only inner deadness, confusion, and ultimately psychosis.

Thomas Ogden (1997), while not writing from the empirical research tradition, has reached conclusions that are remarkably similar to those I have been discussing. He writes beautifully and poetically:

Self-reflective thought occurs when "I" (as subject) look at "me" (as object). Metaphor is a form of language in which I describe "me" so that "I" might see myself. In an important sense, naming and describing "me" metaphorically creates both "I" and "me" as interdependent aspects of human self-awareness (human subjectivity). In other words, the individual (as object) is invisible to the self (as subject) until metaphors for "I" are used to describe or create "me" so that "I" can see myself. This is the mutually creating dialectic of "I" and "me" [p. 727].

Mentalization and Metacognitive Monitoring

In an important series of papers, Fonagy and Target (1995, 1996, 1998; Target and Fonagy, 1996) have described a psychoanalytic model of the development of the "theory of mind," or what they call, more broadly, "mentalization" or "reflective or psychological self-functioning." They believe that this is a "central intrapsychic and interpersonal achievement" and that "this capacity to reflect on feelings and thoughts is built up through an intersubjective process between infant and parent, child and adult, child and sibling." Furthermore, it is their contention that this reflective self-functioning is at the core of the self-structure (Target and Fonagy, 1996, p. 461). Reflective self-functioning implies the ability to understand another's state of mind as a state of mind. It entails the ability to understand mental states as essentially propositional and intentional, that is, entailing beliefs and wishes.

Target and Fonagy (1996) expressly link their contributions to the interpersonal and self-psychological traditions in that these theories have been most explicit regarding their assumption that self-development is an interpersonal process requiring interaction with the minds of others (p. 474). "Unconsciously and pervasively, the caregiver ascribes a mental state to the child with her behavior, this is gradually internalized by the child, and lays the foundations of a core sense of mental selfhood" (p. 461). The caregivers, in their empathy with the child, think about the child's needs and behaviors and thus demonstrate to the child that they think of him or her as an intentional being whose behavior is driven by thoughts, feelings, beliefs, and desires. In so doing, they give meaning to the child's actions and thereby facilitate a sense of mental agency or an intentional stance in the child, who, by thinking about the other's thoughts, comes, like the caregiver, to think about mental experiences.[8]

Fonagy and his colleague's description of "mentalization" builds on the work of Mary Main and her colleagues (Main, 1991; Main and Hesse, 1990), who demonstrated that the strongest indication of the sense of a secure self in adulthood is the person's ability to reflect on experience, a capacity that Main refers to as "metacognitive monitoring." In responding to the Adult Attachment Interview (AAI), people who have this capacity are capable of speaking about their memories of early attachment relationships in a manner that suggests prior reflection and integration as well as the ability to think with some flexibility and openness about the experiences as they are speaking. In a variety of studies conducted by Fonagy and his colleagues, this capacity for metacognitive processing, or reflective self-awareness, has been found to be even more significant in determining health or pathology than is the quality of the attachment experiences that are remembered. Fonagy and his colleagues have been able to demonstrate that children who are securely attached to at least one parent develop a theory of mind earlier than do children who are insecurely attached, and their capacity for self-reflection is less disrupted in emotionally charged situations. Furthermore, the capacity for self-reflective functioning in parents is highly protective of their children's mental health; even parents who themselves suffered loss and abuse in childhood, but who are nevertheless high in reflective self-functioning, tend to have children who are securely attached (Coates, 1998; Fonagy and Target, 1998; Seligman, 1998).

These writers, very much like Auerbach and Blatt (1996), also point to the connection between aggression aimed at the body and failures in mentalization or reflective-self functioning. Just as Auerbach and Blatt suggested that self-mutilation becomes a way for patients who are unable to regulate their reflexive awareness to enhance subjective awareness or to establish some sense of a bodily self, so too Fonagy and Target point out that patients who cannot mentalize may seek identifications or create representations of mental states through the body. "Violence, aggression directed against the body, may be closely linked to failures of mentalisation, as the lack of capacity to think about mental states may force individuals to manage thoughts, beliefs, and desires in the physical domain, primarily in the realm of body states and processes" (Fonagy and Target, 1995, p. 487).

Psychosomatosis, Trauma, and the Self-Reflexive Function: Psychosomatics.

The field of psychosomatic studies has transformed itself in recent years.[9] Beginning with Freud's observations about conversion hysteria— technically not a psychosomatic disease because there is no actual organic dysfunction—psychosomatic specialists were interested in the ways in which social and psychological factors were important in the etiology, development, and maintenance of many illnesses as well as in their treatments. Freud viewed conversion symptoms as expressions of unconscious symbolic tensions, and this became a model for future psychosomatic investigation as it was developed within a psychodynamic framework. Alexander (1950) expanded on the idea that specific illnesses were caused by unconscious, internal conflicts, and a psychoanalytic approach dominated psychosomatic medicine until the 1960s. On the basis of his own clinical psychoanalytic observations, Alexander proposed that each of the classic psychosomatic disorders had its own specific dynamic conflicts or personality characteristics; hence his theory became known as specificity theory.

Beginning in the late 1950s, much dissatisfaction with the psychoanalytic approach arose within psychosomatic medicine because of numerous methodological weaknesses, including that much of the theory was based on clinical observation alone and what seemed like the circular reasoning of psychoanalytic formulations. Perhaps most important, the anticipated efficacy of psychoanalytic treatment for the physically ill failed to materialize. With the publication of Harold Wolff's (1953) *Stress and Disease,* the field began to shift to what he called a psychophysiological approach in an effort to distance his approach from that of the psychodynamicists. Today the field generally refers to itself as the study of psychophysiological disorders, and it studies not just the classical psychosomatic disorders but any physical condition that is affected by psychological factors. A diathesis-stress model of illness is generally used in an attempt to integrate social, psychological, environmental, genetic, and physiological elements of disease (Gatchel, 1993).

In the meantime, in their clinical practices, psychoanalytic clinicians continued to observe and study psychosomatic phenomena and have developed a number of interesting and useful propositions. A few of the recent findings arising within a psychoanalytic framework can be specifically related to self-reflexive functioning.

An important area with which we may begin is the study of alexithymia. The work of a number of French psychosomaticists of the so-called Paris school (researchers in psychosomatic medicine with a psychodynamic orientation) gave rise to the concept of operatory thinking (*la pensee operatoire*), which refers to pragmatic and affectless, delibidinized thinking. Out of the findings of the Paris school emerged further research by psychosomaticists in Boston

(Nemiah and Sifneos, 1970), who subsequently developed the concept of alexithymia, a term that refers to a deficiency in emotional recognition and expressiveness. While these researchers emphasized neuroanatomical considerations, Joyce McDougall (1989), who popularized much of this work on psychosomatics in psychoanalytic circles, emphasized the ways in which alexithymia and operatory thinking, much of which she prefers to call "disaffectation," serve defensive purposes against inexpressible pain and fears of a psychotic nature.

McDougall suggests that feelings that are not processed in language can activate somatic problems. Utilizing an earlier concept of Freud's, McDougall describes these patients as using "foreclosure" to wipe out certain experiences from the mind. McDougall finds that these patients, who appear detached, flat in their affect, and mechanical, robotic, or "normotic" in their presentation, did in fact, experience overwhelming emotions that threatened to attack their sense of identity. Unable to repress or project these feelings, they ejected them from consciousness. These patients are unable to fantasize or even to dream, and they suffer from psychosomatic breakdown. According to McDougall, "emotion is essentially psychosomatic" (p. 95). Thus, when the psychological aspect of an emotion is ejected, the physiological part is left to express itself, leading to "psychosomatic explosions."

This aspect of McDougall's work draws on and elaborates the proposals of Henry Krystal, whose contributions to a psychoanalytic theory of affect development, trauma, and "psychosomatosis" (a term introduced by McDougall, 1989) are crucial. In a breathtaking monograph, Krystal (1988) suggests that affects are initially experienced as bodily sensations and only gradually evolve into subjective states that are verbally articulated. Affects undergo developmental transformation as they become increasingly differentiated, articulated, and desomatized. Very much as we have seen in examining the work of Fonagy and Target on the development of mentalization, Krystal emphasizes the intersubjective origins of these developments: it is the caregiver's empathy and attuned responsiveness that fosters the development of bodily states becoming verbally articulated, leading to the experience of affects as mental and not only bodily phenomena.

Here I want to emphasize Krystal's (1988) understanding of the role of reflective self-awareness in dealing with emotional experience.

> When one is not overly impressed by the physiological aspects of the emotion and is able to pay attention to its cog-

nitive aspects, one observes the self-experience of "feeling," provided one also has the capacity for reflective self-awareness. Attaining this degree of development allows one to "diagnose" one's own emotional response as a subjective state and sets the stage for the optimal utilization of affects as signals to oneself. . . . The more precise the recognition of one's feelings, the greater its utility as a signal to oneself [p. 39].

Krystal underscores that it is this development of "self-awareness of one's affects as signals to oneself," or, as he more dramatically calls it, of "owning one's own soul" (p. 67), that is the key step in the development of adult affect. More broadly, though, the development of affect differentiation, articulation, and desomatization and of affect tolerance is one aspect of a more general development in self-care and self-regulation. For Krystal, "the *keystone* to the whole group of characteristics and problems of alexithymia is the severe prohibition against exercising self-caring and self-regulating functions" (p. 337). Krystal finds that alexithymic and psychosomatic patients never felt that they had the right to usurp the mother's prerogative in exercising caring and soothing functions and so never became capable or willing to sooth or care for themselves. Ultimately, for Krystal, psychosomatic disorders and alexithymic personality traits develop because of a failure in the intersubjective processing of emotions. This failure leads to the inability to symbolize and articulate affect and thus to a defect in reflective self-awareness and to the consequent inability to regulate one's own affective processing, thus a failure to soothe and care for oneself.

Amplifying the earlier work of Krystal and McDougall, Graeme Taylor (1992a, b) has attempted a synthesis of relational psychoanalysis and psychosomatics that emphasizes affect development and affect regulation. Taylor views psychosomatic conditions as disorders of psychobiological regulation. He believes that, with the shift in psychoanalysis away from a purely one-person metapsychology toward a relational model, a modern psychoanalytic approach focuses more on the individual's inability to process emotions effectively and on deficits in self- and object representations.

Psychoanalysis, with its contemporary emphasis on object relations and the development of the self, has increased the understanding of the homeostatic regulatory functions of stable self and object representations; it also provides a way of conceptualizing the apparently greater risk for ill-

> ness and disease in individuals who rely excessively on
> external relationships to compensate for deficits in their
> self-regulating capacities. The psychoanalytic construct of
> alexithymia . . . has focused attention on deficits in affect re-
> presentation and regulation and generated renewed efforts
> to investigate the extent to which unmodulated emotions are
> risk factors for illness and disease [Taylor, 1992a, p. 478].

Nevertheless, this focus on self-regulation should not be taken to imply that people, once mature, no longer need interpersonal contact to aid in self-regulation. Taylor is quick to point out that all the available evidence points to how actual health outcomes are influenced by the availability and the quality of ongoing interpersonal relationships as well as by social, familial, and community ties.

TRAUMA, DISSOCIATION, AND REFLEXIVE FUNCTIONING

The topic of trauma cannot meaningfully be separated from that of psychosomatosis, since we now know that trauma is associated with somatization and self-destructive behaviors (including suicide, self-mutilation, and eating disorders). In the past few years we have learned a great deal about trauma, and, once again, I want to highlight the relationship among trauma, dissociation, self-reflexive functioning, and the body.

In a highly descriptive article on trauma, Laub and Auerhahn (1993) define trauma by the fact that it "overwhelms and defeats our capacity to organize it" (p. 288); it renders our psychological abilities ineffective. Similarly, in his masterwork on trauma, Krystal (1988) defines trauma as follows: "Catastrophic psychic trauma is defined as a surrender to what is experienced as unavoidable danger of external or internal origin. It is the psychic reality of this surrender to what one experiences as an unbearable situation with no escape, no exit, that causes one to give up and abandon life-preserving activity" (p. 154). Krystal describes how, at the peak of distress, a variety of "special protective devices" are engaged, including derealization, depersonalization, and trancelike states of modified consciousness resulting from a constriction and blocking of mental functions, such as memory, imagination, association, and problem solving. Thus, the blocking of affective responses, psychic numbing, is accompanied by cognitive constriction resulting in self-surrender to psychogenic death.

Laub and Auerhahn's (1993) outstanding article may be read as a subtly nuanced exploration of the "many levels of remembering and preserving the horror of atrocity, all of which range along a continuum of differences in the degree of presence of an observing ego and its synthetic functions" (p. 299). Basing their work on the study of holocaust survivors and their children, they articulate eight shades of dissociation in survivors of trauma. Laub and Auerhahn conclude that knowing about the trauma requires the preservation of a "detached sensibility" and that it is precisely this ability to articulate, analyze, elaborate, and reformulate experience that is destroyed by trauma. Trauma disrupts, or to varying degrees destroys, self-reflexive functioning.

One of the leading researchers in the trauma field has asserted that it is the failure to process information on a symbolic level which is at the very core of the difficulties that result from trauma, and it is because these traumatic experiences cannot be processed and integrated that "the body keeps the score" instead of the mind (van der Kolk, 1996, p. 214). It is precisely for this reason that so much interest has arisen recently in the topic of dissociation. Dissociation refers to a way of organizing information in which there occurs a compartmentalization of experience. Elements of a trauma are not integrated into a cohesive sense of self. In primary dissociation, traumatic experience is split into its isolated somatosensory elements without being integrated into a personal narrative. In secondary dissociation, a split occurs between the observing and the experiencing egos such that people experience depersonalization and derealization, leaving them anesthetized, out of touch with their feelings and emotions. In tertiary dissociation, distinct ego states are formed consisting of complex identities with distinct cognitive, affective, and behavioral patterns. This is the realm of dissociative identity disorders (van der Kolk, 1996). Examining the complex psychobiology of posttraumatic stress disorder, van der Kolk concludes that "these patients are unable to integrate the immediate affective experience with the cognitive structuring of experience. Lack of integration resulted in extreme reactivity to the environment without intervening reflection" (p. 234), and van der Kolk has documented the underlying neurophysiological basis for this dissociation.

The cumulative impact of psychoanalytic research on traumatic states has led some relational analysts to revise our general theory of mind from a repression-based model organized around a developmental layering of fixed structures to a much more fluid model. In this newer model, which Jody Messler Davies (1996) has compared to a kaleidoscope, the mind is envisioned as consisting of "intricate patterns, varied but finite, conflating and reconfiguring themselves from moment to moment" (p. 562). This view of what Davies calls a "relational unconscious" is a dissociation-based model of mind rather than a repression-based model. It is organized not by unconscious mind or another, more to the surface conscious mind, but rather by multiple levels of consciousness and unconsciousness—"a multiply organized, associationally linked network of meaning attribution and understanding" (p. 562). This theoretical understanding leads to a re-visioning of the relational psychoanalytic process as a playful and richly evocative "psychic dehomogenization" (p. 566) requiring both patient and analyst to be able to hold, contain, and play with a multi-plicity of states of mind.

Similarly, Bromberg (1996) proposes that psychoanalysis move away from the traditional topographic and structural model of mind "toward a view of the self as decentered, and the mind as a configura-tion of shifting, nonlinear, discontinuous states of consciousness in an ongoing dialectic with the healthy illusion of unitary selfhood" (p. 512). Writing about dissociation resulting from trauma, Bromberg de-fines pathological dissociation as "a defensive impairment of reflec-tive capacity" (p. 519). Conversely, as patients make the structural shift from dissociation to conflict, this movement is seen clinically "as the increasing capacity of the patient to adopt a self-reflective posture in which one aspect of the self observes and reflects (often with distaste) upon others that were formerly dissociated" (p. 525). So, in the work of all the leading theorists of trauma and dissociation, just as in our survey of current work on psychosomatosis and alexithymia, we find an emphasis on the disruption of self-reflexive functioning at the heart of the pathology and the resumption of self-reflexive functioning as central to the cure.

Here I return to the theme of reflexive self-functioning, which re-quires tension between the I and the me, between subjective aware-ness and objective awareness, or a sense of self-as-subject and a self-as-object. What I have been attempting to link together, in this wide-ranging discussion of symbolization, mentalization, reflective self-awareness, self-reflection, and metacognitive processing, is an emerging understanding of how people must maintain tension between various aspects of themselves; or, to use Bromberg's (1996) felicitous expression, how people need to be able to "stand in the spaces be-tween realities without losing any of them" (p. 516). It is this ability to use potential space, to symbolize, to play, that makes analysis pos-sible, and achieving the capacity to use potential space becomes the goal of analysis for those patients who begin an analysis without this ability.

A long-established principle of psychoanalysis is that the analyst needs to form an alliance with the patient's observing ego, which is split off from the patient's experiencing ego. This idea goes back at least as far as Sterba (1934) and is a commonly accepted aspect of classical psychoanalysis, as is the related distinction between the experiential and observational aspects of the ego/self.[10] What I have been developing here, however, moves beyond these insights in a number of respects. First, I agree that Sterba's article was extremely valuable. As a matter of fact, I think that rereading it in the light of contemporary psychoanalytic developments makes it all the more fascinating. Indeed, Sterba recommended the establishment of a therapeutic dissociation, and he was strikingly free in describing dissociative phenomena and double consciousness at a time in the history of psychoanalysis when these terms were rarely used. Furthermore, he quoted Freud in support of his position that dissociation can have healthy, and not only pathological, functions. Freud (1933) wrote:

> We wish to make the ego the matter of our enquiry, our very own ego. But is that possible? After all, the ego is in its very essence a subject; how can it be made into an object? Well there is no doubt that it can be. The ego can take itself as an object, can treat itself like other objects, can observe itself, criticize itself, and do Heaven knows what with itself. In this, one part of the ego is setting itself over against the rest. So the ego can be split; it splits itself during a number of its functions – temporarily at least [p. 58].

Elsewhere (Aron and Harris, 1993), I observed that as early as 1919, years prior to Sterba's paper, Sandor Ferenczi (1919), who was keenly observant of the wide range of states of consciousness in himself and his patients, described the need for the analyst to alternate between "the free play of association and phantasy" and "logical" and "critical scrutiny" (p. 189). This oscillation between experience and self-criticism by the analyst is strikingly similar to the description of the fate of the ego by analytic therapy described by Sterba in 1934.[11]

To return, though, to how current ideas about self-reflexivity and dissociation are an advance over earlier concepts, the capacity for self-observation was taken for granted by classical analysts for it was this very potential that was the determining criterion for analyzability (see Bromberg, 1996). For today's analysts, by contrast, the capacity for self-awareness may be considered more the goal of analysis than a prerequisite for it. Furthermore, contemporary analysts, across a variety of schools and in accordance with postmodern trends, have championed the conceptual power of multiplicity (Harris, 1996). To become self-aware, a person must break the identification with any single aspect of self and engage in the internal dialogue of the multiple voices of subjectivity. Self-reflection, from this point of view, is based on the capacity for internal division and dialogue, healthy dissociation, standing in the spaces between realities, the transcendent, oscillating, or dialectical function. Self-reflection is based on the ability to link up experiences, whereas trauma leads to dissociation as a result of "attacks on linking" (Bion, 1967).

The Transcendent or Dialectical Function of Mind and Reflexive Self-Functioning

Contemporary Jungian theory has built on an early concept of Jung's (1916) that he called "the transcendent function." By way of background, it is important to understand that one of Jung's central contributions was the view of the unconscious as striving to compensate and correct for a one-sided conscious attitude. Thus, Jung viewed the mind as a self-regulating system, an idea that has found considerable support in recent years among psychoanalysts of all schools of thought and that also fits well with modern biological and systems theory. By the transcendent function, Jung meant an internal dialogue in which the boundaries between the conscious and unconscious mind are loosened, thus allowing some mutual influence to occur while still maintaining some dynamic tension between them (Samuels, 1985). Maintenance of the tension between opposites allows a new attitude to emerge, giving birth to a symbol that mediates the tension between these polarities. Jung considered the transcendent function, so clearly related to the capacity for symbolization, as the most important factor in deep psychoanalytic work.

The contemporary Jungian Polly Young-Eisendrath (1996, 1997) suggests that, to achieve individuation, one must draw on this transcendent function.

> In order to reach this goal, one must develop "metacognitive processes"—the capacity to think about and entertain one's own subjective states from different perspectives. To do this, one comes to see oneself not merely from the perspective of the conscious ego complex, not merely from a

complex-related hyperemotional ("gut feelings") perspective. Instead one can find a "third" point of view from which
both of the others can be entertained and looked at without impulsively enacting them. This third perspective is
the transcendent function (comparable to Winnicott's "potential space") from which one can engage in a dialectical
relationship with aspects of oneself [Young-Eisendrath
1997, p. 233].

The transcendent function seems to me to be Jung's way of describing the dialectical way of thinking that I am here referring to as self-
reflexivity.

Donald Kalsched (1996), elaborating a modern Jungian view of
trauma, links it with contemporary object relations theory and describes how the self-care system designed to protect the self from
further injury can instead perpetuate the repetition of trauma. According to Kalsched, the self-care system defensively exploits the in-
commensurability between the mind and the body, resulting in
splitting and dissociation and the inablity to symbolize affective experience. For Kalsched, then, as for Young-Eisendrath (1996, 1997), a
contemporary Jungian approach conceptualizes psychoanalytic treatment as operating by restoring the transcendent function, that capacity to mediate between worlds that was dissocated as a result of
trauma. Sidoli (1993), a contemporary Jungian analyst, suggests that,
with psychosomatic patients, as analysis proceeds and integrative
processes are set in motion, severe psychosomatic reactions often
occur. During these frightening periods it is the analyst who must
sustain the transcendent function and reestablish the broken links
between body and affect that were not properly established in childhood.

SELF-REFLEXIVITY AND THE BODY

Freud's (1923) famous remark that "the ego is first and foremost a
bodily ego" (p. 26) takes on new meaning in the light of the present
discussion. Freud meant, as he went on to explain, that "the ego is
ultimately derived from bodily sensations, chiefly from those springing from the surface of the body" (pp. 26–27). As Freud so often used
the term ego to refer to one's self, this maxim has been taken to mean
that one's self or one's self-representation is first and foremost a bodily
self. One's image of oneself or one's self-representation originates in

one's bodily sensations and is a reflection of one's body image. As Schafer (1997) suggests, "traditional psychoanalysis has centered its theory on corporeality as the starting fact of ego development" (p. 24). [Our bodies, our sensations, particularly the sensations of our skin surfaces (our "feelings") are critical in shaping our images of ourselves.] [In infancy, our bodily sensations are greatly affected by the qualities of the "holding" and "handling" that we receive from caretakers, and so it is not much of an extension to suggest that our self is first and foremost a body-as-experienced-being-handled-and-held-by-other self, in other words, our self is first and foremost a body-in-relation-self.]

Winnicott (1962) specified that a central feature of personalization is the subjective experience of psyche's "indwelling" in the soma. We are not born with a clear sense of boundedness; rather, we only gradually develop a sense of a subjective boundary between self and nonself (other). "The ego is based on a body-ego, but it is only when all goes well that the person of the baby starts to be linked with the body and the body functions, with the skin as the limiting membrane (p. 59). Only gradually do we come to experience ourselves as residing in our bodies.

This state of psychosomatic unity, of achieving personhood, is accomplished under specific relational conditions under which, during early childhood development, the infant's body is handled, stimulated, soothed, mirrored, and held by caregivers.

> The basis for this indwelling is a linkage of motor and sensory and functional experience with the infant's new state of being a person. As a further development there comes into existence what might be called a limiting membrane, which to some extent (in health) is equated with the surface of the skin, and has a position between the infant's "me" and his "not-me." So the infant comes to have an inside and an outside, and a body scheme [Winnicott, 1960a, p. 45].

For Winnicott, under conditions of health the mind is not located in the head but, rather, is experienced as at one with the whole living body, hence the idea that the mind does not really exist as an entity. In a way, Winnicott's famous statement that there is no such thing as a baby, by which he meant that there cannot be a baby without a mother, is paralleled by the related idea that there is no such thing as mind, by which he meant that there is only psyche–soma and that the mind itself exists only in pathology. (He said himself that this was a funny thing for a psychologist to say.) Mind becomes the location of False Self, and the development of False Self is based on a dissociation between intellectual activity and psychosomatic existence (Winnecott, 1960b). True Self, by way of contrast, is rooted in the body, both in the mother's holding the otherwise unintegrated baby (physically and imaginatively) and in the mother's recognition of the baby's spontaneous gestures (which are themselves defined as sensorimotor groupings).

Consider further Winnicott's (1949) discussion of how the mind may come to be localized in the head. He begins with the observation that the body takes in and gives out substances.

> An inner world of personal imaginative experience therefore comes into the scheme of things, and shared reality is on the whole thought of as outside the personality. Although babies cannot draw pictures, I think that they are capable (except through lack of skill) of depicting themselves by a circle at certain moments in their first months. Perhaps if all is going well, they can achieve this soon after birth; at any rate we have good evidence that at six months a baby is at times using the circle or sphere as a diagram of the self [p. 253].

In this imaginative and paradoxical passage,[12] Winnicott speculates on the infant's achieving a rudimentary sense of a core or bodily self based on the differentiation between inside and outside as this is experienced with the skin as the differentiating membrane and symbolized by the image of a circle or sphere.[13]

These considerations regarding the skin as a differentiating membrane are developed in a most creative way by Didier Anzieu (1985).[14] Anzieu's influential body of work centers on the idea that the functions of the skin serve as a rudimentary model for the primitive ego, what he calls the skin ego. Anzieu's conceptualization of the skin ego may be better termed the skin self and may then be viewed as one aspect of what Stern (1985) calls the "core self." It is from the skin, and then the skin ego, that the ego develops the ability to establish boundaries and frontiers as well as filtering exchanges. In the early mother–child relationship, a fantasy evolves of a skin common to both mother and child. In this fantasy, the bodies of mother and child are independent and yet interdependent, located on either side of and sharing the skin. Anzieu (1993) writes that "the fantasy of 'one skin for two' carries along the fantasy of 'one thought for two'" (p. 46). Gradually this fantasy of a shared skin gives way, allowing for separation to take place as the child internalizes both the skin and the mothering environment. The surface of the body becomes internalized as the skin ego, a containing, psychic envelope, while the mothering environment becomes internalized as the internal world of thoughts, images, and affects. The skin ego not only is a containing envelope but also serves as the vehicle of exchange between the mind and the outside world.[15] Here we can observe how and why the erogenous zones, so central to classical theory, may still matter, even if we conceptualize them differently than Freud did and with the understanding that it is not only the erogenous zones, but the sense of the body as a whole, that is important.

As we saw in discussing the work of Auerbach and Blatt (1996), their research and that of others has confirmed the fundamental establishment of a core bodily self as central in differentiating schizophrenic from borderline patients. Winnicott brings to our attention a unique aspect of the "limiting membrane," our skin—namely, that our skin, with its exquisite receptivity to sensory stimulation, has the qualities of a transitional object in the sense that it is experienced as both me and not me. Consider the perimeter of the circle that Winnicott takes to symbolize the self. Is the perimeter on the inside of the circle or the outside? I believe that in this insight lies a finding of utmost importance regarding self-reflexivity. Our bodies, and especially our skin surface, have the quality of being both me and not me, subject and object; and as such it is our skin sensations that mediate between inside and outside, subjective self-awareness and objective self-awareness, self-as-subject and self-as-object. Our experience of our bodies, more than any other experience, partakes of this duality.

As I observe my arm, for example, I recognize it as an object in the world, an object among other objects, subject to all the same forces that affect all objects. It can be pushed and pulled, cut or pressured; it is subject to all the laws of gravity and physics. Simultaneously, though, it is not at all like other objects in the world. It moves at my will. I feel its position. I know where it is without looking. I feel it as warm or cold, at ease or uncomfortable, relaxed or tense. I experience its sensations as a part of me. I experience the sense of bodily movement itself. It is precisely our bodies, and in particular our skin sensations, that are constituted by the two poles in the dialectic with which we began our study of self-reflexivity, self-as-subject and self-as-object.

Once we begin to play with the notion of the skin ego, however, we may be led to other metaphors in an attempt to point to the origins of reflexive self-awareness. Consider, for instance, the image of the breathing self. It is my thesis that the foundations of the capacity for self-reflexivity lies in our bodily sensations. So far I have focused on the sensations of the skin surface, but here I want to add breathing as an alternative model. Eigen (1977), who did a great deal to draw the attention of psychoanalysts to their breathing, pointed out that psychoanalysis has generally focused on the appetite, with its hungers and frustrations as the central feature of the body, but that breathing might also serve as a model, as it does in the East. Eigen suggests that partial identification with the breathing process provides the ego with a model of cohesion and interaction. Comparing Eigen's proposal and that of Anzieu (1985, 1993) might lead to the formulation of a concept such as the breathing self in parallel to the skin ego. At what point is the breath a part of the self, and at what moment is it a part of the outside world? Awareness of breathing points to the dual status of the self, the breathing self, as both subject and object and hence serves to enhance self-reflexive functioning. As Eigen writes, "The ego uses its experience of breathing as a bridge to move safely in and out of the body. In so doing, it strengthens both its capacity for observation and its receptivity to perceived body aliveness" (p. 44). It is precisely for this reason that so many forms of meditative awareness are achieved by focusing on the coming and going of the breath. As Mark Epstein (1995) has described, awareness of breathing and bodily sensations is fundamental to Buddhist mindfulness practice, a goal of which is the deepening of subjectivity, authentic relatedness, and enhanced subjective awareness.

Anzieu's work may also be usefully compared to Ogden's (1989) postulation of an autistic-contiguous position. Ogden proposes that the autistic-contiguous position is the most primitive mode of organizing experience, in which the experience of self is based on the ordering of sensory experience, particularly sensations at the skin surface. In Ogden's scheme of the organization of subjectivity, a contribution is made by each of the three modes of experience. The autistic-contiguous mode contributes the sensory floor of experience. It is important to remember that the paranoid-schizoid mode, which generates much of the sense of immediacy and vitality of experience, is rooted in an experience of the self as an object, with little sense of oneself as the author or agent of one's life. The depressive position, on the other hand, contributes the experience of oneself as an historical, interpreting, agentic self, and thus in the depressive mode the self is recognized as a subject and not only an object.

I read Ogden's schema as providing a blueprint of development and of continued modes of experiencing in which the self is built on bodily sensations, particularly skin sensations and rhythmic sensations, such as experienced in breathing, and gradually acquires the organization of self-as-object and self-as-subject. A healthy person can maintain the tension among these modes, oscillating between a view of self as subject and as an object rooted in the concrete experience of bodily sensations. Ogden (1994), who acknowledges the influence of Anzieu, envisions the infant's primitive self as being formed through the internalization of the mothering function.

> Coming alive as a human being involves the act of being held by and within the matrix of the physical and psychological aliveness of the mother. . . . I am proposing that from the beginning of psychological life (and continuing throughout life), there exists a form of experience in which the mother as psychological matrix is replaced by an autonomous sensory matrix [p. 177].

Ogden (1994) also stresses the overriding importance of the skin as the boundary between inside and outside, life and death. He writes: "Physiologically, it is essential that one's skin be continually generating a layer of dead tissue that serves as a life-preserving outermost layer of the body. In this way (as in Freud's concept of the stimulus barrier), human life is physiologically encapsulated by death" (p. 181). This is perhaps the clearest statement of the meaning of the circle of life, the mandala in Jungian terms, as that which separates inner and outer, life and death, self-as-subject and self-as-object.

If our self is first and foremost a bodily self, then our relational experiences are first and foremost bodily experiences as well. Stolorow and Atwood (1992), following Winnicott, have highlighted how "the caregiver's affect attunement is communicated primarily through sensorimotor contacts with the infant's body." From their intersubjective perspective, "mind-body unity remains linked to a sustaining selfobject milieu throughout the life cycle, although the child's developing use of symbols and images increasingly obviates the need for immediate sensorimotor attunements and concrete mirroring in order to maintain this aspect of self-cohesion" (p. 46). It is through infants' bodies that parents communicate with them, through all of what Winnicott had in mind in describing "handling." It is by handling the child's body, holding the child, reflecting back or mirroring the child's facial expressions and bodily postures and movements that parents convey their affect attunement and recognition of the child as a separate, developing person. If our sense of self is established on the basis of "reflected appraisals," to use a Sullivanian term, it should be clear that these reflections are indeed reflections of our bodies conveyed in turn by the bodily actions of our caretakers.

Self-reflection, then, is certainly rooted in early object relations and continually is regulated through internal object relations; a relational emphasis, however, implicates bodily interaction and somatosensory experience. A relational focus also deconstructs the dichotomy between verbal (mental) and preverbal (bodily) experience; it recognizes the ongoing interaction of language and the body in constructing human subjectivity and intersubjectivity. We need to keep in mind Kristeva's (1980) emphasis on the sensuous materiality of speech and on how closely speech is tied to gesture and to the body, particularly as language first develops in early childhood.

As we have seen, the literature on catastrophic trauma reveals that trauma disrupts the capacity for self-reflexivity by severing the links between the self–as-subject and the self-as-object. Unable to move freely back and forth among different aspects of self, unable to utilize their bodily sensations and their skin membrane to mediate between their subjective and objective awareness, traumatized patients are unable to reflect on their traumatic experiences, self-reflexive functioning fails, and the body is left to keep score. The patients who come to us with psychosomatic illness, self-mutilation, addictions, perversions, and other destructive enactments have used their bodies for the concrete expression of their affective lives because they have no way to process these affects through self-reflection and mentalization. The traditional distinction between conversion reactions and psychosomatic states suggests that conversion symptoms are based on a symbolically mediated expression of unconscious conflict, so that bodily symptoms substitute for some specific unconscious conflict; whereas psychosomatic symptoms follow presymbolic pathways of affect expression. Both disorders are pathological solutions when self-reflexive functioning breaks down. In the case of conversion reactions, there is a capacity for symbolization, but in certain restricted areas the person is not able to reflect on the conflicting states; whereas in psychosomatic states symbolization fails more generally in regard to affective life.

In the course of a psychoanalytic journey, patient and analyst (while generally not literally touching each other's bodies) come to share a psychoanalytic skin-ego or psychoanalytic breathing ego. Within the fluid exchanges of interpretive squiggles and mutual associations between patient and analyst, the question of whose idea that was, patient's or analyst's, who thought of this or that, is often not answerable (Aron, 1996). Gradually, patient and analyst mutually regulate each other's behaviors, enactments, and states of consciousness such that each gets under the other's skin, each reaches into the other's guts, each is breathed in and absorbed by the other. For a while, patient and analyst share a jointly created skin-ego/breathing self.

For patients who have not achieved an ability to symbolize, unformulated affective experiences can be experienced only vicariously by intersubjectively communicating them to another, a process that some analysts describe by speaking of projective identification. Sands (1997) has noted that patients are motivated to communicate these unarticulated experiences to the analyst using projective identification in order to "have one's communication viscerally received, contained, 'lived through,' symbolized, and given back in such a way that one knows that the other has 'gotten' it from the inside out" (p. 699). The patient's unarticulated longing is to have the analyst know the patient "from the inside out" (see Bromberg, 1991). Clearly, the analyst cannot accomplish this without considerable wear and tear on his or her own body/psyche.

Working from within this conjoint analytic skin-ego, the analyst employs his or her capacity for self-reflexivity to process associations with the patient. Where the patient is not capable of using symbolic or metaphoric thought, the analyst may receive communications only nonverbally often in the form of bodily communications, a change in the climate, the air, (mediated by the breath), a change in the feel of things (mediated by the skin). Here the analyst must be attuned to the nonverbal, the affective, the spirit (breath) of the session, the feel of the material, to his or her own bodily responses, so that these may be gradually utilized to construct metaphors and symbols that may be verbally exchanged by the analytic pair, gradually permitting the differentiation of the more primitive shared skin-ego and the construction of a more developed, articulated, and differentiated personal attachment and interpersonal connection. At moments when patients are unable to use reflexive awareness, the analyst must carry much of the analytic work, psychosomatically processing the patient's communications and employ his or her own transcendent function to bring together conscious with unconscious, body with affect, unformulated experience with words and symbols, self-as-subject with self-as-object. At moments, both patient and analyst lose this ability, but, through ongoing oscillations, enactments, role reversals, projections and introjections, they may mutually help each other to regain, reestablish, sustain, and improve reflexive awareness.

CONCLUSIONS

Psychoanalysis is a very specific form of treatment that has for a long time struggled against the accusation that it does not treat symptoms directly or effectively and that other forms of treatment are more parsimonious and cost effective. Historically, analysts have answered that what they provided is more important than symptom relief, namely, insight. It might take longer to get rid of the symptoms than in other treatments, but it is worth it because patients gain important knowledge about themselves that lead to underlying structural change and therefore prevent further symptom development. This argument is not very convincing, especially since structural change seems to be elusive, ambiguous, and hard to document.

I believe that the understanding of self-reflexivity elaborated here leads to a much more refined answer and one that may very well be measurable and empirically testable. Furthermore, it is one with implications for our patient's bodies (as well as our own) that is quite important and dramatic. Specifically, much of the impact of trauma seems to take its toll by interfering with self-reflexive functioning, and much of the psychopathology that we deal with seems to be mediated by this same inability for self-reflection. All dissociation is rooted in the primal dissociation of body from mind, of subjective awareness from objective awareness, of "I" from "me." Psychoanalysis is the only treatment that operates directly to improve the capacity for self-reflexivity. Psychoanalysis involves a process in which patient and analyst set aside a considerable period of time to reflect intensively, deeply, and broadly on their mutual experiences. Analysis is essentially a two-person joint exercise in self-reflexive functioning.

One implication of this formulation is that at the end of an analysis it is not insight or other knowledge or psychic content that demonstrates the patient's growth or the success of the treatment; rather, it is the capacity for self-reflexivity. Analysts have always known this; we have always said that the goal of analysis is the capacity for self-analysis following termination. But we have never succeeded in being able to demonstrate this acquired skill, and, furthermore, not all patients report that they engage in continued self-analysis. But, although people may not deliberately engage in any kind of systematic self-analysis following termination, they may very well have an improved self-reflexive capacity based on a greater ability to maintain the tension between their different selves. In fact, this improvement may be measurable.

Mary Main's work with the Adult Attachment Interview (George, Kaplan, and Main, 1985) seems to me to be the first instrument of its kind to provide a measure of just this kind of metacognitive processing. It does not measure insight, or the content of one's knowledge about oneself, or the content of one's life story; rather, it measures one's ability to think flexibly about and process aspects of one's life. Susan Coates (1998) has called it "the first powerful empirical window on how intersubjective experience becomes transformed into intrapsychic structure." (manuscript, p. 18). Other measures along these lines will undoubtedly be developed that could be used to document changes brought about in reflexive functioning by psychoanalysis.

Another implication of my argument is that analysts need to pay considerably more attention than we have been taught to bodily phenomena in themselves and their patients. A corollary of findings on self-reflection and the body is that, when self-reflection begins to falter, one of the first signals is often a bodily reaction. This is true for both the patient and the analyst, so that an obstacle to self-reflection may become apparent in a change in posture, facial expression, eye movements, respiration, bodily tension, or, more worrisomely, in psychosomatic explosions and the outbreak of illness or deterioration in physical functioning. Analytic patients may often notice these connections themselves in the course of free associating. For many patients, however, particularly those who are less capable of self-reflection, this is an event that may go unnoticed unless the analyst brings it to their attention. Of course, one needs to be careful in bringing the body to the patient's attention, precisely because the body is so central to self-reflection that focusing on it may disrupt a previously established homeostasis and the patient may become self-conscious. This hyperreflexivity is a further demonstration of an impairment in self-regulation in which people cannot regulate the tension between viewing themselves as subjects (of bodily experience) and as objects (of observation).

It is not only patients who may react in their bodies, analysts too must be extremely attentive to their own bodies. That is, much of what we pick up from our patients we may first feel in our bodies and perhaps most immediately in our breathing. Our bodies are the primary arena for the psychophysiological processing of affect. As Fonagy and Target (1998) point out, and as Coates (1998) amplifies in her commentary, many patients, especially those prone to psychosomatic disorders, do not know what they feel. For these patients it is not enough to encourage self-expression, since they know not what to express. Nor is it a matter of interpreting to them their unconscious internal conflicts; rather these patients need to have their affects recognized. Affect recognition first takes place on a bodily level—we feel in our bodily reactions something of what the other person feels, and we convey this recognition through bodily responses. These are often instantaneous and not processed explicitly in language.

In *A Meeting of Minds* (Aron, 1996) I suggested, following Maroda (1995), that analysts need to register their patients' affective experience and convey to their patients that indeed the affective communication had been received by the analyst, recognized, and processed, thus, in Maroda's words "completing the cycle of affective communication." The patient may then feel that he or she has been understood by the analyst "from the inside out" (Bromberg, 1991; Sands, 1997). I believe that there are many ways an analyst may convey this visceral understanding to a patient. It is often done through a good interpretation, but it may also be done by expressing a feeling of one's own, by putting a patient's feelings into words, or even through a more direct bodily response, such as a sudden gasp, a change in posture, breathing, or facial expression. I find that for many patients the most important function of the analyst is to register, acknowledge, and put into words the patient's unformulated or unsymbolized affective experience (Stern, 1997).

Fonagy and his collaborators suggest that analysts invite the patient to consider the therapist's mind. I view this advice as quite compatible with my suggestions regarding how we may focus on "the patient's experience of the analyst's subjectivity" (Aron, 1991). Here I might add that one of the ways in which patients routinely gain some understanding of the analyst's subjectivity is by attending to and noticing aspects of their analyst's body. And, of course a great deal is observed about the analyst's body even when the analyst is behind the couch and out of sight.

Our minds and our bodies are self-regulating systems, and self-reflection is one psychosomatic process that we use to regulate our states of awareness.[16] Maintaining state-constancy or an awareness that we are our same self even as we move between an enormous variety of states of consciousness is an important developmental achievement that is disrupted by trauma (see Bach, 1994, and Aron and Bushra, in press). The transcendent function that Jung (1916) referred to as maintaining a balance between the conscious and unconscious minds has been extended to include maintaining a careful balance among a variety of states of consciousness and a multiplicity of selves. Psychoanalysis is a process that promotes fluid movements among these states of consciousness by facilitating an internal dialogue among these selves. It does so by establishing a setting in which patient and analyst can think together, slowly (without rush), deeply (without coming to quick conclusions), and broadly (covering a wide range of affective experiences) about mental states, interpersonal interactions, and bodily phenomena. It is by creating a shared skin-ego or breathing ego, a "potential space" where one does not have to decide if an experience is subjective or objective, by maintaining a dialectical position between self-as-subject and self-as-object, and by both patient and analyst engaging in a psychoanalytic form of "playing" with multiple selves and multiple relational configurations as these configurations are passed back and forth intersubjectively between patient and analyst, that people develop or strengthen their abilities for mentalization and self-reflexive functioning and transcending limited, constricted, simplified, or caricatured versions of themselves.

NOTES

[1]I am indebted to Damon and Hart's (1988) outstanding scholarship on self-understanding for the following summary of James's theory of the self.

[2]Freud's use of the term *das Ich* included both the idea of the self and the idea of the ego. Thus Freud maintained a dialectical view of a nonunified self in a state of tension or conflict. This aspect of Freud's conceptualization (that the ego and self are dialectically related) is obscured when *das Ich* is officially translated as "the ego." It is for this reason that I begin the paper using James's language, which is both experiential and clear.

[3]James specified four core features of individuality that together constitute what we mean by subjectivity: (1) agency, which leads to a belief in the autonomy of the self; (2) distinctness or uniqueness, which leads to a sense of one's personal individuality; (3) personal continuity, which leads to a sense of the self's stability: and (4) reflection, or awareness of one's own awareness, which leads to self-consciousness and to the subjective meaning of one's identity.

[4]James's distinction between the "I" and the "me" has been echoed by interpersonal psychoanalysts as well. Barnett's (1980) distinction between the "representational self" and the "operational self" refers to the self-concept and the self as the center of agency. Wolstein's (1974) differentiation of the "I" and the "me" similarly follows James. For a comprehensive review of interpersonal theories of the self, see Lionells (1995). In a related vein, Hermans, Kempen, and van Loon (1992) elaborate James's original distinction between the "I" and the "me" by reformulating the differentiation between them in narrative terms as that between the "author" and the "actor."

[5]Bion's (1967) notions of "Vertices," the necessity for "binocular vision,"

and the phenomenon of "reversible perspective" are all ways of conceptual-izing the importance of being able to view a situation from divergent angles.

[6]As I said previously with regard to William James, I think that Bach's terms for these states (subjective awareness and objective self-awareness) are somewhat unfortunate in that they easily lend themselves to misunder-standing. It seems to me that staying with the terms self-as-subject and self-as-object is clearer, more precise, and closer to experience.

[7]This is based on Auerbach and Blatt's (1996) expatiation on the struc-tural differences between borderline and psychotic patients. They suggest that borderline and psychotic patients alike have difficulty with reflexive self-awareness. Whereas borderline patients have achieved a sense of em-bodiment, or a core self, however, psychotics have not. When cognitive de-velopment takes place during adolescence, particularly with the advent of formal operations, one can think about one's own thinking, and this growth heightens the importance of self-reflection. "One becomes schizophrenic, on this perspective, when one looks inward to discover oneself and finds nothing. Thus, schizophrenic hyperreflexivity, according to traditional psy-choanalytic views, may follow from failure to establish or find a bodily sense of self" (p. 306). Schizophrenic hyperreflexivity, which is defined by Sass (1992) as manifest in exaggerated inwardness and self-consciousness along with alienation from the body, emotions, and the social world, is an example of the disregulation of the reflexive function. As Sass (1992), like Bach (1985), has demonstrated, in hyperreflexively attempting to regard their inner states as objects of observation, that is in treating subjective experience too exclu-sively as objective, schizoid individuals experience a sense of inner dead-ness. In contrast, borderline and narcissistic personalities have attained a core, embodied sense of self even if such a self is fragile under conditions of stress. Thus, borderline patients, compared with schizophrenics, have achieved better preverbal boundaries between self and other. "Thus, when borderline personalities introspect, they may be confused about what they see, but they know that there is something there to be seen" (Auerbach and Blatt, 1996, p. 306).

[8]Here, Fonagy's views dovetail with those of Jessica Benjamin (1995), who conceptualizes the development of intersubjective recognition as the basis for the emergence of a personal sense of agency. For Benjamin, recog-nition of the other as an equivalent center of experience "begins with the other's confirming response, which tells us that we have created meaning, had an impact, revealed an intention" (p. 33). From the point of view of rela-tional psychoanalysis, "mother's recognition is the basis for the baby's sense of agency" (p. 34).

[9]The topics of psychosomatics and trauma are each enormous and com-plex, and so I will not attempt any systematic review here. Instead I will be touching on a few recent contributions in these areas in an effort to link up certain key developments that have in common a link to self-reflexive func-tioning.

[10]Consider, as an example, the work of Jacob Arlow, long viewed as the

dean of American mainstream psychoanalysis. In his classic article on depersonalization and derealization, Arlow (1966) describes these phenomena as representing a defensively motivated dissociation between the function of immediate experiencing and the function of self observation, distinct functions which usually are integrated. He notes the common clinical finding that patients describe a split between one self, which appears to be standing off in the distance in a detached and relatively objective manner, observing a second, separate, and estranged self in action: two selves, two centers of awareness. The emphasis that he puts on these two modes of thought, subjective awareness and objective self-awareness, may be seen in his creative observation that hysterical hallucinosis may be viewed as the opposite of depersonalization in that, whereas in depersonalization the awareness of self-as-object is heightened but the experience of the self as an active agent is minimized, in hysterical hallucinosis there is the maximal investment in the function of immediate experience with an almost complete obliteration of the function of self observation.

Arlow suggests four developmental phases that may be activated during the regression that occurs in depersonalization. I describe them here in order to highlight the bodily emphasis in all of these descriptions. He first notes that two of the central characteristics of dreams are the sense of unreality and a split between the observing and the experiencing self, sometimes represented by two different people. Arlow comments on those aspects of dream psychology in which people are alienated and estranged from their body. Second, Arlow evokes Winnicott's idea of a phase of transitional objects in which the limits of the self and the nonself are not yet clearly demarcated. Third, Arlow describes the relation of the child to his or her own fecal matter as the prototype for the split between the experiencing and observing self, in that the fecal matter has qualities of the inner self and of being an object in the outside world. Fourth, Arlow describes the split between the experiencing and observing self as rooted in the early phase in which the self is discovered in the mirror. Each of these descriptions may be viewed as a bodily based prototype or metaphor for the split between the experiencing self and the observing self.

[11]It should also be noted that the Sullivanian notion of participant-observation points to a similar oscillating function between participation, engagement in the immediate experience, and observation, that is, reflection from the perspective of an outsider. Although contemporary interpersonalists may question the possibility of "objective" observation, or of removal of oneself from the immediate experience even momentarily—while they object to Sullivan's positivism—they nevertheless retain an emphasis on this oscillating movement between enactment and reflection.

[12]I refer to this passage as "imaginative" because I either do not take Winnicott literally here or I disagree with his inference. I doubt that preverbal infants can create the symbol of the circle to indicate their boundedness. Symbols and transitional objects require language and self-reflexivity. The

circle more likely comes to represent the bounded self only with the later developments sometime in the second year of life.

[13]Winnicott's idea that the self is symbolized by the circle or sphere strongly reverberates with Jung's notions of how the archetype of the self is symbolized by the mandala.

[14]For a review of Anzieu's ideas, see Chabert (1996).

[15]My reading of Anzieu, like my reading of Winnicott, is to take his ideas as imaginative and suggestive rather then literal. Infants are not self-reflexive until about 18 months and therefore do not self-reflexively understand their boundedness and separateness until then. A preverbal sense of bounded-ness—the skin self—or Stern's preverbal "core self" is formed through contingency detection and does not require self-reflexivity. Winnicott and Anzieu may be reading back into infancy aspects of psychic fantasy that are elaborated only later with the development of verbalization and symbolization.

[16]Viewing the psyche as a self-regulating system is a quintessentially Jungian idea.

REFERENCES

Alexander, F. (1950), *Psychosomatic Medicine*. New York: Norton.

Anzieu, D. (1985), *The Skin Ego*. New Haven, CT: Yale University Press, 1989.

———— (1993), Autistic phenomena and the skin ego. *Psychoanal. Inq.* 13:42–48.

Arlow, J. A. (1966), Depersonalization and derealization. In: *Psychoanalysis: Clinical Theory and Practice*. Madison, CT: International Universities Press, 1991, pp. 137–154.

Aron, L. (1991), The patient's experience of the analyst's subjectivity. *Psychoanal. Dial.,* 1:29–51.

———— (1996), *A Meeting of Minds*. Hillsdale, NJ: The Analytic Press.

———— & Bushra, A. (in press), Mutual regression: Altered states in the psychoanalytic situation. *J. Amer. Psychoanal. Assn.*

———— & Harris, A. (1993), Sandor Ferenczi: Discovery and rediscovery. In: *The Legacy of Sándor Ferenczi*, ed., L. Aron & A. Harris. Hillsdale, NJ: The Analytic Press, 1–35.

Auerbach, J. S. (1993), The origins of narcissism and narcissistic personality disorder: A theoretical and empirical reformulation. In: *Empirical Studies of Psychoanalytic Theories, Vol. 4*, ed. J. M. Masling & R. F. Bernstein. Washington, DC: American Psychological Association, pp. 43–108.

———— & Blatt, S. J. (1996), Self-representation in severe psychopathology: The role of reflexive self-awareness. *Psychoanal. Psychol.,* 13:297–341.

Bach, S. (1985), *Narcissistic States and the Therapeutic Process*. New York: Aronson.

———— (1994), *The Language of Perversion and the Language of Love.* Northvale, NJ: Aronson.

Balint, M. (1950), Changing therapeutic aims and techniques in psychoanalysis. *Internat. J. Psycho-Anal.,* 31:117–124.

Barnett, J. (1980), Interpersonal processes, cognition, and the analysis of character. *Contemp. Psychoanal.,* 16:397–416.

Benjamin, J. (1995), *Like Subjects, Love Objects.* New Haven, CT: Yale University Press.

Bion, W. R. (1967), *Second Thoughts.* London: Heinemann.

Bromberg, P. M. (1991), On knowing one's patient inside out: The aesthetics of unconscious communication. *Psychoanal. Dial.,* 1:399–422.

———— (1996), Standing in the spaces: The multiplicity of self and the psychoanalytic relationship. *Contemp. Psychoanal.* 32:509–536.

Chabert, C. (1996), Book review essay: *Introduction to the Work of Didier Anzieu. Internat. J. Psycho-Anal.,* 77:601–613.

Coates, S. (1998), Having a mind of one's own and holding the other in mind: Commentary on paper by Peter Fonagy and Mary Target. *Psychoanal. Dial.,* 8: 115–148.

Damon, W. & Hart, D. (1988), *Self-Understanding in Childhood and Adolescence.* Cambridge: Cambridge University Press.

Davies, J. M. (1996), Linking the "pre-analytic" with the postclassical: Integration, dissociation, and the multiplicity of unconscious process. *Contemp. Psychoanal.,* 32:553–576.

Eigen, M. (1977), Breathing and identity. In: *The Electrified Tightrope.* Northvale, NJ: Aronson, 1993.

Epstein, M. (1995), *Thoughts Without a Thinker.* New York: Basic Books.

Ferenczi, S. (1919), On the technique of psychoanalysis. In: *Further Contributions to the Theory and Technique of Psycho-Analysis,* ed. J. Richman (trans. J. Suttie). London: Karnac Books, 1980, pp. 177-197.

Fonagy, P. & Target, M. (1995), Understanding the violent patient: The use of the body and the role of the father. *Internat. J. Psycho-Anal.* 76:487-501.

———— & ———— (1996), Playing with reality: I. Theory of mind and the normal development of psychic reality. *Internat. J. Psycho-Anal.* 77:217–233

———— & ———— (1998), Mentalization and changing aims in child psychoanalysis. *Psychoanal. Dial.,* 8:87–114.

Freud, S. (1923), The ego and the id. *Standard Edition,* 19:3–68. London: Hogarth Press, 1961.

———— (1933), New introductory lectures on psychoanalysis. *Standard Edition,* 22:5–182. London: Hogarth Press, 1964.

Gatchel, R. J. (1993), Psychophysiological disorders: Past and present perspectives. In: *Psychophysiological Disorders,* ed. R. J. Gatchel & E. B. Blanchard. Washington, DC: American Psychological Association, pp. 1–21.

George, C., Kaplan, N. & Main, M. (1985), The Berkeley Adult Attachment

Interview. Unpublished manuscript, Department of Psychology, University of California, Berkeley.

Grotstein, J. S. (1997), "Mens sane in corpore sano": The mind and body as an "odd couple" and as an oddly coupled unity. *Psychoanal. Inq.*, 17:204–222.

Harris, A. (1996), The conceptual power of multiplicity. *Contemp. Psychoanal.* 32:537–552.

Hermans, H. J. M., Kempen, H. J. G. & van Loon, R. J. P. (1992), The dialogical self: Beyond individualism and rationalism. *Amer. Psychol.*, 47:23–33.

James, W. (1890), *The Principles of Psychology*. Cambridge, MA: Harvard University Press, 1981.

Jung, C. G. (1916), *The Structure and Dynamics of the Psyche. Collected Works*, 8, 1969.

Kalsched, D. (1996), *The Inner World of Trauma*. London: Routledge.

Kohut, H. (1977), *The Restoration of the Self*. New York: International Universities Press.

Kristeva, J. (1980), *Desire in Language*. New York: Columbia University Press.

Krystal, H. (1988), *Integration and Self-Healing*. Hillsdale, NJ: The Analytic Press.

Laub, D. & Auerhahn, N. C. (1993), Knowing and not knowing massive psychic trauma: Forms of traumatic memory. *Internat. J. Psycho-Anal.*, 74:287–302.

Lionells, M. (1995), The interpersonal self, uniqueness, will and intentionality. In: *Handbook of Interpersonal Psychoanalysis*, ed. M. Lionells, J. Fiscalini, C. H. Mann & D. B. Stern. Hillsdale, NJ: The Analytic Press, pp. 31–62.

Maroda, K. (1995), Show some emotion: Completing the cycle of affective communication. Presented at meeting of the Division of Psychoanalysis (39), American Psychological Association, Santa Monica, CA.

Main, M. (1991), Metacognitive knowledge, metacognitive monitoring and singular (coherent) vs. multiple (incoherent) model of attachment: Findings and directions for future research. In: *Attachment Across the Life Cycle*, ed. C. Parkes, J. Stevenson-Hinde & P. Morris. London: Routledge, pp. 127–160.

———— & Hesse, E. (1990), Parents' unresolved traumatic experiences are related to infant disorganized attachment status: Is frightened and/or frightening parental behavior the linking mechanism? In: *Attachment in the Preschool Years: Theory, Research, and Intervention*, ed. M. T. Greenberg, D. Cicchetti & E. M. Cummings. Chicago: University of Chicago Press, pp. 161–182.

McCallum, M. & Piper, W. E., ed. (1997), *Psychological Mindedness*. Mahwah, NJ: Lawrence Erlbaum Associates.

McDougall, J. (1989), *Theatres of the Body*. New York: Norton.

Nemiah, J. & Sifneos, P. (1970), Affect and fantasy in patients with psychosomatic disorders. *Modern Trends in Psychosomatic Medicine*, Vol. 2, ed. O. W. Hill. London: Butterworth, pp. 22–34.

Ogden, T. H. (1989), *The Primitive Edge of Experience*. Northvale, NJ: Aronson.
────── (1994), *Subjects of Analysis*. Northvale, NJ: Aronson.
────── (1997), Reverie and metaphor: Some thoughts on how I work as a psychoanalyst. *Internat. J. Psycho-Anal.*, 78:719–732.
Samuels, A. (1985), *Jung and the Post-Jungians*. London: Routledge & Kegan Paul.
Sands, S. H. (1997), Protein or foreign body? Reply to commentaries. *Psychoanal. Dial.*, 7:691–706.
Sass, L. A. (1992), *Madness and Modernism*. New York: Basic Books.
Schafer, R. (1997), *Tradition and Change in Psychoanalysis*. Madison, CT: International Universities Press.
Seligman, S. (1998), Child psychoanalysis, adult psychoanalysis and developmental psychology: Introduction to Symposium on Child Analysis, Part II. *Psychoanal. Dial.*, 8:79–86.
Sidoli, M. (1993), When the meaning gets lost in the body. *Anal. Psychol.*, 38:175–190.
Sterba, R. (1934), The fate of the ego in analytic therapy. *Internat. J. Psycho-Anal.*, 15:117–126.
Stern, D. B. (1997), *Unformulated Experience*. Hillsdale, NJ: The Analytic Press.
Stern, D. N. (1985), *The Interpersonal World of the Infant*. New York: Basic Books.
Stolorow, R. D. & Atwood, G. E. (1992), *Contexts of Being*. Hillsdale, NJ: The Analytic Press.
Target, M. & Fonagy, P. (1996), Playing with reality: II. The development of psychic reality from a theoretical perspective. *Internat. J. Psycho-Anal.*, 77:459–479.
Taylor, G. J. (1992a), Psychosomatics and self-regulation. In: *Interface of Psychoanalysis and Psychology*, ed. J. W. Barron, M. N. Eagle & D. S. Wolitzky. Washington, DC: American Psychological Association, pp. 464–488.
────── (1992b), Psychoanalysis and psychosomatics: A new synthesis. *J. Amer. Acad. Psychoanal.*, 20:251–275.
van der Kolk, B. A. (1996), The body keeps the score: Approaches to the psychobiology of posttraumatic stress disorder. In: *Traumatic Stress*, ed. B. A. van der Kolk, A. C. McFarlane & L. Weisaeth. New York: Guilford, pp. 214–241.
Winnicott, D. W. (1949) Mind and its relation to the psyche-soma. In: *Through Paediatrics to Psycho-Analysis*. New York: Basic Books, 1975, pp. 243–254.
────── (1960a), The theory of the parent–infant relationship. In: *The Maturational Process and the Facilitating Environment*. New York: International Universities Press, 1965, pp. 37–55.
────── (1960b), Ego distortion in terms of true and false self. In: *The Maturational Process and the Facilitating Environment*. New York: International Universities Press, 1965, pp. 140–152.
────── (1962), Ego integration in child development. In: *The Maturational*

Process and the Facilitating Environment. New York: International Universities Press, 1965, pp. 56–63.

Wolff, H. G. (1953), *Stress and Disease.* Springfield, IL: Charles C Thomas.

Wolstein, B. (1974), "I" processes and "me" patterns: Two aspects of the psychic self in transference and countertransference. *Contemp. Psychoanal.,* 10:347–357.

Young-Eisendrath, P. (1996), *The Gifts of Suffering.* Reading, MA: Addison-Wesley.

———— (1997), Gender and contrasexuality: Jung's contribution and beyond. In: *The Cambridge Companion to Jung,* ed, P. Young-Eisendrath & T. Dawson. Cambridge: Cambridge University Press.

2

PSYCHIC ENVELOPES
AND SONOROUS BATHS

*Siting the Body in Relational Theory
and Clinical Practice*

Adrienne Harris

This essay explores a relational perspective on the body with particular attention to the experience of *bodies in relationship* within the
analytic dyad. Psychoanalysis is a theory of body–mind integration,
and relational theory must grapple with this project. There are a number of reasons to consider the status of the body in relational theory.
By way of introduction let me just outline three.

First, I think relationalists need to retrieve the body from classical theory. There has been a critique of relational psychoanalysis'
difficulties in integrating sexual life and bodily experience to our theories, our tendency to sanitize and desexualize. André Green (1995,
1997) is concerned that the focus on attachment and its impact on
the emergence of self and object, and therefore on preoedipal life, is
eclipsing the emblematic psychoanalytic project, namely, the constituting power of sexuality. He calls for a reversal of the opposition of
drive and object but would do so with a particular emphasis on sexuality, which is still individually and primarily endogenously founded:
"the drive is the matrix of the subject" (Green, 1997, p. 347). But can
we not rehabilitate the body for relational theory without returning
to a simple or mechanical model of drives or to the centrality of the
oedipal phase as the organizing principle of psychic life? A *relational
body* may be a rather different creature from the body of classical

theory, more inevitably interpersonal and fluid, less reified and static, but no less sexual.

Second, relational theorists (though not alone in this preoccupation) have been increasingly interested in the subjectivity of the analyst. This is perhaps an inevitable consequence of the widening perspective on countertransference and the deepening understanding of the complex interpersonal matrices in which analyses are conducted. The tradition of interest in the analyst's subjectivity can be tracked from Ferenczi (1932) through Winnicott (1947) and Green (1975) and then to contemporary American analysts such as Jacobs (1991), Bromberg (1994) and Aron (1995). In different ways, they all propose that the analytic instrument must have very deep and primitive processing abilities. Analysts must have access to and be comfortable with their subjective affect states and bodily reactivity if they are to experience and metabolize patients' communications. In this concept of an analytic instrument responsive to primitive and archaic interpersonal and intrapsychic experiences, Green and Winnicott were drawing perhaps on Bion's (1961) idea of maternal reverie as the mental state in which conscious and unconscious communication is transferred between people. Given many developments within psychoanalysis and in cognitive neuroscience, we can now see that these primitive mental states will inevitably involve body and somatic experiences. Thus the analyst's body becomes one of the points of registration or representation of experience not verbally symbolizable but nonetheless powerfully dominant in intrapsychic life and therefore projected into interpersonal space.

Third, a theory of the body's potential for the metabolizing and registration of emotional experience must be part of our unfolding understanding of unconscious communication. There is more mystery than clarity in regard to unconscious communication, and this mystery has a long history. In the Freud-Ferenczi correspondence circa 1910–12 there is a lot of shared interest in mediums and psychics (Brabent, Falzeder, and Gampieri-Deutsch, 1993). Judit Mészaros (1994) located the intellectual climate of this interest in 19th-century spiritism and a fascination with the occult. Most clinicians have probably had some experience of the uncanny, inexplicable and powerful resonances that can emerge between patient and analyst, as these brief vignettes illuminate. An analyst began attempts to become pregnant, and in synchrony one of her patients began to produce dreams of babies and pregnancy. On the day the analyst was to learn that she was pregnant but before she actually had the news, the patient was nauseated in session, reporting odd feelings of heaviness and anxiety. In the first trimester of the analyst's pregnancy, the patient's dream life and her physical and emotional state in sessions mirrored much in the analyst's own reveries. Whatever the substrate of such transmissions, they are certainly mutually constructed and often arise in treatments where there are complex bidirectional sensitivities and vulnerabilities. Once, at a point close to a summer break, I listened to a patient's dream of a country cottage, in its landscape and style and interior decor so close to my own as to be quite eerie.

Those unsettled, odd sensations have, of course, long been a preoccupation in psychoanalysis (Freud, 1919). A feeling of the uncanny seems best described as a bodily held, low-grade anxiety, a sign of the press of unconscious material, suspended just out of awareness. It is not entirely uncomfortable, not entirely unwelcome. The pregnant analyst felt an odd mixture of sensations and feeling states. On one hand, she felt invaded, too closely responded to, and, on the other hand, she was entranced and amazed at what seemed like the patient's prescience. Which aspects of the experience of being so seamlessly attached to came from her particularly vulnerable state and situation, which from the dyadic relation in the analysis, and which induced by the patient? Elizabeth Mayer (1997) has been trying to find a language to describe anomalous experience, a task that is difficult and unsettling in itself. In these examples, there is much to speculate about the phenomenon of parallel processing, about the powerful base of knowledge of the other person that emerges in intense treatment dyads, as well as each person's creative, constructive contribution to the shared experience. It is hard to walk a conceptual tightrope conveying the experience of the irrational without being reduced to speaking the language of magic.

In this paper I pursue an extended clinical example of dissociative states produced in treatment and subsequently in supervision. The vignette, like the ones I have just described, illustrates a kind of unconscious communication through shared, induced, and projected body states. Much of how this works seems, as I say, still a mystery, but I am convinced that among the important triggers in these shared body–mind states are certain crucial features of language and speech practices. Speech practices can alter the phenomenological experience of certain states of body–mind. Speech performs an action, and the hallowed split between word and deed, so fundamental to psychoanalysis, no longer always holds. The sedating properties of speech patterns, the impact of mimetically reproduced patterns of breathing and soundings, are features of early sleep induction in infants and in self-soothing and self-regulating speech practices in adults.

Hypnosis and trance induction are probably only the tip of the ice-berg. The sliding space between word and action is a core element in transference and countertransference: "transference is what we have left of possession." (Mannoni, 1980). Although the discovery of trans-ference is supposed to have opened a gulf between hypnosis and psy-choanalysis, all Freud's accounts of how transference works depend on analogies to trance and hypnotic induction. Understanding some of the language processes in such communication and the identi-ficatory ties that promote particularly acute transfers of feeling is part of the understanding of unconscious communications and of the role of the body as a receiving instrument. To quote from Merleau-Ponty (1963), "The perceiving mind is an incarnated body." (p. 3)

A relational theory of the body approaches one of the deepest and most compelling and still mysterious problems in psychoanaly-sis: its foundational project to account for psychic life as a body–mind integration. Freud's commitment was to the emergence of the ego as a body ego, which he thought of as a psychic manifestation of a corporeal projection (Freud, 1923).This is both a complex and a subtle idea. The subjective experience of having a body is not inher-ent or natural but is arrived at as the outcome of a series of interac-tive events with the material, social psychic environment. These events are mentally registered. Freud seems to have used the term projection to indicate a surface of representation. Historically, the psychoanalytic theory of ego formation has used terms like internal-ization as the overarching descriptive term for the taking in of identi-fications (Schafer, 1968). Other terms, such as introjection and incorporation, capture certain other distinctions in the process of ego formation. Along with others working on gender studies, I have come to feel that these terms do not fully do justice to the construc-tion of embodiment or body ego, as they connote too exclusively iden-tity as an "inside" phenomenon . It has certainly been one of the preoccupations of Judith Butler in considering gender identities to think of "surface" as a constructed site of psychic life, a strategy that helps undercut the tendency to see body as given and natural and mind as inner and constructed.

The concept of projection could be taken, as Judith Butler (1990, 1993a) does, to mean a constructed *exterior* surface in mental repre-sentation; or, as Roy Schafer (1968) has, as a mental construction in which a fantasy *interiority* is created (see his work on incorporation). The body is not a substrate of mind or the parallel to mental life. Rather, instead of the body as a natural background, the source of endogenous drives or experiences, the body is constructed, as it were, with a false history. It comes into psychic being and then comes to have the characteristics or features of "always there," "there from the beginning." Both the developmental and the social origins of the body are mystified in the illusion of an inherent material substrate. It is not, of course, that there is not a real body but that it must become sensible. This complex construction, the body ego, is the dialectical engagement of endogenous body experiences with intensely meaningful, charged encounters with a social other. From the beginning, one may therefore read in Freud the inseparability of biology from social relations.

Relational theory can be enhanced by a robust encounter with a tradition of body analyses founded on an anti-Cartesian philosophic tradition. In this essay, I draw on not only the relational theory of Mitchell (1988, 1995), Bromberg (1994, 1997), Aron (1995)—particularly its feminist wing (Dimen, 1991, 1996), Goldner (1991), Benjamin (1988, 1995) and others—but also on the work of Didier Anzieu (1985, 1990), psychoanalysts whose work is strongly rooted in the tradition of psychosomatic medicine in France, and on feminist philosophers of the body (Brennan, 1993; Grosz, 1994; Gatens, 1996).

Relational theory can ground itself within the ongoing history of Freudian thought by rejecting a reified and simple biological base to psychic life and commit itself instead to a view of body states and processes as inseparable from fantasy, interaction, and meaning. I am suggesting that we make a claim for a relational Freud. If the intersubjective and the intrapsychic are simultaneously coevolving processes (Benjamin, 1993), then what illuminates and claims a body state or body site for psychic representation is both material and imaginary. Surfaces, rims, holes, cavities, contours, cues of balance, weight, sound and touch, facial reactivity in gazing and smiling, all become invested in meaning and sensory registration through the child's engagement in the interactive matrix with touching, holding, looking at, talking to, loving, and hating others. The child's body is densely textured in meaning and affect for the parents; the child's material life offers itself profoundly to parental battle, parental excitement and to the family's—and probably also the culture's—conscious and unconscious fantasies. This complex imaginary construction may be underway from the point of conception.

A patient, finally happily pregnant, gives herself over to the fascination of sonograms and the fantasies and dreams they provoke. She describes the sonar image traveling across the interior landscape of her body, and, watching the child moving in the amniotic fluid, says, "She's waving at me." And later she dreams that she is nursing the baby, their eyes locked in a delirious gaze. The mother feels aroused and looks at the nipples and genitals of her baby and sees that the baby is aroused too. Already this baby is a gendered, desiring, and desirable attached subject in the mother's imagination and reverie.

A father leans over the isolette where his very tiny son lies amid tubes and lights and the frightening apparatus surrounding prematurity. He recites all the elements of the Periodic table, tells him about chess and football, and in this way helps himself and his wife make a bridge from frightening tiny creature to "baby" and then to "son," finding (i.e., making and constructing) their child.

In these examples, the complex meanings of the child for the family create grids or networks of body excitements, affects, and anxieties, which are then elaborated in the body ego. For all children to some degree and for some children in overwhelming ways, the body is a contested surface in which inner and outer demands get inextricably tangled. The internally felt subjective experience of agency, for example, is an experience that emerges from being seen, wanted, touched, imagined. This experience is not a passive registration but an active organization. Any body is thus a socially and historically specific site for psychic structure and meaning.

I want to hold two contradictory ideas in mind. First, the body and the forms of identity that arise from an experience of being embodied in a social nexus or in a spatiotemporal grid are never prediscursive. That is, body states—the body ego including the experience of gender—are never knowable outside the matrix of human interaction, symbolization, and meaning making. In claiming there is no body ego before or outside meaning, I need to be specific about what is carried in the term meaning. I include in the concept of meaning a range of representations of experience: linguistic, symbolic, imagistic, perceptual. Wilma Bucci (1997) has developed the most articulated model of multiple coding. Describing three levels of representation—symbolic/verbal, symbolic/nonverbal, and subsymbolic—she sees all three as patterned systems of experience registered and represented in conscious and unconscious memory. Her subsymbolic system is not simply identified with the body, although it has some parallel to procedural memory, an organization of experience that is outside conscious awareness and distinct from a narrated, episodic memory formation. Bucci's multiple coding system clearly is intended to bridge the conscious–unconscious distinction.

These systems of representation, although conceptually distinct, are interrelated and interdependent. Speech always interweaves structures of meaning of syntax and of sound. Speech rhythms, intonation patterns, the suprasegmental elements of language are often disambiguating interpretive parts of speech. It is probably impossible fully to unravel symbolic and subsymbolic aspects of language. Certainly, in clinical listening, there are times when the music and prosody of speech illuminate more than the content or semantics and other moments in which affective life is registered in lexical or grammatical choice.

The second idea moves us in the opposite direction, toward an escape from meaning. Bodily life and experience also escape registration and symbolization. The body is more than language; it exceeds not only symbolization but also subsymbolic registration. Any form of registration, even the analogic, which the subsymbolic system appears to be, must exclude and organize experience. There is material life—some ongoing stream of living activity that is inevitably lost to representation, whether analog or digital. This materiality, which exceeds registration, nonetheless impacts it, and this dialectical nonidentity of body and discourse/representation constitutes one of those spaces Bromberg (1997) has articulated, the space within which the magic and power of psychoanalysis emanates.

In the interactive matrix of early social and emotional life, the body is constituted as both the surface landscape and interior space imaginatively grasped and inhabited.

There is an advantage to abandoning the equation of deepness or innerness with authenticity or "realness" of identity. The usual metaphor or construction of body as "raw," mind as "cooked," maintains the very body–mind split Freud's theorizing of ego was designed to address and integrate. When we think of a body ego, socially and intrapsychically constructed, we need to be thinking of body schemes, sense of boundedness and interiority, experiences of moving through space and nonlinear, nonunitary temporalities. Regimens of diet, exercise, and clothing are participating components in a syncretic, evolving structure in which identity is always both "core" and "surface" and bodies emerge and are known and self is known in relation to other bodies. The registration of body states contributes to and interacts with the creation and elaboration of psychic structure and does so in an interpersonal field. Body style, posture, gait, qualities of mobility or stasis, all forms of mimetic identificatory process, carry and maintain intrapsychic experience.

MIMESIS

The development of a body ego draws on and demands a range of identificatory processes, one of which arises through complex forms of surface contact or imitation. *Mimesis* is a form of identification that involves gesture, the style of being, and external patterns of acting (Borch-Jacobsen, 1992). It is a bodily analog to Bakhtin's (1981) accounts of genres and styles of talk, polylogues. Body styles and speech styles are the lived practice of identity. The term mimesis has an interesting history. Coming from the theory of drama and performance, it is the basis for the production of feelings in actors and for the reproduction of emotion in the audience. Mimetic identifications are thus points of transfer of affective states. Mimesis is not imitation in a behavioral sense, although physical acts are involved; mimesis is a responsive, imitative encounter with another being that can lead to mutually induced affective experiences.

The development of an embodied subject proceeds dialectically. Body and body–mind structures emerge from an encounter with the other. The usual term for this process—mirroring—does not do justice to the constructed and active vitality of mimetic exchange. Think of Fromm Reichman's suggestion, described by Shapiro (1996), that one might imaginatively grasp a patient's affective state by assuming the patient's posture. The other person gives back a vision of the self through transactions and interactive practices imbued with the intense anxieties and feelings states that accompany touching, holding, looking. Mimesis, the experience of merging self in the experience of the other, is an experience both active and passive, creating body ego through a use or appropriation of the other, but an other who is an active seer and constructor, not a neutral feedback apparatus. From the charged social interplay in which self other distinctions are blurred and dissolving, body ego and psychic identity thus emerge as inextricably social and also psychic. Mimesis is an experience in which spatial distinctiveness collapses in an experience of being the other.

Mimesis is one pole of body ego formation: self as other. This is the concept that Ricouer (1992) has deeply and carefully elaborated. Finding the otherness of the other is an achievement, the outcome of transactions and interactive patterns of self and other in which an experience of embodiedness is a prerequisite for the finding of alterity (otherness). Piaget's (1954) account of sensorimotor development notes the developmental necessity for action and sensorimotor schemas in finding/constructing the object. In Piagetian theory, at all levels of development, synthesizing activities become coordinated into schemes which site the body in relation to objects. A number of theorists (Feffer, 1982, 1988; Furth, 1987; Fast, 1992) have been working on integrations of cognitive and psychoanalytic developmental theory, interconnecting the child's discovery of the Piagetian object and the Freudian object. In both theoretical enterprises, identification of the other and elaboration of internal schemas of self and other emerge in a field of sensorimotor, embodied action. The object world and the internal world are thus interdependently coconstructed. Only when you are situated as a body ego can you experience the body ego of the other.

This idea deeply preoccupied Merleau-Ponty (1992), who viewed perception as only imaginable as a human activity sited in a bodily experience, a body whose presence enabled the perception of other bodies. We need to develop the courage and imagination to describe clinical psychoanalytic experience in this way.

IMAGINARY ANATOMIES: BODIES AS SOCIAL HISTORY

Psychic life, including body life and body ego is self-experience socially constructed through intersubjective and interactive dialogues in social life, in family matrices, and certainly in analytic treatments. This is a familiar relational concept applied to the body ego.

From the beginning, the child's body ego is an imaginary anatomy, shaped by the meaning given by the social surrounding and processed by the child (both activities that inevitably distort as they construct). How the baby eats and is fed, how the infant is soothed, how affect attunement, rupture and repair, peaks of excitation are relationally handled come to be actively constructed as an experience of self for the child, as well as an experience of self and other. States of distress and anxiety within the dyad are regulated, understood or ignored, named or silenced, in some way lived in the social matrix and then assigned to and absorbed by the child. Any particular body state is unimaginable outside the historically specific coherences in which human life is constructed and the emotional dynamics in which a particular child comes to be experienced and thus to know and be herself or himself. The work of Susan Coates and colleagues (1991) on boyhood gender identity disorder illuminates how plastic body identity can be, how subtly and astonishingly the body can bend to the relational dynamics within families and within individuals.

The concept of a social and interpersonal body is an application of familiar relational concepts to thinking about the body. But the focus of relational psychoanalytic theories has tended to be dyadic, a dialectically coproduced account of self- and self-and-other-experience that comes to be experienced as individual experience. Relational psychoanalysis has focused in a very finely grained way on the events in the consulting room. It is usually a two-person social theory. A number of writers (Flax, 1990; Dimen, 1991; Goldner, 1991) have been arguing that these relational concepts are congruent with a variety of developments within postmodern discourse in which discursive practices, carrying both local and more generic rules and power interests, come to constitute bodies and persons. Postmodern theories have been more explicitly concerned with situating the individual or the dyad in a network of relationships and experiences in which social and historical forces are in play. Discourse, a layered set of codes, regulatory practices, rules both obligatory and optional, all arise in both local, familial conditions and in wider, ideologically laced practices within the culture and come to be the forces through which experiences of individual life and body life are constituted as subjective experience. These social forces come to be both deeply internalized states and also forms of surface identity and embodiment through which ways of feeling normal, sexual, gendered, real, authentic, and coherent are maintained.[1]

Postmodern and poststructural theories share certain features in common with the French tradition of psychosomatic psychology and with contemporary feminist philosophies of the body. One unifying force is a consistent anti-Cartesian position. The splits between body and mind, the determination to privilege reason over affect and somatic states—what Descartes called the vegetative soul—is the continuing heritage that has so often dominated psychoanalytic thinking and which now unites a variety of theoretical oppositions.

Elizabeth Grosz (1994) is one of a of group of philosophers whose work is described as corporeal feminism. This work draws its theoretical ancestry from Spinoza through Merleau Ponty and Hegel as well as the contemporary work of Foucault. She has been attracted to, and makes a good case for the value of, Spinoza's materialism and monism as an alternative to Cartesian rationalism. Bodies are both relationally and historically constituted, never universally abstractable from the context in which they live and move. Permanence lies in the continuity of process, not in substance or structure. Grosz imbues her work on the body with a materialist and antipositivist spirit, and hers is a viewpoint compatible with relational theory. She is rejecting the Cartesian split of body and mind and the deep, culturally driven system of categorization in which mind is masculinized and body feminized such that woman as category is the embodiment of a natural and unmediated essence.

Grosz is interested in the multiplicity of body states and body types and is attentive to the meaning of body as emergent in context, particularly social and historical context. Although our introspective experiences may usually be of inhabiting one body, it is probably more accurate to see body ego as a set of layered ego states registering a number of spatiotemporal experiences of self, sometimes simultaneously, sometimes successively. Body and mind construct each other; gestures, sensations, experiences create psychic representations, and the psychic structure—the body image—affects the regulation and perception and self-perception of the body.

Grosz deploys Merleau Ponty's phenomonology to counter a more usual view of the body as "ineffable," a natural essence that is prereflective and prediscursive. Merleau Ponty sought to describe embodied existence as a constructed and synthetic experience, not that the body is an unmarked background or substrate to experience. The body is not a thing, but a condition, a context through which I am able to have a relation to objects (and other bodies). This might be one way to think about the function of gender in psychic life. Locating or constructing an experience of having a gender within one's bodyscape creates a psychic experience filtered in and through the body that is an identity, to be sure, but also a mode of perception and sensory synthesis. Gender can be put to use as a mode of seeing, operating as defense, or as a way to regulate anomalies of attachment and interaction. This is probably most clear when the body ego gender appears oppositional to biology. The boy or girl with gender identity disorder—or perhaps any child who alters body type in some actual or psychic way (i.e., body weight, musculature used to fortress or pad the body)—may be both defending psychic life and also creating conditions for seeing and being in the world.

The surfaces of the body, then, are a two-way filtering system, protecting from intrusion and invasion or loss but also shaping what is seen and experienced by the child through the body. Gestures, ways of speaking, practices of body and mind emerge in particular settings under particular conditions of awareness of self and other. At any moment there are multiple possibilities in meaning making and a body–mind schema of considerable plasticity. The particular conditions of emotional and psychic life may shape the fate of that plasticity.

This approach has some interesting theoretical fellow travelers.

There are, as noted earlier in my discussion of mimesis, quite remarkable resonances to Bakhtin's (1981) theories of genres of speech
and the polylog of any speaker, the ability to draw on multiple codes
of expression, style, or gesture both to see the world and to be seen
in it. Bromberg's (1997) concept of multiplicity explores this perspective in clinical experience. This kind of materialist perspective is
also compatible with Thelen and Smith's (1995) dynamic system
model, in which setting, environment, and individual codetermine the
emergent experiences both of body and of psychic life.

Reading Grosz's (1994) meditations on the constituting of bodily
life in context, including interpersonal context, makes me think of my
patient M, for whom the body is a suit of armor. From girlhood, she
managed the memories trauma through a regimen of athleticism and
bodily ordeal. A childhood of repeated, painful surgeries was experienced and managed as a tomboyhood of adventure and enterprise. M
built a powerful defense against pain and vulnerability that became,
somehow, mysteriously caught up with matters of gender. Her anorexic
body was, for her, consciously and deliberately, a nonmaternal body.
She viewed pregnancy and mothering with horror; the inevitably humiliating consequences for anyone trapped in that experience required a stripping of flesh and fat. Magical beliefs and rules for eating
dominated her life. It would be nice, she muses, if eating were not a
totalitarian experience. But she lived terrorized by foods she deemed
dangers, what she termed, ironically, "the demonology of muffins."
Reduced mostly to a regimen of oatmeal and lettuce, she functions as
though fat-bearing food were an inseminating object. Her body's vulnerability and the pressing dilemma she feels concerning its coherence is a complex matter. Invasions could come in the form of surgical
knives, food, or penises, and the threatening passivity with which
she bears these experiences requires a dissociated deadness. The
narcissistic pain of scars and the agonizing memories of surgeries,
reencountered in any experiences of passivity, must be anesthetized
with more and different pain. Is it this same supplanting of one pain
for another that underlies some forms of skin cutting and scarifica-
tion?

M is in a difficult quandary. She can bear to have weight only if it
is muscle. Fat is squishy, disgusting, soft, dangerous. Yet she is aware
that her body presentation is slipping along a continuum toward
oddity that is equally terrifying. Caught between two regimens—her
own mortification of the flesh and the socially driven regulation of
look, gait, gesture, dress—she feels trapped. Between the body she
must structure for personal coherence and the adorned, highly pro-

duced body she must have for social coherence, she is stymied and frightened.

For this woman, the flesh-stripped look is only one feature of the story; pain is also a sought-after state. An agonizing Saturday consisting of a sequence of visits to different gyms across the city began to sound like the Stations of the Cross—the white heat of body pain and ordeal blanching out upset, depression, loneliness. Unafraid of physical ordeal that obliterates the nameless dread of need and vulnerability, she is afraid to feel and she is afraid of me. Although this fear is expressed mostly as contempt. I am identified with softness and warmth and flesh . When I could get a handle on my own narcissistic injury at having to be the fat, humiliated, mothering one, I began to realize that she was organizing intense exercises around session so that she would arrive after a four- to seven-mile run, and by session's end she would be ice cold and shivering, departing to run again. Some measure of the danger of warmth and connection to warm living analytic flesh can be seen in the intensity of the counteracting regimen I devised. I put a little space heater on one morning, and she wept, her face seeming suddenly very childlike and sweet. These moments were important to her, but she avoids them or minimizes them as far as is possible. Later I realized she was also balancing morning analytic sessions with a weightlifting regimen with a physically powerful, well-muscled male trainer whom she carefully told me is the one who is really helping her and who, I note with some irritation, is the only one who can tell her what and when to eat.

M's long and continuing history as a tomboy interests me. In work I have been doing on masculinity in women, I have found that the tomboy aspect in female character serves many functions and is shaped through many different kinds of relationships, object ties, and disidentifications. Some tomboys (M would be an example) live this identity as a defense against trauma. There is an extraordinary passage from Faulkner's (1931) novel *Sanctuary* in which Temple Drake, about to be raped in the barn by Popeye, dreamily imagines that she is turning into a boy. The body ego, as a mimetic activity or structure, may be constructed as a way of forgetting, as an erasure or foreclosure of traumatic memory.

PSYCHIC ENVELOPES: THE SKIN EGO

Another modality for describing the relational construction of body ego is useful in considering clinical material, including my patient, M.

Anzieu (1985, 1990), contemplating the origins of body ego in the sensorimotor enmeshment and interaction of socially handled bodies, uses the medium of skin and the metaphor of the envelope to capture the relational construction of body experience in the process of social development. We can draw some analogies between Anzieu's concept of skin ego and the idea of mimesis and mimetic identifications.

Anzieu imagined that there were multiple functions of the skin: containing; providing stimulus barrier and protection, but also potentially generating excitement and contact; regulating internal and external stimulation; inscribing boundaries and individuation; creating (well or badly) internal structural support and balance; and representing and sometimes amplifying experience. He seems to speak both concretely and metaphorically, like patients. Flesh is spoken of as padding. A patient talks of living with her back to the wall, of the impossibility of feeling supported. Anzieu speculated on the child's experience of being well seated, held against the body of the parent, a structural, postural site of safety and boundedness. Patients talk about leakage, the feeling that substance and energy are flowing out— exsanguinating. A patient repeatedly talks of not being able to get her balance. Although she is speaking of a balance between work and relationships or between family and friends, the language is strikingly about the body. Problems of scale—bigness and smallness—problems of pace, speed, and gait through the world; the psychic dilemma is captured for the patient in images and signification of the body moving in space.

Although skin may seem to be a structure bounding a person, it is, in Anzieu's view, also an envelope. In the fantasy of shared skin, it is a site of dyadic experience. The term envelope is perhaps a curious choice. Anzieu in thinking of the skin ego was suggesting the skin as an organ of containment and contouring; but later, in extensions of his work into other sensory modalities, namely, the envelopes of sound, he seems to be using the term to describe a broad band of experience in which social (particularly dyadic) life is sensorially located and lived. As in so much conceptual work on the body and body ego, one is always slipping along a continuum of symbolic and material phenomena

Anzieu's work adds an important dimension to our current psychoanalytic understanding of early dyadic life, so powerfully delineated in the infancy research literature. The primary focus of infancy studies has centered on visual experience, dyadic, face-to-face play, and the antiphonal interactions through which self and self-with-other come to be registered.

There are sound empirical reasons for the attention to visual gaze, visual attention, facial mimesis, and vocal rhythm matching. Beebe and Lachmann (1994) have drawn from this work salient principles in which patterns of attunement, regulation of joint and single feeling states and the histories of rupture and repair in dyadic interaction are all featured. But it is equally important to remember that facial play and dyadic gaze occur in the context of bodily experience in which the body exists in space and in spatial and temporal patterns in relation to other bodies. Posture, gestures, proprioceptive cues affecting a sense of balance and weightedness, experiences of touch and sound, all form a complex web of experiences in which the body is always a body in social space (and in time, both micro and macro). Sometimes body style can seem like a kind of carbon dating, a freezing of certain physical states and stances that appear relatively unelaborated and unaltered. For instance, a patient described meeting her prospective mother-in-law, a woman whose history or fragility and loss she knew. At the outset she was struck by the childlike walk and a "little girl" quality in the older woman's physical presentation and voice. During the meeting, the mother for the first time told her son and his fianceé of her early traumas. She had been a hidden child in Europe and suffered a terrible postwar reunion with her surviving parent. Vocal style can signal a frozen state as well. As an adolescent, M realized that she was still explaining in a childish syntax, to any inquirer about her scars, "I got bit by a dog."

Didier Houzel (1990), elaborating on Anzieu's idea of skin ego as envelope, stressed both its function as boundary marker and its function as adhesive relational structure. For Houzel, the theoretical precursors for the concept of envelope are Klein's (1975) account of projective identification and Winnicott's (1971) transitional space. I would add the work of Bion (1961) both because he was explicitly interested in container as metaphor and as material registration of identity and also because Bion saw a dynamic dialectic between container and contained. Houzel and Anzieu are trying to theorize a particular form of representation and structure that is not organizable along the conventional categories of primary/secondary; symbolic/ nonsymbolic; verbal/nonverbal. Looked at carefully, I think Winnicott's concept of transitional objects and transitional space spans contradictory dichotomies: symbolic and material, both fetish and symbol, changeable and unchangeable. Here the skin ego, or psychic envelope, is a trace, registered psychically, in which patterns of living and body experience are encoded, whether inscribed as surfaces or organized as knots of action, gestalts of sensorimotor experience. Yet the point of creation and elaboration for such structures includes Bion's (1961) concept of maternal reverie: the gazing preoccupation of the parent (and later the analyst) organizing, making coherent the shapes and patterns of material and social life. This gaze is never ideologically neutral; it must always see certain coherences at the expense of others and inevitably at the expense of some qualities of sensuous life.

Discourse and dialogue are also containing envelopes in which self and other are constituted and in which the body comes to be experienced. Naming, coordinated with sense experience and affective life, creates the body ego, often siting it retrospectively as a natural, always there but actually developed and emergent only in social processes. When we look at language as a envelope or as an aspect of skin formation, however, some very complicated things are happening. It is important to reassert Bion's (1961) dialectic of container and contained and to see that in language this encircling interpenetration is always occurring. Speech functions in this dual way. Speech practices function both as transitional objects and as sites for transitional space: container and contained. Lecourt (1990) proposes the concept of the sonorous bath—that the materiality of speech, its rhythms, patterns, its prosodic tones and tunes function as internal regulation, as internally represented object relations and as external forms of cohesion and adhesion.

Somewhat shyly, a patient describes a bedtime ritual in which she gets ready to sleep, padding around her apartment, involved in many bodily preoccupations, cleaning, washing, quietly talking a kind of babytalk to herself. Putting herself to bed, she calls it, and in the murmuring sounds she plays both parent and child, speaking and being soothingly spoken to. Living alone and discovering in her treatment an understanding of her profound aloneness as a child have made her acutely aware of this speech practice. She and her mother now speak to each other in this way. It has been reparative for them to recognize the patient's deep body needs for maternal care. Interestingly, this body care is provided mostly through language. To say that these murmuring words are a sonorous bath is to speak metaphorically and metanymically and to be describing experience as slipping along a continuum of symbolic and presymbolic process.

The synthesizing accounts of the neurobiology of affect reported by Schore (1994) describe a parallel physiological substrate to these complex, multisensory regulatory experiences. The integrative experiences of dyadic life may alter and shape integrative brain circuitry, such that the term regulation is relevant at many levels of description.

The contemptuous phrase "show and tell," with its infantilizing nod to the activities of preschoolers, exists in the vernacular of clinicians as a kind of hidden code to describe a certain kind of process in which the patient seems to be just reporting events. Sometimes there is an elaborate detailing of symptoms and self-state experiences, sometimes apparently just a listing of events in a spatiotemporal pattern. But what if we saw this activity as identity contouring, drawing the gaze and attention of the listener (in hostility or boredom or fascination) through the routines of body, material life and transactions? If we saw this dialogue as a shared skin, then the mirroring analytic listener's feeling tone and associative processes enter the fabric of words, which become the contouring skin ego of the speaker. If one acknowledges the mixture of contempt and irritation that may accompany our listening to these lists and detailed accounts of daily events, one could think of this listening as the installation of misattunement. But certainly another way to think of the interactive matrix in this context is to see the dyadic construction of masochism, a skin of pain and suffering in which the gaze of the other is a crucial ingredient in the construction of a masochistic envelope.

Anzieu (1985) used the term masochistic envelopes to describe the psychic representation of certain modes of connection in which the adhesion or glue connecting self and other is shared experiences of pain, crisis, or anguish. Experiences and talk of pain come to constitute a social frame, a tissue or web of experiences through which identity is secured, maintained, formed. Drawing on his detailed work on body ego, which focused initially and primarily on the skin as a complex, socially reverberating register of psychic structure and interaction, Anzieu extended his analysis to experiences of pain as identity forming and body contouring. Talking, complaining, naming are the delineating experiences of body state and body distress, the traffic through which the body comes to be psychically represented and experienced for all participants in the discursive scene.

Exploring the power of pain and the discursive practices that surround and frame pain to constitute self as instantiated body ego is not unique to Anzieu and the tradition of psychoanalytically informed psychosomatic medicine in which his work is situated. Ogden (1989) writes of the power of crisis and anguish to act as a congealing, fusing element in interaction, often through the autistic contiguous position. The analytic dyad is merged in response to crisis, as the following vignette suggests.

A patient is describing a hard-won triumph in her professional life. The session has a calm, sweet quality. Tentatively she is hopeful, and I allow myself an experience of happiness and pride, a lightening of the weather in a treatment marked by ongoing crisis and despair. One abiding image we have attended to comes from a dream: the patient wedged on a tiny ledge, holding her family. There is danger if she moves; she is on the edge of a precipice and in that state we have lived together a long time, she frozen in terror and I agitated and helpless. Later she reports a sense of melancholy. Has she lost forever our shared skin of agitation and, along with it, the memories (charged with pleasure and pain) of familial connections in which one's pain and another's anxious worrying attention secure fragile identities and fragile ties?

A number of feminist theorists have been attentive to the function of pain in the elaboration of gender as psychic structure.[2] From work on body scheme in studies of hysteria and neurological accidents, a picture emerges. Pain can amplify sensory and body experience or drain it of meaning and feeling. Bodies can be evacuated, or, alternatively, body states and structures can acquire a limenal status. Kristeva (1992) used the term abject to describe such body experiences, which were often taken as points of horror and disgust but certainly of fascination. A term like *jouissance* suggests a surplus to enjoyment but enjoyment and investment can come in many forms— the frisson of terror, the luxuriating preoccupation with the details of an illness. Infection, injury, certain limenal sates of physicality—mucous, vomit, feces, urine, breast milk—may function as an intermediate state, a contradictory ineradicable foreignness and familiarity, simultaneously alienated and cherished. This site of marginality was extensively theorized by the anthropologist Mary Douglas (1965) in analyzing the dietary laws in Old Testament texts as structures to control forms of ambiguity. Kristeva and others have made psychoanalytic use of these ideas by looking at the power of the culture to regulate the body, to exile its impurities and force certain coherences and orderliness. The plasticity of the body holds a great potential as a site for meaning. Body talk, particularly the litany of descriptive complaints, is one of these masochistic envelopes, a fabric constituting identity formation and transformation.

These concepts and metaphors of shared skin and psychic envelopes can be used to underwrite an intriguing clinical problem. The following vignette illustrate the occurrence and function of shared dissociative states, the sort of transference and countertransference experiences (some solo, some shared) of sleepiness, confusional dissolves, disorganization, and sometimes odd and disturbing somatic disruptions. These shared states draw on some forms of mimetic iden-

tifications and imitations between patient and analyst. These interpersonal states may also function to buffer shared skins, as forms of
the skin ego Anzieu and others have described.

SHARED DISSOCIATIVE STATES

Much of the contemporary discussion of induced countertransference depends on a perspective of intersubjectivity, the psychic envelope of the analytic couple. This vignette describes the play of a
powerful force field with a treatment that replayed in supervision and
that led me to think about the sonorous bath of sound as a mechanism
for inducing dissociated states across various dyads.

An analyst is talking in supervision about a difficult experience
she is having with a patient. The long treatment has been both involving and perplexing for the analyst. Despite intensive careful work,
the patient often appears flat and disconnected from her own experience of her material and from the analyst. Sessions often appear to
be beyond or untouched by any of the history of the treatment. Both
patient and analyst became dazed and appear to be virtually anesthetized from time to time. The analyst is alternately worried and
angry. She is caught in the painful contradiction of knowing the deep
damage to the patient's mental, emotional, and material life while
spending sessions feeling stalled and immobilized.

One day, while she is introducing me to the patient's history in a
violent and confusing family, I realize I am not following her and that
there is something she just said that I can't quite wrap my mind
around. I dimly realize that, minutes earlier, she described a characteristic scene. At some point in childhood, the family's sleeping arrangements changed. The patient was sent to sleep in her parents'
bed while they moved to a living room sofa. The analyst is detailing
the patient's daily experience of adolescence. In a morning ritual, her
father would come into the bedroom, lie down on top of her, and
caress her. Hearing this, I realize that the supervisee has already told
me this, that these events are of central importance to the patient
and are discussed from time to time in the treatment, but in a desul-
tory way. In somewhat enigmatic, passive language, I am told by the
supervisee that it is not clear what, if anything, happened. It's sort of
foggy. And I can feel the fog inside me, transmitted within my analytic
spaces. The supervisee and I then begin to talk about getting fogged
out, a signature experience for her in this treatment and a palpable,
shared state for both us at that moment in the supervision. We notice

that if we can turn our attention to the fog and acknowledge the confusional state, our heads clear.

The analyst and I track the frequency of these dissociated states
and begin to speculate about the conditions and triggers for what
feels like an altered body–mind state. The experience is of a disruption in synthetic thinking, in cognitive processing, and in memory as
well as a cocooning of feelings and emotional reaction, very much
like Bion's (1961) attacks on linking. It occurs to me that our shared
fog is connected to the increased anxiety and ambiguity in our field
regarding the handling of clinical material involving abuse.

The analyst tells me about an active, good hour with the patient.
She is speaking to me in a lively way, wanting to tell me about an
amazing dream the patient had and the vivid session of work that
followed the dream report. The dream is striking. The patient is in a
bed, hiding under the covers and surrounded by her family and a
person who is perhaps the therapist. The therapist is to explain to
the parents why the patient is under the covers.

The analyst then rushes on to tell me about the confusion and
disorganization in the following session, when the patient spent a
muddled, muddling hour describing a friend's husband who is possibly psychotic. I interrupt and ask the analyst to go back and tell me
about the work on the dream. She looks blank, then distressed, and
realizes that she has lost the entire postdream session. She has no
notes and not a glimmer, not a shard of working memory of the session. At this moment she is fogged and very upset. I feel alive and
interested. It occurs to me that one clue to the lost dream work and
to our currently different mental states is in the quality and material
of the next session, which the analyst was in the midst of reporting.
The muddled talk, the confusing preoccupation with the disturbed
family friend (perhaps a displacement of the madness she fears in
her father) erases the lively, clear experience. It is a miniversion of
the sequence of clarity and confusion, the assault on the sense of
reality and a posttraumatic trance induction that retrospectively alters
the encoding and remembering of traumatic events.

I think about the power of speech, its performative functions, in
the creation of body–mind states in which experience is encoded.
Something in the quality or tone of the speech induces an altered
state in the listener. A sonorous bath can soothe you into stupor, and
the content of speech flows by unremarked. Some weeks later the
supervisee describes another vivid dream, this with some strikingly
sexual imagery. I ask about any associations, and the analyst responds
in a casual and flatly declarative voice, mimetically reproducing the

tonal speech patterns of her patient. It is an association to date rape, graphically rendered. Again we are minutes along in the conversation before the quality or content of this quotation registers on either of us. We then both realize that this casual, chatty, understated communication style from the patient was reproduced by the analyst just moments before in our working session. We had been talking about the traumatic impact of the repeated bedroom scenes on the patient's oedipal fantasy. The analyst had spoken in an uncharacteristically flip way, tossing off a casual comment about oedipal guilt and the patient as an oedipal winner. Something in the rhythms and styles of speech was undermining the complexity and seriousness of the semantic content of the material. As in the association of the dream image to the patient's dating experiences, the material flowed between the analyst and me without either of us feeling, or even registering, what we were saying.

With the patient's permission, the analyst began to tape sessions and we began to be able to stand outside the flow of speech and therefore became able to think. Some of the time. I found that I could not listen to the tapes in my car for fear of falling asleep on the highway. We began to notice that, although the patient spoke extensively and volubly, it didn't exactly seem like free association. Her speech did not seem to be addressed to the analyst, and I began to feel that part of the analyst's dissociation was a result of being erased in a stream of speech that only appeared to be spoken to her. The patient also spoke as though nothing had ever been securely known in the long treatment. The same questions were asked and reasked, the same wonder and confusion repeatedly voiced.

The analyst began to speculate about the function for the patient of nothing being clear or known, the advantage of never being sure of what was real and what mattered. Whenever the analyst began very carefully to summarize or clarify something known or shared between them, the patient became extremely anxious. The patient's talk seemed designed to maintain muddle and uncertainty. All of this was quite subtle. The session might appear flowing and full, but the syntax, the pragmatics of the speech and content were oddly disconnected, and the coherence of a narrative was really quite fictive. Listening to the tapes, we could hear that, when the analyst spoke, the patient went on as though nothing had occurred. Soporific, prosodically looping, and either repetitively pleading or flat, the patient's speech was inducing trance states in the analyst and often in me, the supervisor. The theoretical points commented on in the supervision and the clinical data as they appeared in sessions and reported in supervision were flattened out and deadened in a way that would powerfully inhibit any listener from feeling and thinking. Induced countertransference as a communication from and for each of us created an imaginative inhabiting of the patient's experience, but along with the induction came a paralysis of thought.

One interesting sidebar to this: While the analyst and I were tracking the speech practices that were disrupting us, and for some time prior to this, the patient had been making substantial progress in her treatment. This program continued. She was in an important and quite new kind of relationship with a man and was struggling to find the courage to marry and to confront her family with her new-found happiness and contentment. She was getting better in real-life ways while her treatment team often felt that we were falling asleep or falling to pieces.

As I think about these shared dissociative states and mutually altered consciousness across the dyad, I find that there is much still to theorize and understand. Certainly any clinician has the familiar experience of feeling a patient's affect split off from content, and usually this rupture or split between content and affect gives some traction for psychological work. Here something radically different was occurring; the material seemed to be accompanied or surrounded by speech practices that altered the listener's receptive capacities. Speech is functioning as a shared skin, as a soothing and state-inducing container, but this envelope simultaneously connects and disconnects. Dissociative processes are induced in the listener in some form of mimetic imitation and identification.

An analyst may be generically the kind of listener who is particularly attuned to or susceptible to this process. Louise De Turburay (1996), writing about an analyst's difficulty with separations, talks about the power of the analyst's projections and investments in the interior spaces and psychic structures of patients. The psychic envelope of the consulting room perhaps heightens receptivity and connection; the fantasy of shared skin of sonorous baths of words and sounds makes the mutual induction of trance states and altered receptivity to language a likely feature of intense treatments.

CONCLUSION

Most of the theorists I have drawn on for this essay are exploring new ways of imagining body mind integration. Dissatisfied with a Cartesian- based split of reason and emotion, the idealizing of cognition, and the simplification of the body as natural given, they search for metaphors, for theoretical apparatus and for evidence in neurological and clinical studies. One unifying framework is to see all this work under the rubric of a general systems theory, where complex processes of human skill and human interaction are the flexible, plastic, and multivariable outcome of interactions across persons and within body and mental life. Across different disciplines one can see what we might call two-person biologies that appear to match and interact with two-person psychologies. In contemporary developmental theory, set on a strong tradition of empirical research, the principles of multiple pathways, emergent process, variation, and plasticity can help psychoanalysts live in less rigid and deterministic models, appreciating the "surplus of meaning and density" that work with patients always entails.

In so much of this work one feels the struggle to describe limenal experience, states of being and knowing and perceiving that seem sometimes extradiscursive, sometimes marked by discourse, and sometimes on a continuum of representation. Perhaps because we are in this interesting, speculative phase of our understanding, we are proliferating a rich set of metaphors, which we don't think of solely as metaphoric—skins, baths, solutions, infiltrates, musculature and skeletal frames, rhizomes and Mobius strips—I prefer to think of social and relational life as a "continuum of interacting embodied subjectivities" (Merleau-Ponty, 1962 p. 162), we are moving away from the body as machine and towards a more plastic and complex "body," where inside and outside fold around each other and distinctions like inside and outside are abstractions.

NOTES.

[1] I have used the term social to stretch from dyad to family to culture and have invoked historical specificity as an inalienable feature of bodily life. But this has been more a rhetorical strategy than a worked argument. How to write about the impact of the larger social structures on psyche has been a problem for psychoanalysis throughout its history. If often seems either to take the writer away from psychoanalytic ideas and into another discourse or, speaking in linguistic metaphors, to default one descriptive system to another.

Kenneth Gergen's (1997) wide-ranging discussion of social constructionism (1997) offers a useful introduction to the ways in which social formation enters and constitutes scientific and intellectual projects through the densely layered experience of social life and interpersonal dynamics. He also locates

this analysis in an intellectual and philosophic tradition. A full incorporation of these ideas in clinical psychoanalysis and in our theory is a major
but as yet unrealized project.

Another one of the most useful forms of this kind of integration is found
in contemporary cultural studies, particularly work on the cinema, which
focuses on the spectator (Penley, 1988). In that work, the power of certain
iconic and mythic forms to shape psychic life is explored through the use of
ideas of transference and theories of identification.

²The concept that pain initiates body ego and body coherence is the
linchpin idea through which Judith Butler (1993) launched her account of
the constituting of the body through its discourses. She was drawing on
Freud's famous metaphor of the toothache as as the foundational experience of ego states. In Butler's work, gender is founded on and through the
melancholy reaction to loss and pain. Femininity, then, is a body-ego state
and a psychic reality in which the repudiated longing for the mother reposes.
If that early desire must be scarified to ensure identification, and if that desire is repudiated and prohibited in the course of oedipal and preoedipal
sexual organization, these foreclosed loves must remain in some form in
conscious or unconscious life. Gender identity is one site of those aspects of
early love and desire that can never be fully repudiated. Gender is the melancholy residue of loves that have come to be forbidden. One is what one
cannot love, in this argument, but pain and loss are at the epicenter of psychic
identity.

REFERENCES

Anzieu, D. (1985), *The Skin Ego.* New Haven, CT: Yale University Press.
———— (1990), *Psychic Envelopes.* London: Karnac Books.
Aron, L. (1995), *A Meeting of Minds.* Hillsdale, NJ: The Analytic Press.
Bakhtin, M. M. (1981), *The Dialogic Imagination,* ed. & trans. M. Holquist. Aus-
    tin: University of Texas Press.
Beebe, B. & Lachmann, F. (1994), Representation and internalization in infancy:
    Three principles of salience. *Psychoanal. Psychol.,* 11:127–165.
Benjamin, J. (1988), *Bonds of Love.* New York: Pantheon.
———— (1995), *Like Subject, Love Object.* New Haven, CT: Yale University Press.
Bion, W. (1961), A theory of thinking. *Internat. J. PsychoAnal.* 43:306–310.
Borch-Jacobsen, M. (1992), *The Emotional Tie.* Stanford, CA: Stanford Univer-
    sity Press.
Brabant, E., Falzeder, E. & Gampieri-Deutsch, P. (1988), *The Correspondence of
    Sigmund Freud and Sandor Ferenczi, Vol 1. 1908-1914.* Cambridge, MA:
    Harvard University Press.
Brennan, T. (1993), *History After Lacan.* London: Routledge.
Bromberg, P. (1994), "Speak that I may see you": Some reflections on dissocia-
    tion, reality and psychoanalytic listening. *Psychoanal. Dial.,* 4:517–542.

Bucci, W. (1997), *Psychoanalysis and Cognitive Science*. New York: Guilford.

Butler, J. (1990), *Gender Trouble*. New York: Routledge.

——— (1993a), *Bodies That Matter*. New York: Routledge.

Coates, S., Friedman, R. C. & Wolff, S. (1991), The aetiology of boyhood gender identity disorder: A model for integrating psychcodynamics, temperament and development. *Psychoanal. Dial.*, 1:249–272

De Turburey, L. (1995), Countertransference effects of absence. *Internat. J. Psycho-Anal.*, 76:683–694.

Dimen, M. (1991), Deconstructing difference: gender, splitting, and transitional space. *Psychoanal. Dial.*, 1:335–352.

——— (1995), On our nature: Prolegomenon to a theory of sexuality. In: *Disorienting Sexualities*, ed., T. Domenici & R. Lesser. New York: Routledge, pp. 29–52.

Douglas, M. (1965), *Purity and Danger*. London: Routledge & Kegan Paul.

Fast, I. (1992), The embodied mind: Toward a relational perspective. *Psychoanal. Dial.*, 2:389–409.

Faulkner, W. (1931), *Sanctuary*. New York: Cape & Smith.

Feffer, M. (1982), *The Structure of Freudian Thought*. New York: International Universities Press.

——— (1988), *Radical Constructionism*. New York: New York Universiy Press.

Ferenczi, S. (1932), *The Clinical Diaries of Sándor Ferenczi*. ed. J. Dupont (trans. M. Balint & N.Z. Jackson). Cambridge,MA: Harvard University Press, 1988.

Flax, J. (1990), *Thinking Fragments,* Berkeley: University of California Press.

Freud, S. (1919), The uncanny. *Standard Edition*, 17:217–252. London: Hogarth Press, 1955.

——— (1923), The ego and the id. *Standard Edition,* 19:12–68. London: Hogarth Press, 1961.

Furth, H. (1987), *Knowledge as Desire*. New York: Columbia University Press.

Gatens, M. (1996), *Imaginary Bodies*. London: Routledge.

Gergen, K. (1997), *Realities and Relationships*. Cambridge, MA: Harvard University Press.

Goldner, V. (1991), Toward a critical relational theory of gender. *Psychoanal. Dial..* 1:481–523.

Green, A. (1975), The analyst, symbolization and absence in the analytic setting. In: *On Private Madness*. London: Hogarth Press, 1986.

——— (1995), Has sexuality anything to do with psychoanalysis. *Internat. J. Psycho-Anal.*, 76:871–873.

——— (1997), Opening remarks to a discussion of sexuality in contemporary psychoanalysis. *Internat. J. Psycho-Anal.* 78:345–350.

Grosz, E. (1994), *Volatile Bodies*. Bloomington: University of Indiana Press.

Houzel, D. (1990), The concept of the psychic envelope. In: *Psychic Envelopes*, ed. D. Anzieu. London: Karnac Books, pp. 27–58.

Jacobs,T. (1991), *The Use of the Self.* Madison, CT: International Universities Press.

Klein, M. (1975), *Envy and Gratitude*. New York: Delta.

Kristeva, J. (1982), *Powers of Horror.* New York: Columbia University Press.
Lecourt, E. (1990), The musical envelope. In: *Psychic Envelopes*, ed. D. Anzieu. London: Karnac Press. pp. 211–236.
Mannoni, O. (1980), *Un Commencement qui n'en finit pas.* Paris: Le Seuil.
Mayer, E. (1997), Subjectivity and intersubjectivity of clinical facts. *Internat. J. Psycho-Anal.,* 77:709–738.
Merleau-Ponty, M. (1962), *The Primacy of Perception.* Evanston, IL: Northwestern University Press.
Mészáros, J. (1994), Ferenczi' pre-analytic world. In: *The Legacy of Sándor Ferenczi,* ed. L. Aron & A. Harris. Hillsdale, NJ: The Analytic Press, pp. 41–51.
Mitchell, S. (1988), *Relational Concepts in Psychoanalysis.* Cambridge, MA: Harvard University Press.
——— (1993), *Hope and Dread in Psychoanalysis.* New York: Basic Books.
Ogden, T. (1989), *The Primitive Edge of Experience.* Northvale, NJ: Aronson.
Penley, C. (1988), *Feminism and Film Theory.* New York: Routledge.
Piaget, J. (1954), *The Construction of Reality in the World.* New York: Basic Books.
Ricouer, P. (1992), *Oneself as Another.* Chicago: University of Chicago Press.
Schafer, R. (1968), *Aspects of Internalization.* New York: International Universities Press.
Shapiro, S. (1996), The embodied analyst in the Victorian cunsulting room. *Gender & Psychoanal.,* 1:297–322.
Schore, A. (1994), *Affect Regulation and the Origin of the Self.* Hillsdale, NJ: Lawrence Erlbaum Associates.
Thelen, E. & Smith, L. (1995), *A Dynamic Systems Approach to the Development of Cognition and Action.* Cambridge, MA: MIT Press.
Winnicott, D. W. (1947), Hate in the countertransference. In: *Through Paediatrics to Psychoanalysis.* New York: Basic Books, 1958, pp. 194–203.
——— (1971), *Playing and Reality.* London: Tavistock.

3

POLYGLOT BODIES

Thinking Through the Relational

Muriel Dimen

THE SIGNIFYING BODY

The psychoanalytic body is going through changes. Once upon a time, it was real, substantial, finite, mapped by excitable but containable erogenous zones. Recently, however, it seems hardly corporeal or sensate at all. Thanks to Jacques Lacan and Michel Foucault, what was for Sigmund Freud a biological entity has become, in postmodern thought, a linguistic/cultural coproduction, always unstable and contingent, deeply theorized in literary, feminist, queer, and culture studies.[1] The instability of the psychoanalytic body is most prominent in the feminist critique of gender, where the body's classic theoretical services, as the raw material of desire and the fount of epistemic certainty, seem no longer to be required. A dilemma ensues: absent biology, what becomes of the body? Postmodern thinking resolves: See it as language, as construction, as process, as representation. How convenient for psychoanalysis, a practice that, trafficking so heavily in the symbolic, can uniquely assess, if not yet remedy, two linked problems central to the postmodern solution: the consignments of the body to the Real and of the self to the Imaginary.

Current writings on the social construction of the body take critical advantage of this exciting juncture of psychoanalysis, feminism, and postmodernism. Noteworthy is the dizzying array of languages they use: classical, relational, deconstructionist, feminist, Lacanian, even Marxist and New Age. This profusion of language registers the proliferation of the body, the body as discourse. It also expresses the excess of meaning the body stands for, contains, generates. Rethought as significance, the body stirs, as much as when it is flesh. The ideas and implications spinning off it become nearly overwhelming. You feel you can hardly speak for the excitement. (I note how, in this essay, I frequently write in phrases, do not finish sentences. It is hard to speak the body, which, so much an actor, interrupts speech with a language of its own.) One is reminded of the haunting excitement of erotic countertransference. Too much, really. The excess of body. The body as excess in session. The body Freud (1905) dispatched from the room into Dora's absent, cowlike mother, the "housewife" whose "psychosis" cleaned it up for him. The brutely physical body that Jacques Lacan situates in the Real, "that which is outside language and inaccessible to symbolisation," putatively unknowable (Evans, 1996, pp. 159–161).

The body is not only excessive, it is also deep. Patients, like their analysts, often consider as superficial much concern with physical appearance. Far from it, I say. The very appearance of surface in their worries signals its latent opposite. The fathoms of the unconscious are "written on the body" (borrowing the title from Jeannette Winterson's 1993 novel about obsessional love). This torsion between the visible and the invisible, the seen skin and the unseen psyche, has been particularly wrenching for women in our culture. "Unbearable weight," in feminist philosopher Susan Bordo's (1993) phrase. In regard to eating disorders and women's preoccupation with beauty, body matters are profound, not superficial.

The body is, in this sense, almost paradigmatic for psychoanalysis. Body matters are so weighty, so deeply important, they often cannot be spoken. Untellable, they can only be shown—like much that happens in consulting rooms. "Show, don't tell," this is the instruction given to aspiring writers. "Write what you know," goes another. Or, as writer Grace Paley (1985) advised once in a speech, "Write what you don't know about what you do know." This, I think, is what analytic body talk is all about; it is what the analytic session is about. We try to say what we do not yet, or any longer, know about what we do know. If we know where the session will end up, if we're never surprised or confused or at a loss, we might as well change jobs or go back to school: we're not doing it right. If there is no excess of meaning, nothing either remembered, invented, or discovered in speech, feeling, or relatedness, what are we doing there?

Jonathan Miller (1995), the polymath physician/writer/director/ conductor, expatiates on what he calls "the distinctively enabling view of the unconscious" developed by British psychologists in the mid-19th century and soon overshadowed by the psychoanalytic unconscious. Without debating his distinction between the former as productive and the latter as withholding, I would like to note the role of the body in this other unconscious, or, perhaps, the location of this unconscious in the body. Drawing on an analogy from Noam Chomsky's notion of a linguistic unconscious (which Adrienne Harris [personal communication] has remarked is long overdue for deconstruction, Miller tells us about "mental activity," indexed on/in the body, "of which the individual has no explicit awareness." A critical example is "blindsight," a phenomenon in which "patients blinded by injury to the visual cortex" nevertheless "registered the occurrence of a visual stimulus without being subjectively aware of it." Similarly, "patients whom brain damage has robbed of the ability to put names to familiar faces" but whose language and vision remain intact, still reveal a bodily recognition of those forces

> when such patients are subjected to a variant of the forensic lie detector test, i.e., when their sweating is monitored by changes in skin conductivity, their reactions surpass chance whenever the photo of a well-loved face is thrown onto the screen. Although they are unable to consciously identify the familiar features, their emotional response proves that they have registered its familiarity, albeit unconsciously [p. 65].

I don't suppose we need experimental psychology to verify our thought that body-memory exists. Still, the contemporary recuperation of Freud's castoffs, of, for example, early theories of dissociation, renders data and arguments like Miller's all the more appealing, even if he intends them as an argument against the psychoanalytic unconscious. His examples are suggestive, too, of the relation between trauma and body-memory, of experiences that, preceding or exceeding symbolization, remain outside speech in the Real or were foreclosed from it or even abjected.

I want here to set in active play several topics as an excursus, an expedition into the land of the signifying body. In a preliminary way, I shall be mapping out central sites of discourse and debate, regions bordering on other disciplines, and trailheads for future explorations of new theory. Particularly I shall examine the intersection of embodiment and enactment in postclassical psychoanalytic theory and practice so as to address some underconsidered questions about the intra-psychic and the inter-personal. To forward my subtheme, the resonance between clinical and theoretical practice, I shall be both general and very particular, global in my theoretical reference and local in my focus on the body in its transferential and counter-transferential presence. Four clinical essays from the current relational literature anchor a rather wide-ranging network of perhaps abstract ideas from anthropology to philosophy to Zen Buddhism, to which, in my view, psychoanalysis could profitably refer in addressing the body.

BODIES AND ENACTMENTS SPEAK RELATIONAL

Enactment and embodiment have in common their habitation of the inarticulate. Hence, perhaps, this curious coincidence: as interest in enactment abounds and mounts in the relational and even classical sectors of the psychoanalytic world (Chused, 1966; Ogden, 1996a), the body newly takes shape in psychoanalytic purview. If the body speaks, so do enactments, only not in conventionally familiar language. The work of Philip Bromberg (1994) and others accustoms us to the ubiquity of enactment, its clinical normality. Bodies too may qualify as enactments, not only locally, in psychoanalytic matters (see, e.g., McDougall, 1989), but, as Sue Shapiro's (1996) current argument seems to imply, everywhere and always, for better or worse, in illness *and* in health. Shapiro, surveying the psychoanalytic literature on the body, notes that in many formulations, the body continues as a primitive order, while words seem to remain the province of health and maturity. Contrary to this prevailing inferiorization of corporeal sensation and significance, Shapiro wants to privilege it, elevate its clinical and experiential significance to that of speech. Not the same as speech, bodily communication nonetheless is clinically critical in the flesh of not only patients but their analysts too.

Enactment, conversely, constructs bodies. Bodies do not make minds, nor minds, bodies: rather they are intersubjectively emergent, a density of origin with fascinating clinical ramifications. Adrienne Harris (1996) makes plain a familiar clinical enigma. Sometimes you find yourself speechless with a patient, not because there is nothing to say but because there is too much to say. The body is the site of that excess. Technically speaking, there are often too many clinical roads to take. "In the clinical examples," Harris writes, "the problem in the discourse is that we cannot find a through line. . . ." The body, to put in differently, defeats linear narrative. The "bodies' incoher-

ences and volatility," Harris continues, "are examples of the inadequacy of speech in framing enactment and embodiment" (p. 381).

The body, voluble but incomprehensible, then becomes an actor
in the analytic drama, engaging the analyst's response to make a relationship, a character, and, paradoxically, itself. Harris writes of a patient for whom she is the normality police, the reprimanding
voice-over in a cinematic dream-image of the patient's anoretic body.
Intraphysically signifying, intersubjectively negotiated, the body is
here a destroyer and a creator. In the enacted transference to the
holding but also dominating container, it becomes a bad body, punished for its pain. "The body complaints require and maintain a hos-
tile caretaker-listener, and in this way analyst and patient coproduce
the masochistic envelope and thus make a body surface" (p. 380).

The body thus considered extends and concretizes the relational
and, importantly, exemplifies a dilemma of the relational project. If
the mutual implication of embodiment and enactment is a site of excess, so is the imtimate nexus of one-person and two-person psychologies. To put it another way, the delicate tension between body and
action mimics—contains?—that between intrapsychic and interpersonal, a tension we might label "the relational." Both conceptually
and experientially, the relational is always a provisional space, a precarious net spun and respun among a multitude of binary oppositions. Emerging out of the antithesis between the Freudian and the
Sullivanian/Fairbairnian camps, the relational model announces the
necessity of both/and, as sharply distinct from either/or: internal and
external worlds; the here-and-now with the then-and-there; the simultaneous birth—or, to put it more drily, the coconstruction—of child
and mother in the infant–mother unit; and many other mutual
constitutings.

Things fall apart. Relational tension, designating the complex
interimplication of the two psychologies, sustains a complexity whose
headiness invites splitting, a venerable strategy of simplifying that,
even in the brief history of the idea of the relational (see Aron, 1996),
is alive and well. Not alone among professions in its habit of creating
opposites, psychoanalysis falters before the challenge and implication of the relational paradigm shift: to hold the interpersonal and
the intrapsychic in tension. So often in informal professional speech,
"relational" is employed where "interpersonal"— or, inappropriately,
"interactive"—used to be, leaving the "intraphysic" where it always
was: on top, at the head of the class, the real psychoanalytic McCoy.
Intrapsychic means, once again, only a one-person psychology (Ghent,

1989), relational and interpersonal denote two here-and-now persons only, and the fascinating space where one-person and two-person psychologies slip in and out of one another collapses.

Much more interesting both clinically and theoretically, if also more difficult because of its demans on one's tolerance for paradox, is to take relational tension as a site of excess itself. To put it clinically, relational theory can, in my view, be practiced only in the tension of one-person and two-person psychologies. If you look deeply enough into one, you come upon the other. Here the binary split is overcome: "relational" means both, the simultaneity of a one-person and two-person psychology. Look, on one hand, into the psyche, and you find a universe of object relations. Look, on the other, into the interpersonal, and you find private worlds mapped as one. I think of Fritjof Captra's image in *The Tao of Physics*, in which both physical worlds, the tiny world of subatomic particles and the all-emcompassing universe of black holes, are but opposite sides of a coin.

There are other metaphors for relational doubleness. Projective identification, that Kleinian concept so powerfully augmenting our understanding of transference and countertransference, is the original formulation of relational tension. At first meant to describe the patient's one-person operation on the analyst, it can now, I believe, be reinterpreted as a doubled field, a simultaneous engagement of single parties, a psychic process at once internal and external, singled and doubled (Ogden, 1996b; Sand, 1997). Here I would also call on Maurice Merleau-Ponty's (1962) phenomenology, a philosophy with a capacity as remarkable as Winnicott's psychoanalysis for articulating paradox. His phrasing illuminates the dialectical complexity: "Transcendental subjectivity is a revealed subjectivity, revealed to itself and to others, and is for that reason an intersubjectivity" (p. 361). Note the simultaneity of revelation: one is revealed to oneself—"itself"—through revealing oneself in relation—"to other." Conversely, intersubjectivity emerges only through the mutual self-knowing of individual subjects.

The relational as paradox is now almost a psychoanalytic cliché. Easy to say, it is quite difficult to voice. The resolution of paradox is, Emmanuel Ghent (1989) has proposed, yet another paradox. Are we in the postmodern hall of mirrors? I suggest that the concreteness of embodiment and enactment offers another way out. Paradox, as much as embodiment and enactment, inhabits the inarticulate and the enigmatic. It poses a circuit among knowing, doing, and not knowing that may well be captured by the Lacanian orders of the Symbolic,

Imaginery, and Real. I point out and briefly detour into Lacanian theory here in part because it relishes paradox, a taste that may give rise to its enigmatic though illuminating approach to subjectivity.

Instead of the familiar "epigenetic program involving various developmental stages" (Malone, 1997, p. 416; for a friendly critic who disagrees, see Bowie, 1991), Lacanian psychoanalysis envisions psychic structuring as transected by three "orders of being." These orders are registers of meaning that, by positioning the individual simultaneously in psychic process and in culture, describe both subjectivity and clinical process. To put it differently, each register operates in each of us simultaneously and all the time; we inhabit all three simultaneously; individual subjectivity is the point at which they intersect. The clinical session, in fact, articulates all three orders: there one simultaneously speaks in the Symbolic, with its structuring channels of linguistic reason; inhabits the Imaginary, with its elusive fixities and identities; and embodies the Real, the unspeakable of past, present, and future.

Many sorts of difference distinguish these complexly layered categories, and many interesting debates crystalize around them. Of importance here are their connections to the body and to words. Perhaps it is best to define by example. Slavoj Zizek (1996, p. 24), a Lacanian cultural theorist, reads classical psychoanalytic practice as a knowledge that, situated in the Symbolic, creates effects in the Real. If, he says, you think of the classic psychoanalytic patient—the hysteric—and the classic psychoanalytic treatment—the talking cure—you can see that the psychoanalytic ability to undo symptoms with words operates "in the Real of bodily symptoms." The Real, however, cannot be spoken or ever fully captured; the domain of the body, it exceeds speech and is the site of primordial loss. The clinical wager, as Lawrence Jacobson (personal communication) puts it, is that the Symbolic—the region of speech, reason, and culture—will effect a change in the Real. The hysteric will be cured of her symptoms.

Much contemporary psychoanalytic thinking, including that which accepts the name "relational," may beg to differ here. The disagreement centers on the Imaginary. Lacanian theory posits the Imaginary as the site where a foundationally divided self integrates as a necessary but fictive identity. (The intriguing echo among Lacan's decentered self, Laing's divided self and its progenitor, Winnicott's schema of True and False Selves, and the multiple selves of recent relational thinking [Bromberg, Harris, Davies] deserves a larger discussion elsewhere.) In the classical Lacanian view, the Imaginary is not the location of speech, of "signifying," but only of "significance and signification" (Evans, 1996, p. 82). Only the Symbolic, it is held, can articulate meaning.

Oddly, the Lacanian Imaginary seems to emerge as an intermediate space much like that identified and valued in recent relational thinking. Here in the Imaginary the line between speech and body begins to waver. To capture this ambiguity, Julia Kristeva (1995) invents the idea of "semiosis"—all those necessary, body-related elements of communication without which speech loses half its meaning: "pitch, tone, stress, cadence, and duration" (Bollas, 1997, p. 364), rhythm and timing, diction, prosody, inflection, gesture. The Imaginary, one might put it, situates the excess of speech. Roland Barthes (1975) comes up with an odd, almost nonsensical notion that makes us aware of the physicality of speech. If only, he says, there could be a "writing aloud," which would contain the meaningful physical elements of speech that disappear on the page: "the pulsional incidents, the language lined with flesh, a text where we can hear the grain of the throat, the patina of consonants, the voluptuousness of vowels, a whole carnal stereophony: the articulation of the body, of the tongue, not that of meaning, of language." He rhapsodizes about "the sound[s] of speech *close up* . . . their materiality, their sensuality, the breath, the gutturals, the fleshiness of the lips, a whole presence of the human muzzle. . ." (pp. 66–67).

Clinically situated, the Imaginary may not be the dead end Lacan thought but a place of more possibility then he recognized. Kristeva (1995), recounting the treatment of a little boy in which they composed and sang an opera together, argues the clinical value of the body-based significance constituting semiosis. Across channel and oceans (I am trying and will fail to bridge great gaps here), relational theorists also make a claim for an order in which words, bodies, and acts are interimplicated. Newly emerging in many consulting rooms is, as I will go on to show in the next section, a psychoanalytic trust in the triangular tension among words, acts, and bodies. Relational theory, as though in argument with Lacan, rehabilitates the dyad, stipulating, for example, not a maddening but a creative illusion of identity.

In a sense, perhaps, the Imaginary may use the Real in a way that the Symbolic cannot. At least, I would here like to appropriate the Real for relational purposes. The Real, "that which is outside language and unassimilable to symbolization," is in some ways matter as opposed to mind (Evans, 1996, pp. 159–160). Unknowable, the Real can nevertheless be felt, an absence pressing on the present. An absent presence: past trauma, unknown future, present desire. I suggest that,

however inarticulable, the Real, pressing into embodiment and enactment, leads out of the postmodern hall of mirrors. Enactment and
embodiment incarnate and cut through the ambiguity of clinical space.
Embodiment and enactment confront each other as positive and negative, the single-body, one-person psychology speaking multitudes, the
two-person enactment mumming two psychic spaces in and of one.
One-body and two-bodies see each other in the mirror of themselves.

CLINICAL BODY TALK:
BREAKING DOWN DETERMINISM,
SUSTAINING RELATIONAL TENSION

Bodies, in the new relational view, abrogate many binaries. They
weave back and forth between representation and experience. If, one
wonders, psychoanalytic body talk is so difficult, how is it even possible to think about the body? Or is it because we can/may not think
the body that we cannot speak it? These double-sided questions address both theoretical and clinical matters; indeed, they put that familiar psychoanalytic binary into question. In this section, I approach
this matter through the oscillation between the old-time search for
causes and the new project of sustaining relational tension. Several
braided themes emerge. Novel questions crystalize as we peruse clinical accounts offered by Adrienne Harris (1996), Samuel Gerson (1996),
and Steven Knoblauch (1996), which limn the paradoxes and ambiguities of bodies, acts, and speech on the clinical stage. Does the body's
location in the Real/preverbal (to juxtapose the Lacanian and developmental registers) always qualify somatic experience? If so, does
the Real always inform experiences of sexuality and gender insofar
as they encode the body? Does it thereby produce an anguished if
also excited muteness that impels the body to speak as we sit, pleasurably or painfully, on the analytic hot seat?

What anguish? you might ask. Surely, you may reasonably be
thinking, we have at least one good, solid way to address the body,
the old-fashioned way that Freud used: we are animals, after all, biological organisms about which much scientific knowledge has been
accumulated (to wit, Miller, 1995). Right off the bat in her entertaining essay, however, Shapiro (1996) contests the psychoanalytic use
of biology: "while traditional psychoanalytic theory turned to biological explanations as a last resort to support the truth of its state-
ments, it does not rely clinically on an experiential body" (p. 298).
The body on which psychoanalysis has so confidently relied is not

necessarily the body people experience: it is the scientific body known objectively, the object and creation of much research. As suggested by the postmodern mood, however, the scientific body's correspondence with the subjective body should not any longer be taken for granted. Rather, subjective and objective bodies, or, better, scientific, linguistic, and experienced bodies are a crazy quilt of overlaps, mismatches, and novelty, the stuff of excitement, anguish, sanity, and madness.

Historically, the scientific body is caught in a binary created by the problem of determinism, of Nature versus Nurture, or biology versus psychology, or biology versus culture, or psychology versus anything. In a period of neodeterminism (think of *The Bell Curve* [Hernnstein and Murray 1994]), it is worth emphasizing what I hope is tediously familiar: we need to get beyond determinism, whose power as cultural trope and master regulatory practice is stupendous. In the matter of the body, the seductions of science are well-nigh irresistible. Particularly alluring is the Discourse of Nature (as I have called it [Dimen, 1995]). We think "body," we think "biology," a thought that is a search for grounding and authority. Psychoanalysis is always seeking validation, uncertain of its terms except when authorized by Science. Yet such discursive practices of social control, *uncriticized*, block interpretations of psychic process. Deemed truth, their power to regulate—to imagine, interpret, and even value the most intimate experiences of self—becomes undetectable and unintelligible.

Nor can psychoanalysis find a resting place in cultural determinism. If psyche reduces to waves and particles at the hands of Science, it is rendered but a clone at the hands of Culture. In Freud's time, biological sciences may have reigned supreme in their governance of human truth, but since then the social sciences have challenged that supremacy. Now when we think of the battle between Nature and Nurture, we envision two quite worthy antagonists for the determinist crown. Sociology and anthropology, contemporary culture studies, and postmodern theories of representation contextualize the current psychoanalytic fascination with social constructionism. There is a danger. Nature having been eliminated in social construction, Culture assumes all the fixity, the immutability formerly assigned to Nature (Grosz, 1994, p. 21). Here one needs to be mindful of the Foucauldian (1991) argument that oppositional attempts at undoing disciplinary power risk imitation: social constructionism, a critique of determinisms, threatens to mutate into a new theory of conditioning, throwing out the unconscious and psychic process as distinct in their own right.

Living without determinism by sustaining relational tension, this is the psychoanalytic challenge par excellence, and it is, oddly, exemplified by the clinical body. Here the body comes to occupy a sort of transitional space, a force field much as I have described for gender (Dimen, 1991), where many binaries and determinisms show up and then break down. The body challenges the split between one-person and two-person psychologies. Hearing echoes of Winnicott, Harris (1996), for example, wonders about the body's construction. She puts the objectified, one-person body immediately into question: maybe one body is also always two. "There is no baby without the mother, but at the beginning only the mother-baby ego," Harris says, citing Winnicott. Taking his formulation a big step further or, better, departing from it, she imagines how enactment creates a body through an interface. "There is no meaningful individual body ego without the interface—the holding, looking, touching encounter of the social other" (p. 371). Bringing culture into her formulation of body–mind, she has the baby–body come to be only as it is semiotically and linguistically appropriated, processes whose object-relational situation endow infant embodiment with meaning.

Body is equally meaning and flesh, an intersection productive of many different bodies. Drawing on feminist philosopher Elizabeth Grosz's understanding of the way sexual difference is constituted in a social matrix, Harris reexamines that old Cartesian binary, body–mind. Bodies, according to customary thinking, precede psyches. In a one-person psychology, one thinks hierarchically of a mind in a body, of psychology as grounded in biology, of biology in chemistry, and so on all the way down. A relational perspective permits a more complicated view. Body, like subjectivity, is revealed in a two-person matrix. The psychical and social inscription of flesh, blood, and bone is "the surface and raw materials of an integrated and cohesive totality" that, Harris goes on, gives this bag of guts unity, cohesiveness, and organization.

Different matrix, different bodies. Again, Barthes (1975): "Apparently Arab scholars, when speaking of the text, use this admirable expression: *the certain body*. What body? (We have several of them; the body of anatomists and physiologists, the one science sees or discusses. . . . But we also have a body of bliss consisting solely of erotic relations, utterly distinct from the first body: it is another contour, another nomination" (p. 16). Barthes splits, opposing the scientific to the erotc body. Does the excess of bodies lead him to dichotomize? We might want to add others, say, the clinical body, or the psychic body, or the gendered body, or. . . . one could go on.

The effort to sustain relational tension characteristically breaks down as binaries, with their implications of causality, endlessly rematerialize. Note the ease with which, when the body is considered, the maternal metaphor surfaces, bringing with it the binary of sexual, not to mention parent–child, difference. Developmentalism as regulatory practice—that linear sequence of stages in which health and normality cohere—may be a culprit here, inclining us to fill in the blanks of the Enlightenment metanarrative (Flax, 1990) with ontology: compelled by the question, "Where did it all begin, and why?" we answer, "the family."

Sustaining relational tension requires other initial vantage points, other epistemologies, on the mutual infolding of body and object relation. These are found across the psychoanalytic spectrum. Shapiro (1996) recalls interpersonalist Ernst Schachtel's sense categories, the immediacy of touch and smell, and their simultaneous signification of self and other, emotion and body (pp. 311–312). Others begin with language. Like many French psychoanalytic theorists influenced by Lacan's linguistic focus, Didier Anzieu (1989) begins his account with a consideration of the vocabulary for skin (p. 13); it is on his idea of a "skin-ego," as the corporeal counterpart to psychic space, that Harris's notion of interface draws. With gender critique as ground, I myself am more likely to turn first to the sexual psyche–soma, as did Freud, for a figurative account of the interimplications of body and object-relation. Or think of the body in pain. Judith Butler (1993), as Harris later notes, begins her essay on "The Lesbian Phallus" by referring to Freud's argument that pain originates the body–ego; he "associates the process of erogeneity with the consciousness of bodily pain" (p. 59), a process in which the lines between body and emotion, self and other, blur. In Elaine Scarry's (1985) idiosyncratic *The Body in Pain,* bodily pain enters the world as a source of creativity and enters the body as the route by which society, through such practices as torture, inscribes its power in psyches.

One way of breaking down determinism is to deconstruct it. Body may signify Biology, and Biology may evoke its opposite number, Culture. But what if we look into the opposition between them and summon up "embodiment"? When we do, other binaries cohere and dissolve, other matters of psyche and politics surface. Consider, for example, Harris's (1996) examination of that familiar catch-all "constitution." She argues that, for kids with gender identity disorder, and perhaps marginally for the rest of us, gender performativity, conceived by Butler in the one-person language of Freud and Lacan, is in fact relationally constituted. One boy's Gender Identity Disorder (GID), a problem written on his little body, serves to heal and conceal a loss suffered by the parent, a spontaneously aborted sibling. His problem is to sustain his mother. A dilemma that he cannot speak nor his parent comprehend, it finds a solution in being lived "excruciatingly in splits and fragments in the child's body-ego and in the meaning of that body for the child" (p. 368). There the difficulty can be put into an acceptable, disguising language, that of gender, which adults can interpret even as they misunderstand.

This attempted solution to the inarticulate and seemingly irreducibly biologic body creates, of course, another binarized problem, the danger of femininity for boys. A boy, treated by Susan Coates, wanted to be a lady, an angry and violent lady (Harris, 1996, p. 369). His gendercrossing wish, it turned out, stood in for a far less speakable trauma of maternal separation. Interestingly, his gender trouble begot attention that his anguished selfhood could not. At work in this simultaneously relational and regulatory moment is a gendered construction of the body. For boys, it is only when psychic disorder becomes somatically registered that it begets the healing, disciplinary practice of psychomedical intervention; in girls, GID may be the normal pathology of normative femininity, at least in its milder form. A boy's unruly body is not biology; it is unruliness embodied as a failed masculinity, the order that depends on all the other disorders— femininity, homosexuality, otherness in culture—against which it measures itself.

Breakdowns in determinism also reveal embodiment's other side: enactment. We see it in the boy's body enacting femininity, which can be spoken in the language of disorder. In doing so, it enacts that which cannot be articulated at all and so makes a request of the parent, who responsively takes action by taking the child to therapy. Language as an aspect of body and enactment seems critical here: the child's unspoken wish to shape gender through an act begets action. Merleau-Ponty (1962) insists on an intuitively persuasive figure, the body as the materialization of word, thought, memory. Think, he suggests, of the effort you make to remember a lost name. Where is it lost? In your mind? Or on "the tip of your tongue?" He likens this embodied effort to the aphasic's effort to recover voice, a "genuine effort" like that of a straining, trying body (p. 165). How different from his friend and critic, Lacan. If language is embodied and speech is consequently an action, then the Real is not quite so radically other to the Symbolic.

Nor in the consulting room are speaking and acting always different, an ambiguity further enriching relational tension and simultaneously beckoning the oversimplification of splitting. As body fades into speech, so speech fades into action, we are told by Gerson (1996), who brings a particular philosophy of language to bear on psycho-analytic speech. Like gender-talk, he argues, our speech about trans-ference is performative. Words not only say, they do. To recall Paley's (1985) admonition, successful speech and writing often show what they cannot tell. A vehicle for communication and insight, language also enacts. According to Gerson (1996), both analyst nd patient "em-ploy language as a praxis . . . to expand their subjectivity into the realm of the other" (p. 358). The line between discovery and creation being hard to draw, this expansion is, simultaneously, an invention. It is in this effort to establish the domains of knowing," Gerson (1994) has also said that "discourse creates what it comes to represent." The paradox is here: in establishing a relationship through a mutu-ally constructed discourse of self-knowing, analyst and patient come to be themselves.

A theoretical problem now requires some brief attention. As much as discourse theory contributes to the ambiguity sustaining relational tension, it tends to break the tension too, turning discourse into an old-fashioned lever of causality in a shift to determinism that calls for correction. Different understandings of language are at stake here. Gerson, like Butler, uses a twinned approach that draws on not only Lacan but Foucault. The Lacanian rendering of language builds on Ferdinand de Saussure's (1911) structural linguistics, which stipulates an arbitrary relationship between sounds and meaning. This gap be-tween signifier and signified is evident in the existence of multiple languages, in the (in principle) unlimited number of different vocal representations of the same "thing"—the English, Russian, Greek, and Chinese morphemes for, say, a four-legged, bewhiskered, meowing domestic animal are all different. The relation between a cat and its signifier—or, more precisely, among signifiers, significations, signifi-cance, and referents— is not fixed (hence the slippage between one's necessary but fictive identity over one's fundamental multiplicity). In this perspective, we do not fashion language as individuals. Rather language fashions us. It is by entering the Symbolic order—this system of sound and meaning—that subjectivity emerges.

In the matter of articulating bodies, acts, and speech, however, the Lacanian view of language could benefit from two other perspec-tives, those of Michel Foucault and Pierre Bourdieu. While it contains a powerful critique of reification, Lacanian psychoanalysis erases the self in a fashion that strangely suits all too well certain antecedent determinist social theories against which it implicitly argues. In the Marxist intellectual context in which Lacanian thought matured, for example, individual psyches are the products of, caused by, social conditions. For Foucault, the question is more complicated. He addresses this misreading by taking on the question of domination. Domination, he explains, depends not only on material might. People imprison themselves with a little help from their friends in Freud's (1925) three "impossible professions"—education, government, and psychoanalysis (Ehrenreich, 1989; Foucault, 1991). If oppression consists in the force of law backed up by the force of arms, domination depends on what people tell themselves, both consciously and unconsciously. What we tell ourselves, however, draws on a matrix of assorted claims to truth. Domination derives from constructed cultural or, as Foucault (1991) calls them, "disciplinary," practices that, willy-nilly, people believe reveal the truth about themselves, their lives, their value, and therefore the systems producing those truths.

Domination practices achieve this effect, suggests French social theorist Pierre Bourdieu, by impressing the psyche at the level of the body. Hence the centrality of sex, identified by Foucault as the modern preoccupation. Many practices of symbolic violence, Bourdieu holds, sex us, race us, class us, age us, certify us as sane or mad. The body is constructed not only through language but through representation in the media and many forms of direct and indirect instruction. In contrast to, say, military discipline, in which the enemy is clear, symbolic domination "is something you absorb like air, something you don't feel pressured by; it is everywhere and nowhere," and therefore nearly impossible to get away from (Bourdieu and Eagleton, 1992, p. 115). Indeed, the, more nonverbal the symbolic (and Bourdieu's use of this term is not the same as Lacan's, hence its lower case inscription), the greater its power.

Gerson (1996), and other analysts of like cast of mind, want to comprehend how, in the ambiguities of the psychoanalytic process, the self can make its way out of this prison. How can psychoanalysis, despite its deep participation in regulatory practice, undo the power of all disciplinary institutions to sponsor subjectivity? Thinking about domination, he says "that language itself, when reiterated through the voices of the powerful, is the medium through which human possibility is born and dies" (p. 348). This, as we will see in his vignette, is not untrue. But it is only half the truth. It is as though there were one unconstructed language that is filtered through different class and other positions of social hierarchy. In this reading of the politics of language, the dialectics so necessary to sustain relational tension, as well as to animate political praxis, vanishes momentarily: the voice of the ruling class comes out as the singular ruling voice. How does contradiction slip away? Thinking as a social critic, one wonders, Where, in language thus construed, does resistance lie? Thinking as a clinician, one asks, Where is agency?

We begin to see here how the relational perspective on embodiment and enactment may cut through postmodernist impasse: language may speak the person, but clinically we know also that persons speak language. Gerson's argument, in fact, contains just such illumination, its own argument against determinism. Under conditions of domination, Gerson earlier argues, naming creates prisons: "the naming of bodies, sex, gender, and desire effects the embodiment of oppressive social forces as they invade and diminish the privacy of the individual. Names mark the body and are as resistant to erasure as are tattoos. And like tattooing, naming exhibits the ruthless attempt of culture mind to gain control over the body" (p. 348). Yet, as he goes on to show, we can expect psychoanalysis to contest, respeak, reclaim names so as to undermine authority. Urging us to think of the gay reappropriation of "queer," he proposes that "when spoken with new meaning and intent, names may be reclaimed in a manner which undermines their power to create zones of exclusion and of abjection" (p. 348). Postmodernism would question this novelty of meaning and intent, pointing to the discursive context in and of which we are woven, to the impossibility of finding a language of the body that does not re-create its inscription in biopower. At the same time, one would have to remember that language, like an artist's choice of medium, both constrains and frees.

As clinicians, then—and I begin here to indicate another fly in the postmodern ointment—we know that genuinely new experiences, or at least those that feel absolutely and liberatingly novel, do occur to our patients in the course of treatment. Gerson argues that the body offers escape from linguistic prisons: "The enclosures created by naming permit escape only through the fragmentation of bodily and sexual experience; fragments which can then be fluidly shaped by wish and fantasy and thereby avoid the fate of the named and constrained body" (p. 348). Fragmentation suggests dissociation, the land of the foreclosed or never-known, indeed, the land of the Real, where lives what cannot be thought. Gerson does not cite Margo Rivera's (1989) dictum, but he might as well have: "It is not the multiplicity which the individual with multiple personality experiences that is problematic but the defensive dissociation and the consequent limited awareness and ability to act on that awareness" (p. 29). It is the wisdom of the Symbolic, a Lacanian might say in being true to Freud, to recognize that one is not who one thinks one is. Yet clinically the Real becomes a presence only through the Imaginary.

In keeping with the explicitly historicizing feminist and progressive critiques embedding his essay, Gerson (1996) shows how speaking desire, always transgressive, refuses alienation, but instead insists on reclaiming subjectivity from the deadness of naming (a deadness that, according to Lacan, is the inevitable consequence of a fragmenting, but, according to other students of language, is not inherent). A patient, who hated her genitals, was erotically filled with the sound of Gerson's voice and the sense of his presence. For her, sound and sense amounted to touch. She began to speak of her excitement, eventually of her genitals. Still she could not assimilate *what* he would say to her, only *that* he had spoken. For her, there was one body in the room, a denial that her analyst, for whom there were two bodies, read as a sign of impending stalemate. He felt loneliness and, at a well-timed moment, told her of it, that he wanted her company. Thereby, he inaugurated an intimacy of speech and thought. He grasped her elusive dissociation by juxtaposing words and bodies, by naming his own loneliness, in the face of her voiced but self-enclosed excitement. This disclosure enabled her, after some time, to feel love as well as arousal (pp. 350–352).

UP FROM DETERMINISM: A RELATIONAL THEORY OF SPEECH?

I have suggested a postmodernist dilemma of which relational (and other) psychoanalysts, so excitedly adapting constructivist notions, need to be aware. Once, in social theory, it was economic forces that were said to construct society and psyche; now it is language. It all depends, I have intimated, on what you think language is. Lacan's idea of language derives from de Saussure's distinction between *la langue* and *la parole*, and his founding of structural linguistics on the former. If *la parole* refers to language as used in ordinary life, *la langue* denotes the underlying principles by which speech is structured and organized. Through Saussure and Russian formalist Roman Jakobsen to Lacan, *la langue* becomes an independent and causal vector in human, culture and psyche.

La langue does not, however, always have the last word. Russian psycholinguist Mikhail Bakhtin's (1981) theory of speech differs sharply from the Lacanianism underlying most postmodernist thinking. Formulated in contemporaneous disaagreement with Saussure, it emphasizes *la parole* at the expense of *la langue* (Vološinov [1929–30]). Like his colleagues. V. N. Vološinov and Lev Vygotsky, Bakhtin locates meaning "not first inside or outside, but in constant flux between" (Massey, 1996b, p. 127). Where *la langue* is a structure or code that is in effect "a static, impermeable, inanimate object," *la parole*, in contrast, is unstable, variations on a structural theme.

La parole seems more suited to intermediate spaces. Carla Massey (1996b) describes the interface of body, enactment, and speech for Bakhtin. The real thing here is *la parole*, a matter of voice and speech, "an alive phenomenon of a living person" (p. 126). If language is a set of relations, it also lives, breathes, and changes; it "is a dialogic activity, a mode of being, and a means of transformation, as much as it is also a means of sustaining constancy and defense" (p. 125). If Lacan's *langue* is cerebral, Bakhtin's *parole* is "sensorial, affective, . . . pragmatic" (p. 125); "bodies and language are inseparable" (Massey, 1996a, p. 75). In its attention to process rather than structure, *la parole* is perhaps more relevant to the relational construction of the body, returning us to the body as experienced in intersubjective space. For Bakhtin, language is embodied enactment. Simultaneously intrapsychic and interpersonal, it is always multivoiced, an interweaving of voice, gesture, and selves that constitutes meaning.

When one consults Bakhtin—and Merleau-Ponty as well—one finds oneself crossing the boundaries of many a bodily binary. Drawing on Massey's explication of Bakhtin's dialogics, Steven Knoblauch (1996) shows us the interimplicatedness of embodiment and enactment by situating the body in its psychoanalytically familiar sexual home. Not at all coincidentally, his essay also problematizes affect, which, as I have indicated, arguably borders mind, body, and language. Knoblauch writes of his work with a 20-something man who as a boy had experienced sexual intrusions by men who were his mentors. His sexuality nurtured in the soil of mistrust, Dennis was beginning to emerge from the emotional closet. Through the medium of "body movement and body symbolizing," he began to "focus on the dialogue of affective exchange," creating a safety zone in which erotic feelings as sources and [levers] of power emerged (p. 330).

In one of those familiar transitional clinical moments, as Knoblauch dubs them, Dennis brought his and his analyst's bodies into the room in an act accomplished through speech. As Knoblauch was bent over to pick up a crumpled tissue from the floor before officially starting the session, Dennis said, "Nice buns." Having begun to relate details of his sexual abuse, Dennis was now, Knoblauch recognized, putting out feelers to see whether he might expand his range of intimacy. Caught off balance by his patient's chosen port of entry, Knoblauch was yet able to respond in a similarly light tone to what in fact was a playful poke at his anus. Seeing that Dennis's nip was not a bite, he opined as how he would now have to be more aware of his body in session. This observation led Dennis to relate his own uneasy sightings of the outline of Knoblauch's penis inside his pants. As Dennis's fantasies of their relative penis size and potency intensified their dialogue, Knoblauch's ability to sustain talk about body feelings "without shame, anesthetization, or dissociation" (p. 327) communicated itself to Dennis and permitted their shared comprehension of Dennis's "preoccupation with penises and anuses." Freed up to work in areas Knoblauch saw he "had unconsciously colluded with [Dennis] in avoiding," they found a safe way for Dennis to allow the vitalization of his body sensations to unfold into "a vitalized sense of self-worth."

To talk sex is to do sex too. This ambiguity is what makes erotic countertransference so disturbing, dangerous, exciting, potent, and transgressive and what makes for Knoblauch's success. One principal way of breaking the regulatory hold of discourse is to speak words that are not only words but acts. We return here to Gerson's (1996) concern, the relation of performativity to regulatory practice. Not only judicial speech—philosopher J. L. Austin's "I pronounce you man and wife"—not only hate speech (verbal abuse, racial slurring, on which see Butler, 1997), but sexual speech is performative: to speak your desire is to enact desire. Speaking desire is a performative, a speech act that constitutes the situation it declares but is at the same time *not* an action. As such, it is a paradoxical experience in which a word is not a word, an act not an act. Its very ambiguity is what makes it erotically, affectively, cognitively, therapeutically powerful. Analyst and patient must, therefore, always feel *both* disappointment *and* relief when they find a way out of erotic transference and countertransference by speaking their desire.

Sexuality has an enlivening place in the clinic. In recognition of the Foucauldian critique of the repressive hypothesis, we might ask, Why? Knoblauch (1996) is stirred when his patient talks about his analyst's butt, and when another, Leslie, talks about her panties. Ms. B, another patient of Gerson's (1996), who sports a naughty T-shirt that boldly and repetitively says, " 'whore, slut, tramp, bitch,' " at first asks " 'the lesbian in [him] to love [her],' " but later feels excited by the idea of his " 'manhandling' " her (pp. 352–354). One of Harris's (1996) patients dreams of dead lesbian mice in a nexus of pain, disgust, and excitement that eventually leads patient and analyst to wonder about the patient's sexuality, desire, and creativity.

Foucault (1991) tells us why sex is a privileged site of bodily meaning: reaching hearts by going through bodies, the state achieves its power. Can we reverse the question? Why, to put it the other way around, is sex a privileged site of bodily signification? Knoblauch's (1996) patients, we learn,

> thrust their bodies into the dialogue between us, desperately needing not just as a one-person model would explain, the animation of their self-experience, but rather an experience of vitalization contextualized with the vitalization of another emerging within the dialogue between us, and particularly by the impact of body sensations. For their self-states mediated through body experience to be understood, it was crucial for me. . . .to be penetrated at the level of my body experience [p. 3].

Yes. But why, one wonders, *thrusting*? If the body as experienced had a more central, clinical place, would thrusting be the communicative mode, as Shapiro (1996) makes us want to ask? Why penetration? Is this a stereotypically (heteroesexual?) masculine or, as Harriet Wrye (1996) argues (p. 290), oedipal(ized) experience of the climax-seeking body? One would not wish to contest Knoblauch's therapeutic achievement: his somatic experience countered his patients' felt need for their "body thoughts and feelings to be anesthetized or [to become] the source of anxiety, conflict, guilt, and shame." Still, do we have here what the film "Cool Hand Luke" called "a failure to communicate?" Do patients thrust their bodies at analysts because analysts, like the other (parental) authorities who precede them, don't yet know how to understand body talk? Do they thrust their bodies at their analysts because that is how their analysts think of intimate intercourse, as thrusting? Does, furthermore, the incomprehension of body talk have anything to do with the scientific body spawned by what Evelyn Fox Keller (1985) has identified as the heterosexualized mode of knowing in which a cognizing scientist probes a world of mute female objects?

The interstices of body, voice, and action as produced and linked in *la parole* are escape hatches from the Foucauldian prison: moments of contradiction leading out of impasse to personal and political growth. Consider Vološinov's (1929–30) characterization of verbal interaction: "No sharp dividing line can be drawn between understanding and response. Any act of understanding is a response, i.e., it translates what is being understood into a new context from which a response can be made" (p. 69 *n2*). Perhaps, in other words, our bodies are always already penetrated by and responsive to the other's experience; body states never exactly the "unconstructed" *tabulae rasae* suggested by Wrye (1996, p. 293). Instead, as Shapiro would argue, we are simply not aware of this paradoxical dimension of our bodily states of mind because the construction of psychoanalysis—and, one would have to add, the discursive constitution of selfhood as unitary and one bodied—forecloses it.

No one privileges the clinical body more insistently than Shapiro (1996). In a unique essay, which nearly claims that clinical psychoanalysis lacks a body altogether, Shapiro convincingly argues that the scientific body of classical theory is, in fact, defensive: the "highly theorized 'body' of psychoanalysis reflects the kind of defensive stance described by Mitrani in which patients use words to surround themselves and to substitute for bodily containment in the face of loss" (p. 298). The loss that psychoanalysis has classically sustained is, she contends, of the analyst's body and then by extension the patient's. Shapiro boldly puts it baldly: "I think it accurate to describe conventional psychoanalysis as taking place between two minds that happen to inhabit bodies—bodies which should be counted on to stay under control" (p. 309).

The clinical body is a creation by a disembodied Science. The resulting paradox, which Shapiro sets herself to find a way out of, will be familiar to most psychoanalytic practitioners and patients: "The analytic consulting room is now one of the more formal and physically constricting environments that analyst and patient inhabit" (p. 316). She finds one escape route by critiquing binary models of health and maturity. She distills a usually unarticulated, clinically central, developmental tenet: "The mark of maturity is stillness" (p. 317). Acknowledging the contributions of Anzieu, Ogden, and Mitrani to our understanding of the body in clinical practice, she points out that they "tend to view somatic experience as more primitive and pathological than verbally symbolized experience" (p. 299). She, instead, invites the reader, in a series of fun questions, to inhabit your body as you read, as a way of illustrating how one might go about catching the body's awarenesses while sitting on the analytic hot seat. She breaks the somatic into several dimensions that clinicians might begin to observe and register: "visual, auditory, kinesthetic, olfactory, gustatory and visceral experience." She asks you to think about what your body has been doing; what about, she wants to know, the effects of "alcohol or coffee?"

That regulatory practice strikes once again, however, should alert us to the never-ending story in which we are engaged: It's hard to be asked to think about one's caffeine and liquor consumption without feeling at least a little bit scrutinized and wondering whether one may have been doing something, well, "unhealthy," a signifier that, always in this culture but particularly in these neopuritanic times, betokens immorality. I suppose that, even in what some of us on the left used to call "the good society," regulatory practice will require and generate monitoring (or is my dystopian supposition the product of disillusionment?). In any event, the discourse of the body presently and inevitably invokes pathologizing and moralizing, to which even (therefore?) dedicated hedonists may be vulnerable. In other words, why did Shapiro not also ask us to consider the effects on our current somatic state of protein or leafy greens (these are still thought to be good for you, I believe), not to mention eight hours' sleep, designer water, or, for that matter, sexual gratification?

At the same time, focusing on one's self-report of bodily experience marks a limit to the postmodern critique, which has itself so quickly become rule bound and regulatory. Bodily multiplicity reaches out to multiple models. Roger Lancaster (1995), an anthropologist and queer theorist, argues that currently popular (Lacanian) linguistic and semiotic models emerge out of "a deferral of the question of sense-perception" (p. 2). His suggestion of a return to Merleau-Ponty signals the relation between the sensuous and the semiotic. Mindful of the kinship between embodiment and enactment, Shapiro (1996) herself draws on a variety of other models to consider the fate of the senses in psychoanalysis. Referring to Wilhelm Reich and Sándor Ferenczi, she reminds us clinical readers that we sense our bodies, and so do our patients, and that these senses constitute various knowledges of self, other, and relationship.

That one knows through the senses constitutes a primary challenge to the postmodern constitution of the subject through *la langue*. Clinicians, speaking to people rather than to texts, must contend with the postmodern erasure of the "I." Several psychoanalysts, some of them the very feminists who are introducing postmodernist thought (e.g., Flax, 1990, pp. 24–31), have noticed a critical difficulty in deploying deconstruction in clinical practice; they argue variously that, the multiplicity and instability of subjectivity to the contrary notwithstanding, a central consciousness and a sense of subjective coherence are psychically vital (see also Benjamin, 1994b). As language speaks people and people speak language, so selves are shifting and multiply instantiated at the same time as one can sense a self:

a "central consciousness," in Rivera's (1989) terms, knows its own multiplicity.

In a related move, Lancaster (1995) too emphasizes the radical place of feeling, its challenge to alienation and fragmentation:

> Feeling is precisely what is denied in an alienated performance. Feeling, as a mode of sensorimotor perception, is not the Truth. But it is, in Merleau-Ponty's sense, the possibility of truth, and our access to it. It is not necessarily singular, for its somatic modes facilitate many possibilities of embodiment. Its plural truths are luxuriant and splendid [p. 16].

Lancaster, operating still within what psychoanalysts would call a one-person psychology, does not consider what clinicians will want to take up, that shared sensing between beings can be equally constitutive of truthful moments and can help crack equally the prison of naming and the deconstructive hall of mirrors. His thoughts evoke once again the power of the Imaginary, that location of sense, feeling, and semiosis.

CONCLUSION: FREUD'S BODY, BUDDHA'S BODY

Can psychoanalysts think, then, of body, sensation, feeling, affect, and emotion in a Bakhtinian dialogic process as a route to subjectivity or agency or the sense of central consciousness that can name all dissociated states "I"? It is not far from feeling to affect. Referring to Bromberg's ideas on shared self-states, Knoblauch (1996) writes:

> This excitement constituted by a liberating eroticism, then, exploded the illusion of father and daughter and the constricting effect of thinking of depression as some kind of defective disease/process in my patient rather than a potential affective contour, a self-state with significant meanings to be understood and expressed [p. 334].

Perhaps affect, a body–mind state whose relationality puts into question the body's location in the Real, leads back to the ego, whose location in the Imaginary, and to the Subject, whose location in the Symbolic, belie their own moments of sensed reality (Dean, 1994), their own realness (lower case "r" intended).

The postmodernist suspension of the body has two parallels: the banishment of affect from scientific writing and of the analyst's body from the clinic. Holding my breath (and heeding Shapiro's injunction to note my body-tension as I write), I quote Lancaster's (1995) critique of Butler: "Butler's work makes explicit what was implicit all along: a body amputated of the body; a world where language is real and the body is not. The Cartesian dilemmas of mind and body are resolved—by abolishing the body" (p. 4). Criticizing Butler's radical theorization of the body as social construction—well, it's not quite the Empress' new clothes, but close. One wonders whether this is a case of new wine in old regulatory bottles. What happens if, instead, the body's senses are always already problematized? if the experienced body joins the scientific and psychoanalytic bodies? Dean (1994), yet another queer theorist to put Butler's horizon into question, argues that, if the ego is an effect of the Imaginary and the subject an effect of the Symbolic, then sexuality and the body are effects of the Real (p. 95). The independent body, one might call it. From another anthropologist, Bruce Knauft (1994), we learn that, among the Gebusi of south New Guinea, bodies do matter: material embodiment does not resolve into signification. The idea of "longing" in their culture entails both an intense desire "to reduce bodily separation and [loudly voiced] frustration the boundary between the world of the real but unseen [world of spirits] and the material world of people" (p. 422). Both substantial bodies and bona fide spirits are real. Both/ and, not either/or.

"Holding my breath," I have said, experiencing my body as I think and write. How should we theorize the experienced body? How do we begin to articulate those mute domains of embodiment and enactment that exceed *la langue*? How do we undo the rhetorical status that the body has achieved in queer theory while retaining that theory's critical advantage? Probably it is true that we cannot answer such questions undialogically. Let me then bring forward a dialogue implicit in Shapiro's (1996) essay: that between "West" and "East." While I think it false generalizing to suggest, as Shapiro implicitly does, that all or most non-Western constructions of the body differ in the same way from our own (p. 315), still it is possible to challenge the corporeal canon passed on to us from Judeo-Christianity and the Enlightenment by borrowing bodies from elsewhere, even if we necessarily alter them in translation. As Knauft (1994) argues, "the local construction of desire is a lever for critiquing our own" (p. 421), not only our own desire, I would add, but our own understanding of our own desire (which for Lacan might be the same thing).

In Buddhism, for example, the body is not a hungry body, as it is for Freud. It is a breathing body. This different conceptualization of appetite versus breath has consequences for our understandings of suffering and its surcease. As Mark Epstein (1995), an American psychotherapist and Buddhist, argues, "The usual psychodynamic foundation for self experience is that of hunger, not breath. When this is the case, the body is experienced as an alien entity that has to be kept satisfied. . . ." (p. 145). In Winnicott's account of the not good-enough mother, Epstein reminds us, either there is insufficient food/mother or there is excess, and the child becomes, respectively, either deprived and entitled or engulfed and obliterated. Epstein contrasts the Buddhist view: "When awareness is shifted from appetite to breath, the anxieties about not being enough are automatically attenuated" (p. 145). The body is a site not of demand or need but, simply, of being in the timelessness of the present, which is, indeed, the site of psychoanalytic space. Epstein then quotes psychoanalyst Michael Eigen: "'The self structured by an awareness of breathing. . . . does not run after or get ahead of time but, instead, seems simply to move with it'" (p. 146). A self located in its moment, connected to its past and sensible of its flow into the future, produces echoes not only of "going with the flow" but also of free association. Epstein has earlier said, "It is impossible to turn the river around. Once [Buddhist] mindfulness is developed, there is no avoiding the relentless and teeming rush that underlies our experience" (p. 126). Mindfully inhabiting the breath is, in other words, also to inhabit the body, relatedness, desire, the unconscious.

It will not do, of course, to think of this one suggestion taken from the West's Other as a final, oppositional answer to the scientific or linguistic body. Many questions remain: Would such a body be, any longer, the site, cause, structure, origin of relationship? of sex? How would we want to reconceptualize attachment, desire, intimacy? Reciprocally, if we start with the body as merely breathing, not as endlessly longing, is the body still the site of excess? Or is the body's unspeakability produced by a certain sort of speech? Is it this sort of speech that characterizes the Real? If so, is it really the case that the Real can never be known or spoken? For Lacan, the breath can be a cause of desire, which he sometimes defines as the demand for love minus the appetite for satisfaction (Dean, 1994, p. 98); he speaks of "respiratory erogeneity," and deplores the paucity of its study (Lacan, 1977, p. 315, cited by Dean, 1994). Is Buddhist breathing Lacan's desire? Or is mindful breathing a different sort of knowledge?

The point is to destabilize: As Shapiro (1996) observes, psychoanalytic conventions of the body iron out contradictory wrinkles in the name of scientific legitimacy. Resituating the body in relational tension reveals the wrinkles once more. Good. They help us to appreciate, as we age into psychoanalysis (itself a discipline of maturity), the complexity and paradox that, face-lifted by science and linguistics from the experienced body, characterize what feminist philosopher Naomi Scheman (1993) has identified as the core modern epistemological problem of identifying and then bridging gaps, such as those between masculine and feminine, psyche and society, and, of course, mind and body (p. 3).

One mind–body bridge is pain, another is pleasure, affects also bridging the two bodies posed here, the one that hungers, the other that breathes. Two concluding anecdotes on affects as carriers of paradox: I recall a neighbor girl when I was a child, she was about five and I was ten. When she was unhappy, she didn't cry or scream. She would instead squat down and hold her breath until, blue in the face, she would faint. Laughingly, her father would call her "Sarah Heartburn," much as my father did me, if for different reasons; as we now all know, the female body is not hysterical for no reason. My point is that, whatever unbearable states of relational affairs would lead her to terrorize her family with her tantrums, still, something was intolerable as long as she continued to breathe. Not breathing, she no longer had to feel.

By the same token, if you breathe, you feel, and not only pain. A meditation-minded psychiatric resident, wanting to integrate her two practices, began during our work together to bring her meditative awareness into the consulting room. This interface of psychoanalysis and Zen Buddhism, by helping her to keep thinking despite the anxious tension of uncertainty and inarticulate affect, enabled her to open up rather than foreclose the multiple interpretive possibilities her patients' dilemmas suggested. Neither of us, however, had anticipated the personal spin-off from this professional progress. In our penultimate supervisory session, she rather generously and unexpectedly revealed to me that, during the previous evening's sex-making with her boyfriend, she found herself focusing not on her hungry body's need for what Lacanians see as illusory satisfaction, but instead on her breath, on each inhalation and exhalation, until she found herself, in the end, overtaken by the most extraordinary orgasm of her life.

NOTE

[1]The idea of "queer" originiated in the gay activist reappropriation of a standard pejorative for homosexual desire (see my discussion of Gerson

later). Signifying and valorizing not sexual object choice but that which is opposite to "normal" (you don't have to be homosexual to be queer), queerness also implies action, whether political protest or ethical demand or theoretical critique. Queer studies, reacting to the institutionalization of gay studies in academia, privileges the margin as a vantage point from which to deconstruct the center (the association of queer with postmodernism is implicit).

REFERENCES

Anzieu, D. (1989), *The Skin Ego*, trans. C. Turner. New Haven, CT: Yale University Press.

Aron, L. (1996), *The Meeting of Minds*. Hillsdale, NJ: The Analytic Press.

Bakhtin, M. M. (1981), *The Dialogic Imagination*, ed. M. Holmquist (trans. C. Emerson & M. Holmquist). Austin: University of Texas Press.

Barthes, R. (1975), *The Pleasure of the Text*. New York: Hill & Wang.

Benjamin, J. (1994a), Commentary on papers by Tansey, Hirsch, and Davies. *Psychoanal. Dial.*, 4:193–202.

———— (1994b), The shadow of the other (subject): Intersubjectivity and feminist theory. *Constellations*, 1:231–254.

Bollas, C. (1997), Wording and telling sexuality, *Internat. J. Psycho-Anal.*, 78:363–72.

Bordo, S. (1993), *Unbearable Weight*. Berkeley: University of California Press.

Bourdieu, P. & Eagleton, T. (1992), In conversation: Doxa and common life. *New Left Rev.*, 191:111–120.

Bowie, M. (1991), *Lacan*. Cambridge, MA: Harvard University Press.

Bromberg, P. (1994), "Speak! That I may see you: Some reflections on dissociation, reality, and psychoanalytic listening." *Psychoanal. Dial.* 4:517–547.

Butler, J. (1993), *Bodies That Matter*. New York: Routledge

———— (1997), *Excitable Speech*. New York: Routledge.

Capra, F. (1983) *The Tao of Physics*. Boulder, CO: Shambhala.

Chused, J. (1996), Abstinence and informative experience. *J. Amer. Psychoanal. Assn.*, 44:1047–1073.

Dean, T. (1994), Bodies that mutter. *Pre/Text*, 15:81–117.

Dimen, M. (1995), On "our nature": Prolegomenon to a relational theory of sexuality. In: *Disorienting Sexuality*, ed. T. Domenici & R. Lesser. New York: Routledge, pp. 129–152.

Ehrenreich, B. (1989), *Fear of Failing*. New York: Pantheon.

Epstein, M. (1995), *Thoughts Without a Thinker*. New York :Basic Books.

Evans, D. (1996), *An Introductory Dictionary of Lacanian Psychoanalysis*. New York: Routledge.

Flax, J. (1990), *Thinking Fragments*. Berkeley: University of California Press.

Foucault, M. (1991), *Discipline and Punish*, trans. A. Sheridan. New York: Vintage.

Freud, S. (1905), Fragment of an analysis of a case of hysteria. *Standard Edition*, 7:3–122. London: Hogarth Press, 1953.

—— (1925), Preface to Aichhorn's *Wayward Youth*. *Standard Edition*,19:272–275, 1961.

Gerson, S. (1994), A shared body of language. Presented at meeting of the Division of Psychoanalysis (39), American Psychological Association, Santa Monica, CA.

—— (1996), A shared body of language. *Gender & Psychoanal.* 1: 345–360.

Ghent, E. (1989), Credo: The dialectics of one-person and two-person psychologies. *Contemp. Psychoanal.*, 25:169–241.

Grosz, E. (1994), *Volatile Bodies.*Bloomington: Indiana University Press.

Harris, A. (1996), Animated conversation: Embodying and engendering. *Gender & Psychoanal.*, 1:361–384.

Hernnstein, R. J. & C. Murray, C.. (1994), *The Bell Curve*. New York: Free Press.

Keller, E. F. (1985), *Reflections on Gender and Science*. New Haven, CT: Yale University Press.

Knauft, B. (1994), Foucault meets South New Guinea: Knowledge, power, sexuality. *Ethos*, 22:391–438.

Knoblauch, S. (1996), The play and interplay of passionate experience. *Gender & Psychoanal.*, 1:323–344.

Kristeva, J. (1995), *New Maladies of the Soul*. New York: Columbia University Press.

Lacan, J. (1977), The subversion of the subject and the dialectic of desire in the Freudian unconscious, *Ecrîts*, trans. A. Sheridan. New York: Norton, pp. 292–325.

Lancaster, R. (1995) The queer body: Notes on masculinity, desire, and sexuality, or movies, magazines, and bodies that trade places: A phenomenological triptych. Presented at New York Academy of Sciences, January 22.

Malone, K. R. (1997), Working through the question of the phallus to the other side: Commentary on Bracha Lichtenberg-Ettinger's Paper. *Psychoanal. Dial.*, 7:407–422.

Massey, C. (1996a), Body smarts: An adolescent girl thinking, talking, mattering. *Gender & Psychoanal.*, 1:75–102.

—— (1996b), Cultural and conceptual dissonance in theoretical practice: Commentary on RoseMarie Pérez Foster's "The bilingual self: Duet in two voices." *Psychoanal. Dial.*, 6:123–140.

McDougall, J. (1989), *Theaters of the Body*. New York: Norton.

Merleau–Ponty, M. (1962), *The Phenomenology of Perception*, trans. C. Smith. New York: Routledge.

Miller, J. (1995), Going unconscious. *The New York Review of Books*, April 24.

Ogden, T. (1996a), The perverse subject of analysis. *J. Amer. Psychoanal. Assn.*, 44:1021–1046.

—— (1996b), *Subjects of Analysis*. New York: Aronson.

Paley, G. (1985), Talk given to Columbia University Seminar on Women and Society. April.

Rivera, M. (1989), Linking the psychological and the social: Feminism, poststructuralism, and multiple personality. *Dissociation*, 2:24–31.

Sands, S. H. (1997), Self psychology and projective identification—Whither shall they meet? A reply to the editors (1995). *Psychoanal. Dial.*, 7:669–683.

Saussure, F. de (1974), *Course in General Linguistics*, ed. C. Bally & A. Sechehaye with A. Reidlinger (trans. W. Baskin). London: Peter Owen.

Scarry, E. (1985), *The Body in Pain*. Oxford: Oxford University Press.

Shapiro, S. (1996), The embodied analyst in the Victorian consulting room. *Gender & Psychoanal.*, 1:297–322.

Scheman, N. (1993), *Engenderings*. New York: Routledge.

Vološinov, V. N. (1929–30), *Marxism and the Philosophy of Language,* trans. L. Matejka & I. R. Titunik. New York: Seminar Press, 1973.

Winterson, J. (1993), *Written on the Body*. London: Macmillan.

Wrye, H. K. (1996), Bodily states of mind. *Gender & Psychoanaly.* 1:283–296.

Zizek, S. (1996), Re–visioning "Lacanian" social criticism: The law and its obscene double. *J. Psychoanal. Culture & Society* 1:15–25.

PART II

*Linking the Mind
and Body*

4

THE EMBODIMENT OF DESIRE

Relinking the Bodymind Within the Analytic Dyad

Harriet Kimble Wrye

THE BODY OUT OF THE CLOSET

A century after the Victorian era, and in honor of psychoanalysis' 100th birthday, it is certainly time to celebrate embodiment and bring it to the forefront of our analytic minds. With the evolution of theoretical paradigms emphasizing the transference–countertransference duet, beyond the one-person drive model and with new data sources of infant observation, we are poised to embrace the paradoxes inherent in a mind–body continuum. Embodiment, viewed within the realm of transitional phenomena, invites us to awaken our senses and our own sensual bodily responses to our patients' material, to help us attune as well to the rich data within the realm of body talk. Diane Ackerman (1990) puts it this way:

> Our senses define the edge of consciousness, and because we are born explorers and questors after the unknown, we spend a lot of our lives pacing that windswept perimeter: We take drugs; we go to circuses; we tramp through jungles; we listen to loud music; we purchase exotic fragrances; we pay hugely for culinary novelties and are even willing to risk our lives to sample a new taste [p. xv]. . . .most people think of the mind as being located in the head, but the latest findings in physiology suggest that *the mind* doesn't really dwell in the brain but travels the whole body on cara-

vans of hormone and enzyme, busily making sense of the
compound wonders we catalogue as touch, taste, smell,
hearing, vision [p. xix].

In this chapter, I raise far more questions than I can begin to
answer. Referents of discourse about embodiment have not yet been
clearly conceptualized. It is time to bring mindfulness to these questions about the mind–body dialectic. For this project, we need to continue the deconstruction of aspects of psychoanalysis that are
prejudicially gendered, hierarchical, and dichotomized. We need to
decenter language, to unpack some of the accumulated sedimenta-
tion of speech that impedes accessing the *différence* in Derrida's (1982,
1985) sense, all the enlivened bodily states of mind (see also Shawver,
1996).

WHAT BODY? INSIDE, OUTSIDE
AND SOMEWHERE IN BETWEEN

We know it is time to extend the psychosomatic frame beyond visibly
observable body postures and outlines and classically noted tics and
tears, erections. So, after 100 years of psychoanalysis, how are we to
read and speak the language of the body afresh? Whose body we are
talking about: the analyst's? the patient's? the oedipal/genital body
of fantasy? the sexually experienced adolescent and adult body? Are
we referring simply to the observable body, a fist clenched or a tear
in the eye? Or the body as consciously experienced by the subject
(the speaker who says ,"I have a stomach ache," "I feel hot . . . or cold
. . . or tense")? Or the body symbolized on the dream screen (for
example, the budding excitation of a chase upstairs figuring for a
building of sexual tension prior to orgasm, or where the mind or brain
might be dreamed of as an ocean or the whole body as a car—kittenish
convertible, phallic Jaguar, disabled wreck)? Or the body as defined
and known by its skin surfaces, knowable to the sense of sight and
touch and smell (Anzieu, 1989)?

Or are we talking about the internal, unseen body of the viscera,
involuntary musculature and processes known only through extended
yoga practice, heightened states of consciousness, medicine, or profound experiences such as pregnancy or heart surgery, which impel
our attention to our bodies? More and more of us are going on either
spectacular or frightening visual voyages of our internal bodies
through new medical technology—MRIs, catheterized cameras surf-

ing through our arteries or intestines, ultrasounds revealing our earliest acquaintances with the embryos that will become our children. Joyous, frightening, or heartbreaking, these visual experiences, usually heightened by intense anxiety are being added to our language of the body.

To what extent may language acquisition reify, objectify, and even limit our consciousness of bodily experience and our construction of our gender (Butler, 1990, 1993; Irigaray, 1993)? While psychoanalytic attention has generally focused on the differentiated, more accessible, oedipal/genital body, how can we, and how often do we, access the undeveloped early body *before* words? How can we reach the far more elusive and perhaps terrifying preoedipal body of boundary diffusion and fluid exchanges, my own particular area of interest (Wrye and Welles, 1989), or the intrauterine "shared body" of mother and infant? As Daniel Stern (1985) points out, while language acquisition is a developmental achievement enhancing our understanding of conscious experience, what is lost when the infant, bathed in the sensually delicious warmth and visual brightness of yellow sunlight in her crib and rolling and gurgling and playing in the experience, has the experience labeled and catalogued simply as "a patch of sunlight"? Is the fulsome experience *ever* the same after it has been labeled? Eskimos have a rich vocabulary to describe snow, with close to 20 words for it, while Laplanders reportedly have 100 words for snow to our paltry one. Our analytic consciousness and even vocabulary for somatic experience, like our single word for snow, is comparatively limited and limiting. When we talk about the body, we need at least to be able to be more precise—we need at least the equivalent of those 20 different Eskimo words for snow to specify what we are speaking about when we speak about the body.

When we talk about embodiment in psychoanalysis, what shall we include? Are we talking about the body as a shape, a map in an atlas, an outline of a person, a symbol of the thing, like a map of a country? Or are we talking about the body as experienced, as the country itself, hiked in, mountains climbed, rivers run, scents smelled, the primitive, preverbal terrrain, as well as the urbanely articulated terrain? How apprehended? How sensed? How represented? How described? When and how is it known to the subjects of analysis? What would a regenerative embodiment of psychoanalysis mean?

We must extend the terrain of analytic work to bring the entire body beyond and before words into the mind of analyst and patient. We need, in other words, to relink the entire body and mind in an alive, informative, and potentially transformative way. As analysts, when we bring our own unnoticed bodily states into our conscious-ness, we may enable our patients to bring to life deadened or inac-cessible aspects of themselves. One image I particularly like in this domain of "inside, outside and somewhere in between" is the idea of holding our patients' beleaguered, oftimes deadened bodies in our mind/womb, creating a safe mental and palpably physical space for gestation and psychic rebirth.

JARED:
FROM A DISEMBODIED CLINICAL PRESENTATION
TO EMBODIMENT

With a fiercely cheerless and intense expression, Jared entered psy-choanalysis with me several years ago. A successful stock trader, Jared seemed to be always on his portable phone right to the threshold of my office. Never looking at me, he would push into the room and stride to the couch "ready for work." I became aware that my body would tighten warily, as if sensing danger. At times I imagined un-pleasant smells emanating from him; at others I wondered how his girlfriend could tolerate sex with him. I felt invaded and repelled. I say sex, because what I imagined could not be called lovemaking. Jared had to work through many deep oedipal and preoedipal issues relating to love, work, and play. The following brief selections from sessions late in his analysis particularly reveal my way of working within the primitive level of body-based transferences and counter-transferences. These sessions, several years into analysis, signaled for us both that Jared's long analysis would soon be coming to an end.

Jared said that the night before he'd been watching TV with his girlfriend. Thinking about masturbating, he went into the bathroom to gaze at himself in the mirror. "I was surprised, I look pretty good. My legs are muscular, my penis is nice, my shoulders strong. I think this is not what it seems, like we've talked about my avoiding women, my self-absorption, but I think this is something else you've mentioned, that longing for some real early touch from my mother." Over the years, I had noticed that my own bodily responses to Jared were chang-ing considerably. Feeling newly emerging pleasure in seeing him, I felt much more like reaching out to him. Although he was talking about an isolating experience of masturbation, I felt a visceral response to him that seemed in resonance with his own earliest experience. No longer repelled or guarded, I said, "Perhaps you were longing to feel special—all over beautiful, with a mother's adoring hands and delighted gaze touching her baby all over."

Jared thought for a moment and said, "Yes, but when you said that, instead of feeling all wrapped up and able to enjoy it, I felt anxious, like your interpretation would be a stick, pointed, probing. My mother was so intrusive, so hard to trust. I can't trust that you'd be soothing and not turn it into an angry, cutting comment, as I can be cutting, too." Wanting to highlight his resistance to the possibility of early maternal pleasure and inviting him to reconsider, I said, "As you cut my comment into a sharp pointed stick, not letting yourself feel its roundness, its softness, the pleasure of it. Then you're left with no comfort except masturbation and your own gazes in the mirror, longing to be touched and admired but afraid and alone." He seemed moved, apparently recognizing how my interpretation recapitulated his complaint of chronic isolation.

In the next session, 40-year-old Jared talked about planning his first vacation ever. Studying the map of Africa, he was amazed at "the way the countries fit together—like the pieces of a puzzle." My sense was first that in marveling at the African countries that "fit together" Jared was talking about discovering an early mother who complements, completes, mirrors in a twinship kind of way. This assumption informed my interpretive line, which was not to focus on the perverse distancing of his masturbatory avoidance of his girlfriend, but rather to speak to the early longings he felt for a mother who would be delighted to see him, cherish his whole body, and mirror his gaze. I had come to this interpretive line out of my own bodily identification with him early on, as the needy baby who, feeling poked and undesired, defensively turns his disappointment into an identification with the intrusive object. My interpretation of this earliest body-based desire brought forth his counteridentification with the cutting object, and we could approach the negative body transference states that way, freeing Jared's deeper bodily longings. Jared was very taken with my next interpretation about how the countries fitting together represented what he'd always wanted with his mother—to be able to feel complemented, shaped, and held snug, but separate and not invaded.

After this session, Jared was able to describe freely his heretofore blocked desire: "Over the weekend, I was thinking a lot about us. I was thinking. 'Could I have ever been a really sweet, innocent good baby? Not the messy one I always felt my mother didn't want to touch?' Then I had the most amazing fantasy. I could just feel you holding me. I was really small and I was nursing at your breast. It was round and warm and soft and full. I nursed and nursed, playing with it with my hand, looking at your face. When I was full, you shifted me to the other breast and it was so full. There was so much milk, more than I needed to feel completely satisfied. It was so lovely! You smelled clean and sweet and I felt so safe, so good!' " I was silently reminded of the haunting line from Leonard Cohen's song "Suzanne" : "And she touched your perfect body with her mind." How sapient was Cohen, I thought, to express so powerfully and poetically the idea that one may indeed touch another's body with one's mind. This moment clearly felt transformational to both Jared and me. By imagining my nursing him in a sensually experience-near way, he was able to move from distancing, deanimating, schizoid concreteness with part objects to being able to hold a playful and palpable, bodily based, transformational experience. In his mind. I held him with my body and he held me with his mind.

   This session with Jared touched me so that that night I dreamed of him. We were dancing. He was a strong, attractive, graceful dancing partner. He spun me around the dance floor, swooping and gliding. Then marveling at how we were gliding around, I looked down at my feet; instead of wearing shoes, I was dancing in bright yellow dust mops! I awoke, almost laughing, with a feeling of rhythmic pleasure, delight. I realized that one thing Jared had described about his mother was that she was a fiercely compulsive cleaner, so preoccupied, always scrubbing and mopping. I realized that, in the moment, in place of such a fiercely rigid, intrusive, cutting object, I had become another sort—the complementary, playful dance partner. The fierce work face he had worn in the beginning had metamorphosed, within our encounter in the realm of early bodily states, into the playground of psychoanalysis (Sanville, 1991). We were dancing together and polishing the floor! Here we had Freud's love, work, and play in one parsimonious dream image! I also realized that it was only at the very end of his analysis that Jared could physically immerse himself in the early maternal erotic transference and that, with this full sensual immersion, we were both sprung from the cutting, poking impasse, and the postoedipal resolution was free to emerge and did. Jared soon announced his plans to marry his fiancée.

FREUD'S BODY IN THE VICTORIAN CONSULTING ROOM

When Freud (1915) made his landmark discoveries of the psychosomatic connection, he formally introduced the difficulties facing the analyst whose patient brings her body into the consulting room and untoward erotic feelings present themselves with an urgent demand for response from the analyst. He battled then with the issues raised when the urges of the body break into consciousness, in that case, when a woman patient falls in love with her male analyst and begs that he return her love. He noted that the line between the psychical and the physical is ambiguous and hard to define. He also observed the difficulty of differentiating the meaning of those feelings. They may present themselves as a resistance—such as in the patient's attempt to deflect the analyst from his work, to "knock him off his perch"—or they may be a transference repetition of the patient's infantile neurosis, awaiting insight and interpretation, or they are real in the present situation and require utmost delicacy. While Freud was occupied with the technical management of transference love in his 1915 paper, primarily what we more frequently call erotized transferences (Blum, 1973), he was also attempting to establish a credibility beyond reproach for his fledgling science. On both counts he argued strongly for the analyst's abstinence and refusal to gratify the patient's libidinal wishes. The analyst's body was to be kept out of sight, behind the "blank screen." Sue Shapiro (1995) puts it this way:

> Psychoanalysis is the talking cure. Patients talk, we interpret. We sit quietly in our chairs, seeking to remove our body from the patient's objective experience. The patient may fantasize about our bodily state, but as much as possible our bodily state remains opaque. . . . what began as a liberating environment where one could at least talk dirty, has become a strait jacket for analyst and patient alike.

Though a transcendent genius interested in bridging soma and psyche, Freud was also Victorian, Cartesian, Newtonian, patriarchal, drive oriented, and oedipal. In the classical focus on the differentiated, oedipally desired body of otherness, mapped by symbolic language from the "objective" point of view, many analysts, like Freud himself, miss the body of sensorially lived experience. He was enamored of dichotomies and tended to think in terms of a dualism of body and mind (Carella, 1974), which has, to the postmodern mind become outdated. Following Freud's studies on hysteria, the primary focus on the body within analytic literature has been on the body as the object of sexual curiosity and forbidden rapacious desire. (Or the body has also been viewed classically from the angle of psychosomatic medicine and pathological somatization of unconscious conflict.) Very little attention has been paid to the entire range of normal body experience or to the body as the fundamental primal self-state wherein the ego is "first and foremost a body ego" (Freud, 1923). While the body has languished quietly in the analytic closet, it has never been forgotten. Fenichel (1945), and others early joined Freud's (1923) emphasis that body sensations form the basis of ego development, and Erikson (1956), echoing Federn (1952) and Schilder (1950), has defined identity as "a feeling of being at home in one's body." (p. 74; see also Hagglund, 1980). Contemporary bioenergetics has focused on the body (skin, musculoskeletal system) as the repository of archaic object relations (Shubs, 1996, personal communication).

THE RELATIONAL CONSTRUCTION OF THE BODY: ANALYSTS WRITING ABOUT BODY-BASED TRANSFERENCES AND COUNTERTRANSFERENCES

I would like to draw attention to the kinds of issues emerging in relation to embodiment in psychoanalysis, particularly ways in which we bring our culture-bound, linguistically valenced psychic apparatus to bear on our patients' embodiment and sexuality. My colleague, Judy Welles, and I have been preoccupied for the last decade by the manifestations of very early, preoedipal material—what we call maternal erotic transferences and countertransferences (MET and MEC)—nonverbal phenomena that often present in the treatment by way of very concrete and often viscerally tinged communications, or enactments (Wrye and Welles, 1989, 1993, 1994; Wrye, 1993). When we first started exploring these phenomena, we could find practically no reports of them in the literature.

Recently more reports of analysts' bodily responses and erotic fantasies in the countertransference have begun to appear in print (Ehrenberg, 1992; Davies, 1994). Renewed interest in embodiment in psychoanalysis has been fed by several changes. Disturbances in the field have come from the challenge to the hegemony of the most rigidly classical medical model; the feminization of the field has also made an impact. The ebb and flow of menstrual blood, pregnancies, childbirth, and nursing babies in public places may give women somewhat more freedom to live in their bodies and to talk about it a little more comfortably. Until 1969, however, according to Ruth Lax, there was still such inhibition among female analysts to talk about their patients' reactions to such an obvious bodily event as the analyst's pregnancy that no published reports existed until hers.

Some contemporary analysts are writing more of their use of

their own bodily and sensual responses to patients. Susan Bady (1984) argues eloquently for the development within the therapist of an artistic sensibility whereby the therapist, like the artist or performer, is able to use the "medium of self to create art" (p. 529). Schafer (1959) describes empathy as "a sharing of another person's organization of thoughts, feelings, desires, defenses" (p. 344), and Bady calls it "that *ability* to put *ourselves in the skin of another person* and to *hear, smell, see, taste,* and *touch the roses and the weeds of another*" (p. 530, italics added). A therapist can use projective identification, introjection, and associations to personal sensory memories to increase the permeability of her ego boundaries in order to achieve a closer state of atonement with a patient. Knoblauch (1996), Gerson (1996), and Harris (1996) emphasize conscious attention to relinquishing the embedded intellectual prejudice toward the body carried by analyst and patient alike. Shapiro (1996) urges the reading of the body as a new unprejudiced text. Dimen (1996), citing Lancaster's trenchant critique of Judith Butler's work as a "body amputated of the body; a world where language is real and the body is not." (p. 398), offers a fresh challenge to the postmodern feminist deconstruction of the body.

Jane Burka (1996), marrying Ogden's (1994) concept of the analytic third with Green's (1975) notion of the analytic object, births a creative notion of the analyst's body as an analytic object cocreated and recreated by the intersubjectivity of analyst and patient. Green's *analytic object,* based on Winnicott's transitional object, is neither entirely inside nor entirely outside. It exists, or is created, in the mutual in-between unconscious space between analyst and analysand. Ogden's *analytic third* is "the inter subjectively generated experience of the analytic pair" (p. 94). Expanding on Green's and Ogden's ideas, Burka conceptualizes the analyst's body as an analytic third, illustrating patients' at times cooptive and perverse use and at other times cooperative use of the analyst's body as a creative medium for transference transformation. Burka describes her own wide-ranging feelings about and transference use of her "overweight body" with particular patients and in particular times in the treatment. Her feelings vary dramatically according to transference phenomena: "sometimes feeling dumpy and self-conscious, sometimes feeling voluptuous and racy, sometimes feeling motherly and nurturing, sometimes feeling shriveled and empty. My same body can seem frail in relation to a large man or monumental in relation to a petite woman. With two bodies present and two unconsciouses at play, any experience is possible" (p. 17).

Elaine Siegel (1996) offers her own somatic countertransference reactions noted in her journal during her analytic treatment with four patients in whom clear and corroborated memories of incest emerged during the analyses. A former dancer, Siegel had been trained in such a classical model that for years she believed she must practice abstinence and suppress her own natural bodily acuity: "I then believed that such primary-process phenomena as the ability to understand body language bore the stamp of pathology—in myself and others" (p. 19). Nearing retirement, she felt safe enough to describe vividly her own body-based reveries with several patients whose experiences of incest were discovered in analysis. It was through her interpretive use of these data that she was able to help her patients attune themselves to their own profoundly derailing dissociative states and to help bring them into conscious connection with bodily memories.

PSCYHOANALYSIS AND LITERATURE: THE BODY AS OBJECT VERSUS SUBJECT OF EXPERIENCE

The analytic armamentarium is dull if these data remain unconscious in the analyst. So how can we enhance our analyzing instrument to be more attuned to kinesthetic and sensory cues? One way to bring the body to mind is to turn to literature. Like analysts, writers struggle to get ever more deeply into the depths and viscera of human experience; and they also wrestle with the limitations of the verbal "talking" project, in which language is symbolic and removed from the "real." There is a shift in modern literature from the objectification of the body to the body as subject of experience. As analysts, we share this struggle to come to terms with the subjectively lived body versus the body as objectified "semantic project" (Flax, 1990 pp. 218–219).

For this body, language is first and foremost sound and physical reverberation. When did we first experience words? Long before birth, rocked in the sound chamber of amniotic fluid, our whole bodies physically reverberating to the chords of our mother's vocalizations. In this quadraphonic, no, omniphonic, stereo chamber, this word bath, we first knew our mother's sound. Why do adolescents, struggling so with separateness, at the same time seek out rock bands (yes, the words rock and roll apply perfectly) with a rhythmic drumbeat whose amplification inevitably recreates a virtual physically pulsating sound bath? Why do our analysands sometimes forget so many of our "brilliant" interpretations and remember only having felt lost in our voices? This isn't resistance; this may be the transformational early "attunement" we all seek—access to the deepest bodily states of mind.

How do we open up the channels in our own consciousness to our own bodily states as well as of our patients? In *New Poems,* Rainer Maria Rilke addressed this question by describing a poet's unique way of experiencing he called *einsicht,* or inseeing. Rilke's *einsicht* can be translated in the clinical setting as a way of listening to the body talk without words. Colleague Hedda Bolgar reminded me that *einsicht* may be translated from the German both as "inseeing" and as "insight." Rilke (personal communcation) says:

> I love inseeing. Can you imagine with me how glorious it is to insee, for example a dog as one passes by. *Insee* (I don't mean in-spect, which is only a kind of human gymnastic, by means of which one immediately comes out again on the other side of the dog, regarding it merely, so to speak, as a window upon the humanity lying behind it, not that)—but to let oneself precisely into the dog's very center, the point from which it becomes a dog, the place in it where God, as it were, would have sat down for a moment when the dog was finished, in order to watch it under the influence of its first embarrassments and inspirations and to know that it was good, that nothing was lacking, that it could not have been better made. . . . Laugh though you may, dear confidant, if I am to tell you *where* my all-greatest feeling, my world-feeling, my earthly bliss was to be found, I must confess to you: it was to be found time and again, here and there, in such timeless moments of this divine inseeing.

Poets like Rilke lead us to discover body-based states of awareness. Unlike in classic literature, where the sensual body was described mostly like a painter's nude or odalisque, as the *object* of desire (see Brooks, 1993), Rilke exemplifies the contemporary shift from the objectification of the body to the body as subject of experience.

Similarly, a scene in David Malouf's (1994) evanescent novel, *Remembering Babylon,* depicts a transformational moment when bodily consciousness is altered. The scene occurs in a story describing the clash of cultures when a Victorian community in the Australian outback encounters a shipwrecked English cabin boy raised by aborigines. The colonialists embody the "civilized" fear of the primal; in their paranoia they project their own primitive hatred and aggression onto the aborigines and the lost boy. In so doing, they represent the Victorian split between body and mind, locating intelligence and religious discipline in themselves and primitive bodily states in the natives. The following passage depicts a transformational mind–body moment that occurs when a young colonial girl is swarmed by bees. Just prior to this moment, the wild boy had gently and curiously touched her; this contact with the primordial allows the young girl to contain her panic, surrender to the onslaught and trust the bees:

> Suddenly there was the sound of a wind getting up in the grove, though she did not feel the touch of it, and before she could complete the breath she had taken, or expel it in a cry, the swarm was on her, thickening so fast about her that it was as if night had fallen, just like that, in a single cloud. She just had time to see her hands covered with plushy, alive fur gloves before her whole body crusted over and she was blazingly gathered into the single sound they made, the single mind. Her own mind closed in her. She lost all sense of where her feet might be, or her dreamy wrists, or whether she was still standing, as she had been a moment before, in the shadowy grove, or had been lifted from the face of the earth.
>
> The bees have their stomachs full, her mind told her, they will not sting. Stand still. Stand Still. It was her old mind that told her this. She stood still as still and did not breathe. She surrendered herself. You are our bride, her new and separate mind told her as it drummed and swayed above the earth. Ah, so that is it! They have smelled the sticky blood-flow. They think it is honey. It is. . . . She could hear voices calling to her through the din her body was making. But it made no difference, now, the distance, three feet or a thousand years, no difference at all; or whether she was a girl (a woman), or a tree. She stood sleeping. Upright. A bride. Then the bitterness of smoke came to her throat, and the cloud began to lift. . . . Years later she would become expert . . . at the bee business . . . [from] a bodily excitement that went back to this moment under the trees, when her mind had for a moment been their unbodied one and she had been drawn into the process and mystery of things [pp. 106–107].

Malouf's writing, like the writing in Carlos Casteneda's *Don Juan* series, immerses us in another level of consciousness, the transcendent and mind–altering transformational bodily experience. We can also read the passage as a poetic depiction of how the analyst, surrendering to such powerful, unknown, primitive bodily states in the countertransference, can, through identification with her own dark interior, be transformed and attain new creative awareness. A contrasting powerful scene is depicted by poet/novelist Vargas Llosa (1990). Vargas Llosa creates, in the character of Don Rigoberto, an exquisite ode to anal narcissism, a picture of a man who has honed introspective bodily awareness to an art form. For Don Rigoberto, a hedonist who worships at every orifice in the temple of his body, consciousness transforms the most mundane bodily acts into acts of attention, pleasure and mindfulness:

> Don Rigoberto half closed his eyes and strained, just a little. That was all it took: he immediately felt the beneficent tickle in his rectum and the sensation that, there inside, in the hollows of his lower belly, something obedient to his will was about to depart and was already wriggling its way down that passage which, in order to make its exit easier, was widening. His anus, in turn, had begun to dilate in anticipation, preparing itself to complete the expulsion of the expelled, whereupon it would shut itself up tight and pout, with its thousand little puckers, as though mocking: "You're gone, you rascal you, and can't ever return."
>
> Don Rigoberto gave a satisfied smile. Shitting, defecating, excreting: synonyms for sexual pleasure? he thought. Of course. Why not? Provided it was done slowly, savoring the task, without the least hurry, taking one's time, imparting to the muscles of the colon a gentle, sustained quivering. It was a matter not of pushing but of guiding, of accompanying, of graciously escorting the gliding of the offerings toward the exit. Don Rigoberto sighed once again, his five senses absorbed in what was happening inside his body. [p. 55].

Vargas Llosa offers this extraordinarily sensual and evocative description, a wake-up call to the senses, particularly the "unmentionable" sensuality of anal narcissism. Yet doesn't this autoerotic passage also recreate or evoke not only orgasm or child birth, but a sense of the shared bodily pleasures of the mother and infant in a blissful feeding experience—the baby's sucking, the mother's let-down reflex from pressure to release, the rhythmic flow, the enraptured attention, the mutual sensual absorption with a totally natural process?

In the consulting room, when we fully attune ourselves to the nonverbal world of sensual body communication, for example, the evocation of a sense memory can open up for a patient an extraordinary panoply of associations. "Smells detonate softly in our memory like poignant land mines hidden under the weedy mass of many years and experiences. Hit a tripwire of smell, and memories explode all at once. A complex vision leaps out of the undergrowth" (Ackerman, 1990, p. 6).

Aiming for such powerful enhancement of our patients' experience requires that we travel beyond the epistomophilic to the introspective path. In the inchoate, ungendered, nonverbal sensorium of the body, other ways to reinscribe consciousness may emerge and foster more integrated states of mind–body coherence.

CLINICAL EMBODIMENTS

The following work was with a female patient who had great difficulty being in touch with and at ease in her body; Françoise, like Jared earlier, used her body perversely. This material comes from the ending phase of a typically complex analysis, for it takes time, safety and intense mindfulness to reach this depth; the pathway to mutually enlivening erotic resonance is typically rugged and slow.

Françoise

Françoise, an unmarried professional woman in her 30s, entered analysis with a kind of compulsive sexuality, an erotomania with innumerable partners, mostly married, emotionally unavailable, or otherwise inappropriate. AIDS awareness finally made her realize that her behavior was suicidal. Françoise was tall, glamorous in a uniquely French way, but also driven and manic. She had had prior treatments of various kinds, ranging from behavior therapy, to marathon encounter groups, to Rolfing, and twelve-step groups. Her inability to choose and commit to any one treatment approach mirrored her inability to tolerate intimacy and continued for some time in analysis. Whenever she sensed that our work might touch her too deeply, she would seek compulsive therapy "affairs" and compulsive sexual enactments to take her attention away from me.

From the beginning, I sensed her emotional rigidity and powerful defensiveness. She reminded me of a stiff painted doll, the wooden kind with head and body in one piece and arms and legs attached by internal cords. Françoise's French Calvinist mother had died when she was 16, but not before imprinting her daughter with all manner of rules and regulations about sin and virtue, hard work, thrift, ambition, and a routine of internal scourings by weekly enemas. Her father, a handsome seaman who was frequently away, would appear on the scene as an excitingly seductive but also mean-tempered figure, regaling her with gifts from foreign ports and impetuously lashing her with his impatience and denigrating insults. After her mother's death, he sent her from France to relatives in New England to complete her education. He died when she was in her 20s, and her promiscuity began in earnest.

At the beginning of therapy she had no early childhood memories. She could not recollect a session after it had passed and often experienced lapses of consciousness during sessions. She frequently spoke in disjointed, pressured associations. Françoise became aware of a panic state if she experienced any longings toward me. At 13, her mother had "found" her in bed with another young girl and frightened that her daughter was homosexual, sent her immediately for her first year in a convent. We talked about how panicked her mother had seemed about her bodily longings and functions—officiously purging her with weekly enemas and then dispatching her to a convent in an attempt to expunge her first sexual experiment. Interestingly, *The Narration of Desire* (Wrye and Welles, 1994) evolved out of Judy Welles's and my clinical observations of the perverse erotization of girls who, like Françoise, had been subjected to frequent enemas. I felt that Françoise's primary bodily contact with her mother had felt traumatically intrusive, both over stimulating and distant— in short, profoundly disturbing.

My countertransference to her ranged from strong feelings of anger and frustration to trying to reel her in to get her attention and wanting to find a way through her manically pressured "to do" lists and disconnected enactments with men. I felt like arguing with her that she was missing out by ruling out half the population, women, as unworthy of her interest. On other, at first very rare occasions, I felt tenderness, a desire to pick her up, rock her, soothe her, and kiss her tear-stained cheeks. Most often, however, I felt tense, provoked, and worn out after sessions; often; I would get a stiff neck. It was probably five years into her ten year analysis before Françoise could allow herself even to notice any feelings about me between sessions, and we both agreed that, when she arrived at the point of feeling the depth and richness of our relationship and could tolerate the vulnerability of needing one person and really miss me, she would be approaching capacity for intimacy.

Although she did not look at me directly or refer to me or bodily fantasies in any personal way, she played out much of her maternal transference in relation to my house and office. One day, the wrought iron gate outside my office door was still locked when she arrived and she had to wait for me. When I unlocked the gate, she was beside herself, first with rage at the inconvenience and that it took "one full extra minute of *my* time while you fumbled with the key"; then, as we continued to explore, she described how shut out she had felt, how cold she was waiting, how harsh and unwelcoming the bars looked. This painful episode led to her bringing me a photograph that her father had taken of her mother feeding her a bottle when she was about six months old. The picture was everything I had felt in a bodily way on many occasions. It was remarkable, as it was a "portrait" taken by father and ostensibly proudly enlarged for posterity, but Françoise's mother looked very stern, very buttoned up, almost scowling as she held little Françoise away from her. I felt my whole body stiffen as I looked at the picture of the baby feeding. Mother seemed to be ramming the bottle efficiently into Françoise, whose little fists clenched and whose back looked arched. We were able to talk about how my iron gate had evoked that stiff, forbidding maternal body. Eventually Françoise began to talk about how her sexual foray with another adolescent girl had terrified her as much as it had her mother, although probably in a very different way. She was afraid of the intensity of her forbidden longings to touch the softness of a woman's body.

In a subsequent session she revealed that, in all the years she had been coming to analysis, she had never driven or walked on the hill behind my home/office. Amazed, I queried and she said, "Oh, I'm not allowed to do that. Not ever." I pointed out that she seemed to feel that she could never feel desire or curiosity or be drawn to wander or look around—and how remarkable, as this was a public road, in no way restricted. I said she might be telling me that my house felt like my body; she could not feel like a little Françoise who would be welcome to explore, to touch, to wander, but must keep a rigid distance. Shortly after that session, she said, "Well, I got here early and I walked around the neighborhood. Then I saw that there's a path that goes around your house the other way leading to the office. I wanted to walk there, but I couldn't. You wouldn't like it. Besides you might catch me at it." I said, "You couldn't come close to me even though you wanted to. You were afraid I'd be patrolling the perimeters, eagle-eyed. Perhaps you are telling us about how it felt at my closed gate, or as a baby, or a little Françoise, wanting to reach out to Mommy, but sensing her stiffen and pull away." "Oh, yes, I couldn't get close!" "You have felt sure that I wouldn't be the sort of mommy who would want you close, to let you explore my face or my mommy body, that I wouldn't be the sort of mommy who could be eager to see her baby girl, who couldn't wait to pick her up, kiss her cheeks, stroke her hair, check her little toes, maybe playfully tickle her."

This opened up all kinds of early material, about the enemas, the painfully tight braiding of her hair, and how she longed for her father's ship to come in to break the tension. Even though she knew he might get drunk and explosive, he was funny and he played with her. As Françoise relaxed, she began to notice my perfume, the colors and scent of the flowers in the office, the texture of my clothes; and she noticed that she was going for long periods of time with no interest in dating and was making new friendships with women. She began taking her little niece to the park, taking long baths, and noticing that she was missing me between sessions. I missed her too and found myself looking forward to seeing her: I was able to imagine her not only as a lovable baby but as a very bright little girl and an entertaining friend.

Soon thereafter she came barefooted to her session, her toenails freshly painted. She looked coyly sheepish, apologizing that she'd just had a pedicure. I said, "Well, I guess maybe you also wanted to bring those little toes to me so we could play 'This Little Piggy'!" She laughed and said, "I guess I can finally say there are these ways I'd love to be able to play with you!" The opening of this body-based maternal erotic transference, ushered in by the bars on my gate and tracked through my own bodily based maternal erotic counter-transferences to her, brought a sea change in her relationships with men as well. Françoise became careful in her choices of men and insisted on developing a relationship and friendship first. She began to talk about wanting to marry, settle down, and have her own little babies to play "This Little Piggy" with. The analysis came to life when we were finally able to move from the outside of my house to inside and approach her bodily feelings in a playful, sensual way. It was not, and typically is not, an easy course with a patient as "disembodied" as Françoise. Such material often does not evolve until quite late in an analysis, until well after the analytic playground has been established and tested for safety.

CONCLUSIONS

Analysts of both genders share a myriad of resistances toward immersion in and creative use of primitive, bodily based erotic transferences. I am referring to the entire gamut of the earliest, preverbal,
positively and negatively valenced longings and desire. Many of these
resistances Judy Welles and I have elaborated in our book, *The Narration of Desire* (Wrye and Welles, 1994). It helps enormously when we
recognize these resistances, but that does not make them disappear,
nor does it lead to instant cure. Like the colonialists in David Malouf's
Remembering Babylon, we and our patients are often inclined to want
the messy aboriginal stuff to stay far from us in the analytic outback.

Freud discovered psychoanalysis, the "talking cure," and freed
his fledgling science from hypnotic touch. At the same time, in his
effort to make his scientific project respectable within the Victorian
culture of, and with his own penchant for, Cartesian dualism, he fos-
tered an inadvertent splitting off of the body. A century after Freud's
landmark discoveries, we are now engaging in a lively project to bring
embodiment back into psychoanalysis and to bring bodily states to
the forefront of the minds of patient and analyst alike. We are still
talking about the "talking cure," but a cure that includes profound
awareness of primitive bodily states of mind. Not just the sexual, oedipal body as object, but the subjectively experienced, lived-in whole
body—the inside and the outside and somewhere between—the body
that is relationally created, apprehended, and enjoyed.

But it is not just resistance that gets in our way. Making contact
with this inchoate, preverbal body is hard! We do have some guides,
however. Our own analytic instruments are honed to bodily states
through the increasingly available reports of psychoanalysts describing their own bodily countertransferences and resonances to the body
states of their patients. We can apprehend that body with consciousness enhanced by the increasingly marvelous experiences that inadvertently come to us on trips to the doctor's office or hospital through
medical technology, the journeys we are privileged to participate in
as we observe our own internal bodies (or unborn babies) through
ultrasound, by microscopic cameras projecting their journeys through
our arteries, colons, and hearts, *and* with the help of contemporary
artists and writers like Malouf and Vargas Llosa, who richly describe
bodily states of mind, or with the help of Rilke's "inseeing."

Though it is not easy, we can attune ourselves more to the body–
mind in the analytic dance, if we not only listen with the third ear but

consciously feel with our skin, our bones, and our viscera our patients' narratives of desire. That capacity to resonate with patients' total subjective and sensory experience enriches our patients' self-awareness and contributes to therapeutic change. So much of our psychic health, our sexual identity and expression, and our capacity to function well in love, work, and play—in other words, dancing with our dustmops on—depends on the integration of enlivened, body-conscious self-states that can be retuned in an analysis that relinks this early bodymind.

REFERENCES

Ackerman, D.(1990), *A Natural History of the Senses*. New York, Vintage Books.

Anzieu, D. (1989), *The Skin Ego*. New Haven, CT: Yale University Press.

Bady, S. L. (1984), Countertransference, sensory images, and the therapeutic cure. *Psychoanal. Rev.*, 71:529–539.

Blum, H. P. (1973), The concept of erotized transference. *J. Amer. Psychoanal. Assn.*, 21:61–76.

Brooks, P. (1993), *Body Work*. Cambridge, MA: Harvard University Press.

Burka, J. (1996), The therapist's body in reality and fantasy: A perspective from an overweight therapist. In: *The Therapist as a Person*, ed., B. Gerson. Hillsdale, NJ: The Analytic Press.

Butler, J. (1990), *Gender Trouble*. London: Routledge.

——— (1993), *Bodies That Matter*. London: Routledge.

Carella, M. J. (1974), Psychoanalysis and the mind-body problem. *Psychoanal. Rev.*, 61:53–62.

Derrida, J. (1982), Differance. In: *Margins of Philosophy*, ed. J. Derrida, Chicago: University of Chicago Press, pp. 309–330.

——— (1985), *The Ear of the Other*. New York: Schocken Books.

Dimen, M. (1996), Discussion of symposium, "The Relational Construction of the Body." *Gender & Psychoanal.*, 1: 385–402.

Ehrenberg, D. (1992), *The Intimate Edge*. New York: Norton.

Erikson, E. (1956), The problem of ego identity. *J. Amer. Pschoanal. Assn.*, 4:56–121.

Federn, P. (1952), *Ego Psychology and the Psychoses*. New York: Basic Books.

Fenichel, O. (1945), *The Psychoanalytic Theory of Neurosis*. New York: Norton.

Flax, J. (1990), *Thinking Fragments*. Berkeley: University of California Press.

Freud, S. (1915), Observations on transference-love (further recommendations on the technique of psycho-analysis III), *Standard Edition*, 12:157–172. London: Hogarth Press, 1958.

——— (1923), The ego and the id, *Standard Edition*, 19:1–59. London: Hogarth Press, 1961.

Gerson, S. (1996), A shared body of language. *Gender & Psychoanal.*, I:345–360.

Green, A. (1975), The analyst, symbolization and absence in the analytic setting. *Internat. J. Psycho-Anal.*, 56:1–22.

Hagglund, T. H. P. (1980), The inner space of the body image. *Psychoanal. Quart.*, 49:256–283.

Harris, A. (1996), Animated conversation: Embodying and gendering. *Gender & Psychoanal.* I:361–383.

Irigaray, L. (1993), *Je, Tu, Nous*, trans. A. Martin, London: Routledge.

Knoblauch, S. (1996). The play and interplay of passionate experience: multiple organizations of desire. *Gender & Psychoanal.*, I:323–344.

Lax, R. (1969), Some considerations about transference and countertransference manifestations evoked by the analyst's pregnancy. *Internat. J. Psycho-Anal.*, 50:363–372.

Malouf, D. (1994), *Remembering Babylon*. New York: Vintage Books.

Ogden, T. (1994), *Subjects of Analysis*. Northvale, NJ: Aronson.

Sanville, S. (1991), *The Playground of Psychoanalytic Therapy*. Hillsdale, NJ: The Analytic Press.

Schafer, R. (1959), Generative empathy in the treatment situation. *Psychoanal. Quart.*, 28:342–73.

Schilder, P. (1950), *The Image and Appearance of the Human Body*. New York: Wiley.

Shapiro, S. (1995), The embodied analyst in the Victorian consulting room. Presented at meeting of Division of Psychoanalysis (39), American Psychoanalytic Association, Santa Monica, CA.

———— (1996), The embodied analyst in the Victorian consulting room. *Gender & Psychoanal.*,1:3 297–322.

Shawver, L. (1996). What postmodernism can do for psychoanalysis: A guide to the postmodern vision. *Amer. J. Psychoanal.*, 56:371–393.

Siegel, E. V. (1996), *Transformations*. Hillsdale, NJ: The Analytic Press.

Stern, D. (1985), *The Interpersonal World of the Infant*. New York: Basic Books.

Vargas Llosa, M. (1990), *In Praise of the Stepmother*, trans. H. Lane, New York: Farrar Straus Giroux.

Wrye, H. K. (1989), Hello the hollow: from deadspace to playspace. *Psychoanal. Rev.*, 80:1. 101–122.

———— (1993), Erotic terror: male patient's horror of the maternal erotic transference. *Psychoanal. Inq.*, 13:240–257.

———— & Welles, J., (1989), The maternal erotic transference. *Internat. J. of Psychoanal.*, 70673–684.

———— & ———— (1994), *The Narration of Desire*. Hillsdale, NJ: The Analytic Press.

5

THE BODY–MIND

Psychopathology of Its Ownership

Linda Gunsberg and Isaac Tylim

The body has begun to reclaim the central position it occupied earlier in the development of psychoanalysis. Contemporary focus on the body aims at revisiting Freud's psychoanalytic discoveries in his work with hysterical patients. Freud constructed a theory and a technique capable of healing the rift between the body and the mind, affect and ideation. For our purposes, the body is a psychological construct; aspects of the body or somatic functions that do not achieve psychic representation do not exist. Ownership of the body and the mind, then, refers to representations that allow a transformation of the "bio-logic" to the "psycho-logic" (McDougall, 1995). To own, one must name. In this chapter we primarily address the pregender body.

Trusting that they will be cared for and loved, babies offer themselves to their parents unconditionally even before birth. The "imagined body" of the child-to-be is complemented by the fantasy of the body image, which represents not just the anatomical or biological body (Aulangnier, 1991), but also the "imagined" body in the parents' internal world. The child is bound to occupy a unique place in the psyche of the parents. Love and other parental affects are communicated through touching the baby's body and through gestures and

---

Portions of this chapter were published in Gunsberg and Tylim (1995). Adapted by permission of the publisher.

verbalizations. A parent's fantasies about the child and his or her relationship with the baby are also communicated, often unconsciously. A mother can do to, and for, the child what she wishes. She can be gentle and loving, or she can be cruel. In some societies she can even kill her child if she wishes, with social approval of her act. The infant is hers, her product, her possession (A. Balint, 1939).

This power of possession is inexplicable, but we can see from our patients in treatment how difficult it is for women and men alike to extricate themselves from the primitive, archaic love relationship with mother. Although some mothers permit this separation to occur better than others do, this dilemma is universal for all children with their mothers. Because of the regressive pulls of this relationship, mothers are often experienced as villainous or witchlike, partly owing to an externalization of the regressive pulls and, in some cases, to the sheer power and psychopathology of the mother.

Thus, the preoedipal mother has a hold on the child's preoedipal internal world that the father rarely has. This is reassuring, but at times frightening. Many fathers are anxious about the physical nature of the early father–infant relationship. They report fantasies of injuring their infants during the wife's pregnancy (Gurwitt, 1976; Herzog, 1982) as well as once the baby is born. They view the baby as fragile and prefer to engage the child when he or she is older and physically sturdier (Ross, 1979). Because of the father's fears of hurting the baby, a certain preoedipal physical and psychological distance can emerge between the father and the baby, which makes the baby even more the mother's possession.

MATERNAL AND PATERNAL ROLES: NORMAL FUNCTIONS AND POTENTIAL DISTURBANCES

McDougall (1980, 1989), Fain (1971), and Balint (1939) have offered very meaningful formulations for understanding the necessary maternal and paternal roles in early child development. McDougall (1980) states that the mother's role is to offer the child an interpretation of his cries and gestures. The mother gives her child the words for his bodily zones and thus offers the baby a framework of meaning for his body. She conveys to her baby the extent of the "fantasy space" that these bodily zones occupy and the nature of the connection between the bodily zone and the "complementary object." Thus, the mother is responsible for offering the child the beginnings of a body image that contains erogenous zones, feelings, and sensations, all of which become part of the symbolic process and the symbolization of the body. Alexithymia is the result of failure to symbolize the body. Owing to their failure to symbolize the concrete body, alexithymic adults and children need the mother continually to interpret affective experiences and to name the emotional states.

Fain (1971) has referred to *la mère calmant,* as a tranquilizing mother whose baby forms an addictive relationship with her. That is, she does not allow the baby to make a primary identification with her so that he can take his own self-satisfaction in the form of auto-erotic activities and later achieve symbolic representation of the self. Instead, the baby is totally reliant on his mother and stays in the concrete realm of action rather than in the realm of psychic activity and mental representation. These children are made to believe that the mother is the only person who can satisfy them physically and emotionally. Reliance on the mother excludes the possibility of the child's feeling that he can satisfy himself physically and emotionally or that father and other significant adults can do this. The child remains in a constant need-state for the mother, and the mother in a constant need-state for the child. Further fantasy development, when it does occur, has a "need" level quality to it rather than a "want" level.

In addition, McDougall (1980) states, babies who have been given too much or too little psychic space are in danger of failing to develop a meaningful body representation. That is, a mother who is too far from or too close to her child is unable to act as a shield or a stimulus barrier for her baby. She fails to interpret his nonverbal communications and give meaning to the child's experiences, which the child then uses to represent psychically in the symbolic chain.

One may ask why the mother is so prone to this failure. Balint (1939) believed that this maternal failure may come from the natural state of affairs in the love relationship between mother and baby: they both share an unreal sense of the mother's self-interests or ego interests. That is, the child does not recognize the separate identity of the mother, nor does the mother recognize the separate identity of her child. The mother looks upon her child as part of herself and of the child's interests as being equivalent to her own. Balint felt that all mothers have a touch of this archaic loving relationship and that it is the mother's responsibility to rise above it and help the child become a separate individual.

THEORETICAL FRAMEWORK

Parenting is a vehicle for the unconscious of the parents. Through the parental function, unconscious fantasies of both parents are set into motion, providing the first external reality of the baby. It is as if the mother's or father's fantasy life anchors onto the infant's body and mind. The body and mind of the child are borrowed by the parents to externalize their own anxieties and to serve other functions as well.

Mother's and father's unconscious fantasies may or may not complement each other. For example, a mother may be exclusively interested in the body of her child; she may ignore the child's mind or not be attuned to it. The father, wanting to possess the secrets of the infant's inner world, may bypass the body field of his child. It is also possible for both parents to overemphasize the internal, thus invading the child and robbing him or her of it. The child must own his own body and mind before he can share it. The infant will begin to relate to his body zones as partial substitutes for the object. The mother's overemphasis on the infant's body functions and misfunctions, however, may create a link between her body and the infant's that is not easily broken. She could regard her infant's body as an extension of her own, invading it from within and from outside. She may try to fill the empty spaces while attempting to cleanse the fully occupied ones. She may strive to possess what the infant's body produces, as if its contents belonged to her. Hence, she attempts to preclude the attribution of meaning to the body and its zones by denying its existence as an external object beyond her domain. The infant's body ego will become atrophied, so to speak, and the mind will fail to integrate the body in the gestalt of the self-representation. The split between the mind and the body appears, then, as the final expression of the surrender of the infant to the object by way of the body. The body never becomes a true possession of the child and remains attached to the mother, who will care for its well being; the mother becomes the fountain of air for the asthmatic child, the vacuum cleaner/enema of the ulcerative colitis patient, the soothing cream for the skin-rashed infant.

The body that has been closed to meanings is unable to open the doors to the internal world. The lack of fantasies centered on the erogenous zones, the vast holes of the body/self with no monsters to speak for the mysteries and the unknown, leave the infant's ego to expand in a factual, affectless material world (McDougall, 1980).

PSYCHOSOMATIC ILLNESS AND PERVERSIONS

Psychosomatic illnesses can be regarded as crystalized byproducts of parenting functions. The body, through its signals, manifests the failure of internalization. The psychosomatic signal allows the individual to hold on to concrete, action-oriented means of protection and survival. This holding on to the concrete seems to develop out of the threat that another person, whether caregiver or parent, exerts a double and contradictory power over the child. The caregiver insures life and well-being, yet in such an intrusive and overbearing fashion that the child is bound to be destroyed by this distorted parenting.

In psychosomatic illness, the body becomes the stage on which the action for survival is played out. Mind and body split, and self-caring functions follow the same fate. While the self cares for the mind, the body remains too attached to its owner, the mother. Since the mother owns the body, caring for it could be equated with destroying the mother. To protect the mother, the self renounces its body and the responsibilities attached to it.

The mind, split from the body, will attempt to save a sense of self by isolating the affects and depleting the thoughts from any affective or energetic tone. The operational mode of thinking, the flatness and concreteness of the psychosomatic verbalizations, could then be regarded as false self formations (Winnicott, 1960). It is as if the true self fuses with mother through the body. Mental life is hidden, kept secret, and unconnected to the body. The body cannot be used to link the infant's fantasies because the body is the link to the parent's fantasies, not the child's. The self is not experienced as the vital agent. Rather, life is experience.

We concur with McDougall (1980, 1989) and Krystal (1988) that work with patients with psychosomatic conditions must attend to those aspects of the transference that actualize the patient's early self-representation. The absence of fantasy should not discourage the analyst, who must then respond to the signs of distress emitted from the body in multiple forms. Krystal, and McDougall to a certain degree, rely on their own fantasies of the patient's world in order to understand what the patient needs.

Krystal (1988) tends to be more prescriptive than McDougall is regarding the modifications in technique with psychosomatic patients. He advocates a quasi-didactic approach in which he carefully explains to his patients their affective and cognitive problems. He insists on the analyst's attentiveness to patients' ability (or lack thereof) to take good care of themselves. Once the analyst becomes aware of the patient's difficulties in self-caring, he must "be involved continuously in explanation, elucidation, interpretation of the blocks in self-regulatory, self-preserving, and self-solacing functions" (p. 336). While Krystal attempts to create and formulate an adult reconstruction of early traumatic experience, deconstruction, or breaking down, of the adult patient's interpretation of the child experience must take place. The traumatized child's main experience is one of prohibition against full autonomy.

Although we are in agreement with Krystal and McDougall theoretically, we offer two new contributions to psychoanalytic work with patients. First is the concept of "ownership" of both the body and the mind; we believe that this "ownership" must become an achievement during the psychoanalytic process. Second, we bring the analyst's body and mind into the analytic arena; the nuances of the analyst's body and mind are listened to along with the patient's. The immediacy of the two bodies and minds in session is never ignored. We believe that the ownership of the patient's body and mind occurs within a psychoanalytic context that requires not only the analyst's engagement but also the willingness of the analyst to own, reown, and at times surrender his or her own body and mind. Although these ideas are compatible with the contributions of both McDougall and Krystal, we put emphasis on the necessity of this kind of inclusion of the analyst's body and mind in the psychoanalytic process which allows for the patient's ownership of his or her body and mind.

In summary, somatic symptoms, while pointing out the archaic connection with the primary object, highlight the failure or the inability to own the body and the mind. The body and the mind are not separate entities. Cartesian dualities have biased psychoanalytic thinking about the connection between the body and the mind, thus offering a schematic and fragmented perspective on their interrelationship. Rather, mind and body are better understood as operating within a dual track, a "Siamese twinship," a "mind–body" that is one although it seems to be two (Grotstein, 1997).

Some specific conceptualizations by patients about the ownership of the body and the mind may be helpful to clinicians when listening to their patients from this framework. First, some patients actually physically tighten or tense their bodies in order to give the body boundaries, for fear that a relaxed body state would be equivalent to fusion with the powerful object. For example, Malcolm, a 45-year-old man, was preoccupied with tight, firm "butts," both his own and that of the woman with whom he was involved. In the transference, he was preoccupied with the degree of firmness of the analyst's "butt." If two firm "butts" come together, there was no fear of fusion; but if one "butt" was not firm, even if his was, body boundaries would disappear and he would fuse with the powerful object, the woman.

Second, affects that are localized in the body in a concrete way are real and therefore preferred. John, a 30-year-old single man suffering from ulcerative colitis, displayed the alexithymic trait of being unable to name affects and claimed ignorance when attempting to elaborate on his feelings. Inner life was practically nonexistent during the early stages of treatment. Only while talking about his illness did John become alive, as if the diseased body existed in ways his mind did not. To John, the body's affliction was a sign of life.

Third, the psychic body exists if one does not admit loneliness. If loneliness or need for another person is acknowledged, psychic structure crumbles. Margaret, a 32-year-old woman, spent much of her time in analytic sessions caressing and stroking herself, particularly when the analyst was actively engaged with her (interpretations). Her attention was less on the interpretations offered by her analyst than on strengthening the boundaries of her own body. Fantasied relations with men were available to her 24 hours a day; she was never left in a state of loneliness or need for another person. Her ultimate desire to remain in mother's womb, and later to remain in analysis for the rest of her life, was the solution that warded off psychic disintegration.

Fourth, there can be a temporary mind–body dissociation when the body is experienced by the patient as failing him. Sam, a 48-year-old man, felt that his body had been weak since childhood. He described posture problems and not feeling balanced on his feet. He felt that his backbone could not keep him erect. During the analysis, Sam attempted various strenuous physical activities to try to correct this sense of his physical body. Each activity would start with hope and end in despair. His feelings about his weak body affected his feelings about his mind: weak body, weak mind. Unfortunately, during the course of the analysis, Sam developed a slowly degenerative physical condition that took away any hope of his having a strong body and, with it, a strong mind. Sam might have progressed if he could have separated the weak body from the strong mind. Instead, his anger at his weak body preoccupied him, and his mind was filled with attacks on his weak body. His mind was also filled with fantasies of his being an Olympic skier or a famous basketball player. He had two minds, one belonging to the weak body and split off from the other mind, which was full of potent, hopeful fantasies.

Several female patients who were experiencing physical difficulties felt that the body was their enemy, motivated to defeat them, that it was a "foreign body" with a mind of its own. Here we note a feeling of betrayal of the self by the body. This can, however, be a temporary state. Alice, a 52-year-old woman, and Margaret, 32 years of age, were enraged with their bodies when they experienced serious difficulties in their pregnancies and were unable to have their own children. They were particularly envious of their analyst's body for being able to produce not only one baby but two (twins). They each had two bodies—their real bodies, which did not function as promised by their mothers, and their fantasied bodies, which worked perfectly and allowed for childbirth. For Alice, going through her pregnancy and childbirth in the analytic sessions led to her being able to buy a kitten to nurture. Margaret, who carried in her womb a baby who had to be aborted, was unable to mourn the loss. She continued to remain heavy—"pregnant"— even after the adoption of several children.

Fifth, the body realm is often used to avoid relationships. It serves to keep internal object relations a secret and ongoing while there is an actual avoidance of establishing new, real relationships. Andrew, a 41-year-old socially withdrawn single man, complained of an unusual sensitivity to temperature changes in the analyst's office. He would remove his jacket and put it back on several times during a session. Andrew was convinced of the "biological reasons" for his condition, ignoring the analyst's attempt to address his social isolation. Only at home, in the privacy of his bedroom, was he successful in regulating the temperature, which he maintained unchanged through the entire year. His preoccupation with his cold or warm body served as a buffer against relating. He ignored the analyst's interventions and devalued both personal and professional relationships.

Sixth, psychosomatic concerns are often defenses against sexual and aggressive impulses, wishes and fantasies. Julia, a 27-year-old graduate student, tended to develop severe migraine headaches during sessions that she described as "heavy" or "difficult." She would sit up on the couch, reach for her purse, and get her medication. She would then apologize, spending the rest of the session attending to her headache by pressing her temples with her hands or massaging her head. The analyst became a passive, useless observer, lacking the "touch" to soothe his patient's pain.

In addition, concerns in both women and men about potency have hidden body-ownership aspects. For example, women may be concerned about whether or not they can have babies and whether or not their bodies will work. What may lie behind these concerns are issues of who owns the mind and the body if one is pregnant, having a relationship with another, or having intercourse with a man. Men, frequently are concerned about whether their sperm is strong enough to fertilize an egg and whether or not they can have an erection and hold off ejaculating prematurely. Here again, concerns reflect body ownership; that is, there is the question of who owns the body of the man who is having the erection, the ejaculation, or providing the sperm to make a baby. Margaret (who has lost her baby) was delighted that artificial insemination meant that she did not know who had impregnated her. She did not have to have intercourse in order to become pregnant, and the father of her baby could remain her own fantasy construction, and therefore an extension of her own body. John felt reassured about the integrity of his body when his wife got pregnant for the first time. The expansion of his wife's womb affirmed his body, instilling hope and a longing for a healthy body, his and his baby's.

CLINICAL ILLUSTRATIONS

John

John, whom we mentioned earlier, relates to his body as a physical object devoid of any meaning or fantasy elaboration. The early stages of his analysis were devoted to scientific descriptions of the vicissitudes of his illness. He reported his wife's being unable to tolerate his demands for bodily attention, and his grieving about his illness in the middle of the night. Being alone with and within his body was too painful. He wanted the analyst to become familiar with the illness that perturbed his body and, keep him away from the contents of his mind; he hoped that the analyst would become *la mère calmant* (Fain, 1971).

A premature baby, John was placed in an incubator for several weeks. His mother, fearing that she might get too attached to him and then she would have to deal with a painful loss, refused to visit him in the hospital. She was convinced that her child was not going to survive. She refused to name her child, and only at the hospital's insistence did the father name the child so he could obtain a birth certificate. Although John lived, his mother never overcame the fear of losing him. She became overprotective of John's frail body. She used enemas, vitamins, and oils to assure herself of her child's survival.

As an adult, John truly felt that he could not live without the assistance of others. He demanded from his analyst a complete recognition of his bodily illness. He wanted the analyst to care for his body, to listen to its noises, and to observe its movements. To John, the condition of his body was a matter of life and death. He was not sure whether he was going "to make it," as his mother felt toward him.

The analyst felt that he needed to be cautious owing to John's serious physical condition. The transference repeated an early archaic connection to the maternal object. The patient's concrete physical preoccupation left no room for psychological elaborations. The analyst, like mother, often felt he could lose the patient, and he wondered how the analysis could be of help to anyone suffering from colitis.

In the early stages of treatment, the patient succeeded in reinstating the original collusion established between himself and his mother. The analysis became the incubator that was sustaining John's life. John felt that he would never be cured of his illness, and he wondered whether he might need analysis for the rest of his life. The threat of losing the analyst was acute prior to the analyst's vacations. It manifested itself through fantasies of dying while the analyst was away. John could not imagine the analyst during his absence, as he lacked internal representations of both himself and the analyst. While the analyst was away, it appeared as if both the self and the object ceased to exist. The analyst's absence was not unlike his mother's inability to cathect her baby left alone in the hospital. John could never take for granted his survival or that of the object. Just like his mother, who was unable to build an internal representation of her sick baby, John was incapable of building his own self-representation. Thus, the analyst's absence brought up the threat of psychic dissolution and actual death.

It was from his father that John got a glimpse of hope and survival. Father had named his child and in the biblical sense conferred life. Having a name was an assertion of life over death. Similarly, the analyst, by naming affects, putting words to silences, and reading between the lines of dreams and fantasies, acquired the power of the father in the patient's struggle for survival.

John was unusually sensitive to the body of the analyst. He expressed concern about minor colds or changes in the analyst's voice. On one occasion, he reported having watched the analyst walking on the street; he commented on the analyst's body, "erect, self-assured posture always looking forward." John seemed impressed with the analyst's ownership of his body.

John desperately wanted the analyst to own his (John's) body but resisted the analyst's entering his mind. He misunderstood that interpretations were in the mental realm between analyst and patient. Rather, he tended to experience the contents of the analyst's interpretations.

As the analysis progressed, the patient was able to interrupt the sessions in order to use the bathroom. At those times, he revealed feeling embarrassed or self-conscious, paving the way to bring the body into the session and transforming a physical experience into a psychological one. The dissociation between the body and the mind permeated his experience. He was convinced that his body was damaged beyond repair.

Preoccupation with concrete bodily experiences served the purpose of keeping aggressive impulses under control. The body needed doors to contain the bad objects, the "shit" threatening to come out. When the patient informed the analyst that his wife was pregnant with their first child, he felt relief, assured of "pieces of goodness" in himself. The body was functioning, producing life.

Countertransferentially, the analyst became more aware of his own body as a potentially fragile object, which, like his patient's, could be easily attacked by forces beyond his control. A recurrent fantasy emerged while the patient was reporting vivid details of an endoscopy he had undergone on a previous day. The analyst found himself speculating about how his body might look if a camera were able to record inside his body. He pictured himself taking a trip through arteries and veins, further associating to the film *Invasion of the Body Snatchers*. The analyst's interventions were accompanied by unusual body actions and movements. His tone of voice, modulations of verbalizations, and a more pronounced accent seemed to catch him by surprise. It was as if words were coming independently out of his throat rather than forming in his mind. He became increasingly aware of the presence of his body in sessions.

The analyst was uneasy about the patient's reports about painful bowel movements; the analytic space seemed smelly at times. He often noted hypochondriacal concerns during or after sessions. Listening to the patient's physical pain evoked tension and distress within the analyst. He could not find a comfortable position on the chair; he motioned or gestured while attempting to address his patient's experience.

Dan

Dan, a 38-year-old twin, came to treatment experiencing severe depression and periods of intense anxiety. He also was concerned about a chronic skin rash, which a friend had categorized as a "nervous manifestation."

He had suffered an early traumatic separation from his twin brother when the latter was sent to another country to be treated for a severe case of asthma. Dan recalled having to cheer his mother, who became very depressed upon losing her favorite son. Shortly after the separation from his twin brother, Dan developed a skin disorder on his chest and neck. Dan remembered how involved his mother had become with his condition, dragging him from doctor to doctor. Dan seemed to have relinquished his body for the sake of his depressed mother. In Dan's own words, "Mother had my body to worry about."

In analysis, Dan often feared the analyst was not interested in the material he was bringing to the sessions. To Dan, the analyst's silences were signs of indifference and boredom. Dan felt he could do nothing to move the analyst out of his "depressed analytic posture," not unlike his inability to cheer up his mother. The analyst became Dan's depressed mother, seclusive and isolated, thinking about other twins/patients.

Countertransferentially, the analyst felt the patient was demanding a kind of attention that could only be translated into physical terms. Since the analyst was not asking about the current state of his skin, Dan felt that he did not know what might be "appropriate to talk about." Dan knew only one way of connecting to the object, namely through the body. Through his body, Dan attempted to repair his wounded mother as well as his own self. The physical symptoms served the double purpose of healing mother and the split twinship. The skin rash evoked the absent twin in a most concrete, bodily form. Coming into analysis and fantasizing about other patients sharing the analyst was a less concrete and more symbolic or abstract attempt at repairing the object.

For Dan, father had occupied a secondary position. Unable to cope with his wife's depression, he withdrew from her and spent extra time working, indulging himself in sporadic drinking. Dan felt that he could not count on his father. Father was a bystander, unwilling to pitch in or offer a hand. The transference in this case repeated the patient's early connection to archaic objects. Once again, Dan was offering his body (by delving into his skin condition) to mobilize his depressed analyst. In so doing, he encountered the father as well, with his passivity, uninvolvement, or blunt indifference. Other patients/twins were more important than Dan, despite his offering a skin disorder to heal the analyst/mother.

Dan trusted and relied on signals from his body. His diseased skin had the quality of a "presence" he could hold on to. Unlike the unnamed affects, which betrayed the longing for his absent mother and twin brother, his body offered the immediacy he needed to ward off the fear of psychic disintegration. The overinvolvement with his skin precluded the establishment of object relationships. Dan avoided social functions, complaining about his skin irritation, which he referred to as the "irritability of the boundaries between me and others."

In the analytic process, both patient and analyst became silent voyeurs of the other person's skin, especially variations in tone and color. When Dan entered and exited sessions, and while he was lying on the couch, his and the analyst's eyes would surf the areas of exposed skin as if in search of concrete signals emanating from the body. The treatment reenacted Dan's primitive mode of relating to the object.

Dan was the only analysand who detected the grief "by the color of your eyes" after the analyst cancelled a week's sessions because of the death of his father. Through the use of the analyst's body (eyes), Dan was temporarily taking possession of the analyst's body, both in an empathic response to the analyst and as a resistance against owning his own partially damaged body.

The impact of the patient's skin condition on the analyst became acute during the summer months. Dan wore long sleeves in the middle of July in an attempt to conceal "the redness that plague my arms." The analyst recalled feeling itchy, rubbing his legs or upper arms and producing noises that made the patient wonder about the analyst's body. The analyst's body seemed to be colluding with the patient's body. Dan complained of feeling distracted by the analyst's movements, thus putting the analyst's body on the spot. The analyst's hypochondriacal concerns increased. He was fearful that he might have contracted something contagious from his patient, a bug that took residence on the pillow or the rich fabric of his couch. Dan began to entertain the thought that something was wrong with the analyst's body. The analyst wished he could reveal how healthy he was feeling at that moment.

Margaret

Margaret, whom we also referred to earlier, has been in a rather long analysis. Interpretations within the framework of psychosexual stages and self psychology have been made with limited success. Outstanding in this case is a lack of developmental thrust, that is, a lack of the wish to move forward and progress developmentally. The analyst has sensed that this patient never wanted to be awakened; she was essentially refusing to leave her mother's womb, wishing to be an appendage of another person. Her mother was not sufficiently interested in her mind and thoughts. In addition, her mother touched her mentally and physically in ways that were gratifying for the mother but not for Margaret. Relatives had told her that, when Margaret was a child, her mother kept her constantly at her knee, caressing and fondling her. At the same time, her father was too involved in her mind and attempted to control every mental activity; for example, Margaret's father required her to adopt his political views.

One of Margaret's gestures was self-touching, a physical contact with her own body that was extremely agitated and constant. She did this during her analytic sessions without abatement. In understanding the self-touching from the possession of mind and body framework, what emerged was that, when she touched herself while listening to the analyst, she was both soothing and affirming the existence of her body. That is, in the transference she was defending against the analyst's ownership of her body, repeating her mother's and father's excessive and agitated physical and mental "touch", this time as the active rather than the passive agent.

Margaret reported fantasies of boyfriends touching her. She seemed more interested in these illusory boyfriends than in real ones. She felt that if she touched herself while she thought of an illusory boyfriend she could be who she wanted to be, think what she wanted to think, without interference.

When Margaret experienced herself as separate, her image of herself was that of an "ice princess," reflecting the idea that no one could touch her and that she owned her self. Her feeling was that, if she exposed herself to loneliness, that is, if she needed another person, she would melt.

Free association was difficult for Margaret. She felt that the analyst was forcing her to be separate and leave the analyst's "womb." Her marked resistance to free association represented resistance to the evolution of her own body and mind.

During the analysis, Margaret often stared at the analyst's body and clothing, as if looking for clues to show her how to connect to her own body. Her stare made the analyst self-conscious, as if Margaret were reaching beyond the surface of the analyst's body. Margaret's preoccupation with the analyst's appearance evoked the same persistent attention on the part of the analyst toward Margaret.

It became apparent that Margaret wished to go beyond the boundaries of the analyst's body and enter the analyst's womb. Her eyes ultimately turned to the analyst's abdomen. Her fantasies were that she had a chance, before the analyst became pregnant, to enter and remain in the analyst's womb. After it became obvious to her that her analyst was pregnant, she felt that the analyst was pushing her out of the womb to make room for her own babies. Thus began Margaret's long journey to wanting a child of her own. However enjoyable this idea was, it was colored by dangerous, aggressive fantasies toward the analyst for not letting her remain inside the analyst's body. By becoming pregnant (though having to abort the pregnancy), she created a fantasy that her dead baby was still inside her forever. She would "parade" into sessions, forcing the analyst to view her body and wonder what was inside. She felt she had outdone the analyst by remaining pregnant forever, never having to separate from her baby or have the baby separate from her. She would focus on the fantasy that the analyst took hormones in order to become pregnant and that the analyst's body was indeed defective.

Knowing first-hand the joy of being pregnant, carrying to term, and enjoying motherhood, Margaret's analyst felt tremendous compassion for her. Margaret's desire to enter the analyst's body, however, at times felt like a forcing, a pushing to enter the analyst's womb. When a patient comes close to the analyst's body with her own body, the analyst can feel temporarily invaded in a way that is different from invasion by the analysand's words. There is an intrusion in the analyst's own personal, private space. Analysts may have more difficulty dealing with this kind of intrusion in the transference and countertransference. Countertransferentially, this analyst found herself trying to peer inside Margaret's body in the same way, intrusively. Margaret welcomed this intrusiveness, which was interpreted as a reenactment of her relationship with both her mother and father. A tension was experienced between the analyst and her patient in that the patient welcomed the intrusiveness while the analyst's discomfort with it was noticeable. Ultimately, the analytic work led to the patient's giving up her fantasy that she would live inside the analyst and the analysis, and she would become more separate. As carefully as this process of separation and individuation was handled, she still felt rejected by the analyst.

Alice

Alice, a 52-year-old woman, grew up with a mother and a father who did not validate her feelings and thoughts. Her mother would tell her what she was supposed to feel or what she was thinking or feeling. She denied anything bad that happened to Alice and wiped out portions of Alice's identity, in terms both of Alice's actual experiences and of her symbolic processes. The mother virtually owned her daughter's mind and body and decided unilaterally what was and what was not going to be part of Alice's life experience. She would read Alice's diaries and snoop in her drawers. Alice felt that her father joined in disavowing her feelings, thoughts, and sexuality. In order to have a relationship with her father, Alice had to remain a little girl.

After Alice's first marriage, which ended in divorce, the mother decided to burn Alice's wedding pictures. After Alice's second miscarriage in her second marriage, Alice's mother took her maternity clothes away from her so that she would not be reminded of the miscarriage. Alice talked about the "past" Alice, parts of her that were no longer hers. Her mother had "bamboozled" her. She did not have respect for the intelligence of her child. She would give her aspirin in a red glass and not tell her what it was she was giving. In the transference, Alice felt that the analyst too had "bamboozled" her through her free associations. Alice remarked, "I have to watch you so that I don't get humiliated by you and have you feel that I don't know what you are doing to me."

Both parents rejected Alice's wishes to give the "gifts" of her body and her thoughts—to accept her hugs, kisses, and verbal affection would require her parents to feel their bodies in relationship to her. Alice was denied these avenues of self- and object knowledge. Alice's need for these avenues of self and object knowledge emerged in the transference in a very unusual way. Recall that Alice had had two miscarriages in her second marriage. The second miscarriage was particularly devastating since she carried this baby for almost seven months. In the treatment, Alice gained considerable weight over a period of nine months. She essentially reexperienced this miscarriage but this time experienced a "real childbirth" with a "real product" as the outcome. During the course of this nine months in treatment, the transference was stormy and there was considerable regression. The whole journey, however, was one in ownership of the mind and body. She called friends and told them that she was undergoing labor pains, and in some ways she was thrilled that her pain was getting worse. She felt that she was allowed to feel what she was feeling.

Alice stated that the only other time in her life she had felt that she was free to feel what she felt was the three days and three nights when she was in labor in the hospital. This time, in the treatment, she could have the birth experience and enjoy it. She did not enjoy the pain but did enjoy the latitude of her affects, which were the basis of her self. In the "analytic birth process," she was psychologically reborn.

This nine months in treatment followed the analyst's own pregnancy and birth of twins. Shortly after the analyst gave birth, Alice bought a cat, which she felt was a "lunatic" thing to do. In fact, the cat was her first real baby to nurture. Prior to her "analytic" birth experience, she expressed both envy of the analyst's well-functioning body and her desire to own the analyst's body. She wanted to hug and kiss the analyst, the very thing once offered to her parents and rejected.

Alice's need to know how the analyst was feeling physically and emotionally was exacerbated during the analyst's pregnancy but was persistent throughout the analysis. She was also preoccupied with thoughts about how the analyst was feeling about her, physically and emotionally. Did the analyst like her? Did she think the analysand was fat? What did the analyst think of her clothing? When the analyst was pregnant, Alice could focus on the real changes in the analyst's body and imagine what the corresponding psychological state of the analyst was. After she felt that the analyst had allowed her to witness her pregnancy and childbirth, she could allow herself to invite the analyst to relive with her her own pregnancy and childbirth. Alice reenacted on the couch the delivery of her stillborn baby. She was sweating, screaming, and delirious. She yelled with her labor pains. Her feet in stirrups, she pushed her baby out.

Although Alice bought a cat and nurtured it after this birth experience in analysis, she retained fantasies of sharing the analyst's children with her; afterall, the analyst had two babies, not one. Even though analyst and analysand could share these intimate body experiences, however, Alice continued to refuse to let the analyst help her understand what was happening in her professional life. To Alice, her professional life was her mind. This attempt—essentially to deny her mother access to the privacy of her diary—had disastrous consequences. Her business, once thriving, became over time a complete financial loss. She left analysis prematurely, in a negative state of transference and feeling that the analyst had robbed her of her body (all the money she had paid for analysis).

Shortly after the premature termination, Alice sent the analyst a letter that the analyst experienced as a dagger in the analyst's body.

The accusations could not be discussed or worked through since the treatment was over. They remained piercing. As the patient experienced the analyst as robbing her body of its contents, she sought revenge by aggressively piercing the body boundaries of the analyst.

CONCLUSION

We have found that resistances in analytic treatment are often not to specific content, but, rather, to yielding ownership of one's mind and body. In analysis, there is always the issue of who owns the patient's mind and body as well as the patient's fight to hold on to his or her own mind and body. Patients who struggle to own their minds and bodies manifest subtle attunement to changes in the analyst's body and affects. Although, in the course of treatment, they navigate from the concrete to the symbolic, they continue to rely on and trust the immediacy of their sensory experiences. Given freedom in the patient–analyst/mind–body field, these patients are bound to become "body–mind readers" of the analyst. The analysand's involvement with the analyst's body may, at times, be experienced by the analyst as a bombardment.

As analysts, we must be alert to how we are involved with our patients' bodies and minds (our fantasies, conscious and unconscious) and how our patients are involved (patients' conscious and unconscious fantasies) with our bodies and minds. In addition, we must keep track of how both we and our patients are involved in the shared patient–analyst/mind–body field. The qualities of the analyst's ownership of his or her own body and mind will largely determine a patient's ability to express curiosity about the analyst's body and mind and to share a mutual mind–body/body–mind field (Gunsberg and Tylim, 1995; Looker, this volume; Balamuth, this volume). This is a crucial framework within which to look at transference elaborations and transformations.

REFERENCES

Aulangnier P. (1991), *Remarques sur la structure psychotique*. Paris: Payor.
Balint, A. (1939), Love for the mother and mother love. In: *Primary Love and Psychoanalytic Technique*, ed. M. Balint. New York: Liveright, 1965, pp. 91–108.

Fain, M. (1971), Prelude a la vie fantasmatique. *Rev Franc. Psychoanal*, 35:291-364. Excerpted in McDougall, J. (1980), *Plea for a Measure of Abnormality*. New York: International Universities Press, pp. 362–367.

Grotstein, J. S. (1997), "Mens sane in corpore sano": The mind and body as an "odd couple" and as oddly coupled unity. *Psychoanal. Inq.*, 17:204–222.

Gunsberg, L. & Tylim, I. (1995), Ownership of the body and mind: Developmental considerations for adult psychoanalytic treatment. *Psychoanal. Rev.*, 82:257–266.

Gurwitt, A. (1976), Aspects of prospective fatherhood: A case report. *The Psychoanalytic Study of the Child*, 31:237-271. New Haven, CT: Yale University Press.

Herzog, J. (1982), Patterns of expectant fatherhood: A study of the fathers of a group of premature infants. In: *Father and Child*, ed. S. Cath, A. Gurwitt, & J. Ross. Hillsdale, NJ: The Analytic Press, 1994, pp. 301–314.

Krystal, H. (1988), *Integration and Self-Healing*. Hillsdale, NJ: The Analytic Press.

McDougall, J. (1980), *Plea for a Measure of Abnormality*. New York: International Universities Press.

———— (1989), *Theaters of the Body*. New York: Norton.

———— (1995), *The Many Faces of Eros*. New York: Norton

Ross, J. (1979), Fathering: A review of some psychoanalytic contributions on paternity. *Internat. J. Psycho-Anal.*, 60:317–328.

Winnicott, D. (1960), Ego distortion in terms of true and false self. In: *Maturational Processes and the Facilitating Environment*. New York: International Universities Press, 1965, pp. 140–152.

PART III

*The Material Body
in the Relational Matrix*

6

CANCER AS A FACTITIOUS DISORDER (MUNCHAUSEN SYNDROME) RELATED TO BODY SELF-IMAGE AND OBJECT RELATIONS IN A BORDERLINE PATIENT

Kerstin Kupfermann

This chapter presents the case history of Eva, a young borderline patient with occasional psychotic breakdowns, with whom psychoanalysis and techniques aimed at strengthening her sense of body and self-image, were used. During the last three years of eight years of analysis, Eva claimed to have colon cancer. That her cancer was an invention of her mind was unknown to me and the physicians working in some of our most prestigious hospitals whom she contacted for control of "the side effects of cancer treatment." Her case offers important insights into her reason and purpose for the development of a factitious disorder, often referred to as Munchausen syndrome.

Munchausen syndrome (or factitious disorder) was first described by Asher (1951), who took the name from Freiherr von Munchausen (1720–1797), a German officer who gained fame for his tall tales. Factitious disorder is characterized by physical and psychological symptoms that a person invents (American Psychiatric Association, 1994, Kaplan and Saddock, 1975). Bursten (1965) and Greenacre (1958) express the idea that the term impostor is important in regarding psychodynamics of this disorder insofar that there is a lack of a sense of solid identity and the "impostor" is then used to create such an iden-

tity. Grinker (1961) and Spiro (1968) suggest that the symptom reflects an attempt to master past trauma and feelings of helplessness
in response to separation anxiety. This symptom has a compulsive
quality, but the concealment, the judgment of timing, and the intellectual planning suggest voluntary control. Most patients are females
who share a history of emotional deprivation in childhood. The symptoms serve the purpose of securing attention and care. Many such
patients are addicted to narcotics. Most of them are diagnosed as
borderline with conversion symptoms, along with suicidal ideation
(Nadelson, 1979). These characteristics were all present in the case
of Eva.

   This chapter not only describes why Eva developed a factitious
disorder but offers a unique opportunity to follow her use of the syndrome as well as her recovery. In a metaphorical way (Sontag, 1979),
she expressively described her bad body image and her perception
of her environment as "a cancer." She used the factitious disorder to
express herself in a more deeply personally meaningful way than during her initial phase of treatment, before the onset of the disorder.
She gave herself a last chance to work through her conflicts and traumas. After the termination of analysis, when she disclosed that she
did not, in fact, have cancer, she was able to give up the Munchausen
syndrome. The process of successful psychoanalytic treatment of this
very troublesome and resistant syndrome, to my knowledge, has never
before been described in the literature.

   From the time she was about five years of age, Eva was able to
depict her experience of her situation in hundreds of drawings, and
this ability turned out to be an extremely helpful resource during her
analysis. She never drew during her sessions but brought with her
drawings, depicting her body self-image and her past and present
situation, her self-termed "mental biopsies." As we found out, they
depicted early childhood traumatic events the verbal and emotional
expressions of which had been blocked. Associating to her drawings
in my presence, Eva became increasingly able not just to recall her
past with feelings, but also gradually to apply her secondary-process
thinking to the distorted part-object figures of the primary process;
they came alive for her as entire outer and inner experiences of an
adult looking back at the horrors of her past. No longer could she
fend them off with defense mechanisms like denial, repression, dissociation, and isolation. (A detailed discussion of the use of the drawings in the context of treatment not related to Munchausen syndrome,
has been presented elsewhere [Kupfermann, 1996].)

   The cancerous-body self-image Eva had of herself expressed powerfully how she felt herself to be "the bad seed," "the cancer of her family." In her mind, she deserved nothing but imprisonment. Cancer was also a way of describing the abusive conditions she had lived through during a traumatic childhood. She had been the victim of extensive physical abuse (mainly of a sexual nature) by her parents and their friends. Later in her analysis these object relations were seen by her as "her cancer," meaning that the abusers were now located inside of her, as expressed in the Munchausen syndrome, a gratifying sadomasochistic fantasy.

For Eva, the temporary development of this factitious disorder, and the special and intensive care she thereby gained from all of us who had contact with her during the three and a half years she claimed she had cancer, had a definite positive effect psychologically. The concrete experience of care, not just the use of "the talking cure," had a major influence, solidifying her good self-image. She developed a deeper sense of self and gained control of her formerly frequent and severe self-destructive behavior. By living the role of a cancer patient, she gave herself the opportunity on "a gut level" to sense and gradually come to know more about her true self (Winnicott, 1960; Miller, 1981). She more intensely experienced and worked through her deeply ingrained negative feelings about her body and her self-image and the impact that destructive relationships from the past had had on her.

EVA AT THE ONSET OF ANALYSIS

At the onset of her psychoanalysis, which began in the mid-70s, Eva suffered from hallucinations and severe headaches for which she consumed about 18 aspirins a day. She complained about her distorted view of reality, about seeing people and objects as sexual organs, their body image being totally contorted. She had a brittle mental representation of her body image and a poorly developed object constancy. She often referred to herself in the third person. Her social relationships were characterized by instability. She was prone either to idealize or to devalue other people as well as taking advantage of them for her own needs, and her friends were likewise self-destructive. Since childhood she had made frequent suicide attempts. Self-damaging acts like cutting herself were a daily event. The experience of pain and the sight of blood made her feel alive. She was addicted to work and kept herself going on amphetamines. She had been a drug user since her teenage years. She had an identity disturbance and a chronic feeling of emptiness and boredom. Her voice could instantly shift from that of a mature woman who was in charge to the voice of a helpless little child. She was impulsive and had inappropriately intense feelings of anger, sometimes becoming rage. Fluctuations of mood occurred frequently. I diagnosed her as having borderline character disorder (Gunderson and Singer, 1975).

EVA'S CHILDHOOD AND ADOLESCENCE

Eva's family life was complex and filled with perverse and torturous abuse, criminality, and catastrophes of various kinds. Most of Eva's recollections were based on verifiable facts.

Born to a heroin addict, Eva had to remain, for her first four months of life, in a hospital to be treated for withdrawal symptoms. Coming home, she was cared for by relatives, but mainly by an adolescent sister who disliked her. Eva's mother was a well-known performer who relied heavily on her husband for her drug supply. As an adult, while in psychoanalysis, Eva learned that she was a child of doubtful paternity, although her mother's husband had brought her up as his child. He had psychomotor epilepsy and was a very violent man, perverse and feared.

While growing up, Eva had a couple of positively cathected love objects, her grandmother and a nursemaid, Star, a young North American Native woman. She was with Eva from the time she was three years of age until she was eight. Star fulfilled many functions, that of a nanny and a lover of Eva's mother. Star never abused Eva but gave her a feeling of security, predictability, structure, and fun. She taught Eva motor as well as basic educational skills to counteract Eva's learning difficulties.

Eva lived with her mother until her mother died, as consequence of medical incompetence, when Eva was 15 years old. Her father had stayed at home until Eva was eight, at which time he was imprisoned for seven years on drug charges. After her mother's death, her father offered Eva the chance to remain in the home, provided she assumed the position of his late wife. When Eva refused, he sold all their possessions and home. Suffering mental illness and claiming paralysis, he spent the remainder of his life, about 15 years, in a Veterans' Hospital, where he died when Eva was in her 30s.

After her mother's death, Eva went to live with her then married sister, an unsuccessful arrangement. Eva then moved in with one of her teachers and her family, getting room and board in exchange for doing household chores and baby sitting. Eva went to college and earned a degree in art and later added another degree in counseling. She was married for a year, but the marriage broke up because of her difficulties adjusting to sex. After sharing a household with various people, Eva decided, after two years in psychoanalysis with me, to live by herself with her dog. With the support of psychoanalysis, Eva was all along capable of holding a job as a counselor and later was promoted to director of the agency. Because she so convincingly presented herself as a cancer victim, however, she lost her job. In spite of this tragedy, she fared well.

THE FIRST PHASE OF EVA'S PSYCHOANALYSIS, INCLUDING PARAMETERS AND MODIFIERS

My first contact with Eva occurred during a course I was giving in child development and parenting, which she attended. Eva asked me to be her therapist after hearing me speak about the transitional object (Winnicott, 1953). It was my description of the transitional object (so crucial for her) that impressed her and allowed her to experience some sense of trust. She remained in analysis with me five hours per week for eight years.

I chose different therapeutic techniques during the phase before and after the development of her factitious disorder. I will describe the treatment techniques only as they relate to her body- and self-image, since technique is not the primary focus of this chapter.

Considering her borderline characteristics, I presented her with firm rules for her sessions to induce a feeling of safety and a sense that I would not allow her to act either on her sexual or on her aggressive impulses. The rules for analytic work had to be stated repeatedly. Any attempts to act out, such as her initial seductive overtures, were interpreted (she had been seduced by her previous female therapist and needed to test me out).

My aim was to form a strong therapeutic alliance based on a positive transference, where I would empathize with the patient in any of her conflicts. Paul Federn (1943a, b) urged the modification of psychoanalytic technique to adapt to patients with severe emotional problems and reported good results. He emphasized the vital importance of positive transference, which, if dissolved, would cause the analyst to lose all influence over the patient. Federn (1947) saw positive transference and identification with the analyst as gratifying and directly influencing the patient's body- and self-image, channeling libido away from an exaggerated narcissism. The patient thus becomes less vulnerable, more able to use his libido to maintain his imperiled functioning.

In the beginning of treatment, when Eva was greatly hampered by a lack of object constancy (the ability to maintain an internal representation of the loved object even in its physical absence). Experiencing panic when a sense of unreality overcame her, she needed reassurance of my presence. I had to employ and also invent techniques to make her feel supported and safe, with the aim of developing basic trust and object constancy (Erikson, 1950). I tried to create an atmosphere of understanding and validation of her comprehension and feelings related to her experiences. My listening, clarifications, and interpretations gave her feelings of my being attuned to her—in its extreme, a sense of the state of symbiosis she had always longed for but never had experienced. For the symbiosis to be experienced as positively as possible and not as a threat of loss of sense of self, however, I was always careful to let her know that I could make my interpretations only because of what she had told me about herself. That is, I presented myself as a guardian of autonomy (Blanck and Blanck, 1974).

To counteract regression, fragmentation, confusion, and panic, I resorted to the technique of the complete interpretation; I delivered to her, in their entirety, the resistance, defenses, transference, conflicts, her past and present experiences, and future expectations. To strengthen her self-image further, I focused on how her present life was different from her past, with specific references to the fact that, in contrast to her childhood, she now had an opportunity to make choices.

Not to be underestimated is the importance of action in psychoanalysis with severe borderline and psychotic patients, action that will eventually correct the past detrimental experiences with the original love object. These experiences have affected and interfered with the patient's ability to incorporate and identify with a caring attitude toward herself as compared with the experience of the analyst, who is a distinct personality and is experienced, in the here-and-now situation, as such (Alexander, 1954, 1958, 1960). For example, shortly after Eva had begun analysis, I suspected that her symptoms were not just psychologically based on conflicts but also heavily related to early traumatizations. She refused to go for a regular medical checkup. In good conscience, I explained, I could not continue to see her unless she also saw a physician. She broke down in panic. Her association was to an incident when she was five years old: when her mother forgot to close a car door, causing Eva to fall out and be severely injured. Instead of taking the child to a hospital, her mother called a relative and continued to her rehearsal studio. Realizing that Eva's panic about going to a doctor by herself was insurmountable, I agreed to accompany her on her initial visit. Subsequently, Eva was able to follow through with recommended medical check-ups and treatments on her own.

Considering how vulnerable these patients are to rejection and object loss, I had to be creative in preventing any further suicidal attempts as one that occurred after my first brief vacation. Helpful here were the writings of Sechehaye (1951). She describes in detail the necessity for analysts to furnish patients with the experience of satisfaction in cases where basic needs have not been sufficiently met early in life. Object constancy can be developed only if the therapist is willing to furnish proof of "maternal love." Doing so will serve the purpose of counteracting the introject of the bad object and promote neutralization of the aggression and the emergence of the good self-image based on the introject of "the good image." Since the patient has not developed emotionally beyond the nonverbal phase, when the original traumas occurred, she needs a nonverbal, concrete experience for the early fixation to dissolve and for the libido to attach itself to other objects. Owing to the experience of symbolic fulfillment of needs through the analyst's "maternal love," the patient feels relief and becomes able to adapt to reality. For example, in order to supply a corrective experience, the analyst will occasionally give the patient an object that relates to the developmental phase at which the patient was emotionally arrested. What counts is not the object as such, but the meaning it takes on for the patient in relation to the mother substitute, the analyst.

In my experience, it has been of vital importance that this object be chosen so it can match and connect with an original good experience with the mother or her substitute(s) and thereby be cathected with a feeling of "good-enough mothering" (Winnicott, 1953, 1960). This makes the transitional object introduced later in life more effective in helping the adult patient hold on to "the good mother image" and feel cared for in the absence of the love object, now represented by the analyst.

With the qualities of Star's mothering of her and to promote the stabilization of the introjected concretely felt "good love object," promoting a good body- and self-image, so she would no longer be in danger of suicide, I made Eva a pillow and a sleeping bag (referred to by Eva as the papoose). One more object of "symbolic realization," though, turned out to be necessary, this time connected to her mother. Prior to my leaving, Eva phoned me incessantly. It became clear that her calls were not just acts of aggression, but rather, expressions of a desperate need to hold on to and introject "the good love object" so that she would be fully able to be self-caring during my absence. The need to listen to my recorded telephone message turned out to be a vestige from the past, when Eva had listened to her mother's recordings during her absences. A transference interpretation diminished the frequency of phone calls but was not entirely effective in putting a complete stop to her acting-out behavior. I proceeded then to make a tape for her of special personal significance. After Eva had undergone the basic experience of corrective symbiosis by way of symbolic realization and I saw emerging signs of the capacity for differentiation and separate functioning, the time had come to promote this capacity, and again a concrete symbolic experience of separate functioning was called for.

Another therapeutic procedure that Eva herself initiated while working on "her puzzled self" and fragmented body- and self-image was what I would call "Eva's enactments." She considered them to be of vital importance in her work on "piecing myself together." During these enactments, with me as the passively observing audience, Eva deliberately closed herself off from my attempts either to clarify or to interpret what she seemed to be doing; she explained that they interfered in her struggle to relive, to get fully into her past by letting herself get the missing piece: her intense feelings. Her solo enactments could be seen as introductions to making the foundation for the process of working through her traumas verbally.

Eva's behavior must not be construed as her unconscious need for the repetition compulsion, which leads to discharge of tension, Eva had not repressed the traumatic events the way Freud (1914) described. It seems to me that people like Eva, with very severe pathology, sometimes need to resort to a concrete reliving of the original trauma if they are ever to have a chance to get fully in touch with the feelings connected with it and consequently later be able to absorb the trauma, to let go of it to a sufficient degree so that it no longer interferes in their everyday functioning. For example, Eva rated as the worst among many devastating abusive experiences the time when her mother forced her, then a 14-year-old, to have facial surgery that would make Eva's face look like her own (her mother had a realistic sense that her life was coming to an end and wished to survive through her daughter by making her daughter an exact replica of herself). Eva referred to that day as "the day my mother crossed me out." Eva's mother's behavior had always been a puzzlement to Eva to the point that Eva at times had felt dead, robbed of her sense of identity and individuality; she had no sense of her self.

Eva needed concretely to reenact this experience in her urge to work it through. For example, one night her landlord made an emergency call, asking me to come over. Eva had been running back and forth for some time, violently banging her face on the wall. Well knowing her need for no interpretation at such time, I seated myself quietly on the floor. My countertransference was that of witnessing the self-inflicted process of death, a death more horrific than I had ever experienced in my own life. At the same time, in my countertransference, I also trusted that it would contribute to a healing experience. At this moment, Eva was the active one; no longer the passive victim, she was giving herself a new face. I wordlessly and empathically validated her experience (Barbara Eisold, 1997, personal communication). Finally Eva exhaustedly collapsed on the floor next to me.

During the following sessions, Eva was able, with great pain and with great emotion, to describe the impact that her facial surgery (performed under local anesthesia) had had on her; she had lost a sense of self and body, for example, hearing pieces of her chin-bone thrown like garbage into the metal disposal receptacle. Eva talked about the utter puzzlement and devastation of having had—as an adolescent—her own face erased. She cried, "A face is supposed to be the mirror of one's soul" (the mental representation of the most important part of one's body). I said that her face, with its expressions and emerging wrinkles, would always reflect her individual, unique experience of herself.

My conjecture is that the facial surgery became specifically traumatic because in her early life her parents had so blatantly failed to create an environment in which not only basic trust but also a sense of her body-ego and self-image should have had a chance to develop. Eva had always taken great pride in her high intellectual capacity and was set on making use of her brain, to piece herself (her situation) together, literally, into a coherent, comprehensible picture so that she could become a person with her own specific uniqueness, regardless of and differentiated from what others had imposed on her in the past. No longer did she have nosebleeds and headaches at the time around the anniversary of this event (Pollock, 1970). In conclusion, Eva's body no longer became the scene of her acting out her tragedy through bodily symptoms (McDougall, 1989).

In her treatment, not just her traumatic past but also her constitutional strength for survival came fully to life. To prevent herself, however, from getting totally lost during her parents' overwhelmingly abusive acts, which caused confusion and unbearable excitement, she used to focus on an object in her environment. Her parents' daily and extensive sexual abuse of her seemed to have caused Eva to distort reality to the point where people and things invariably appeared to her as sexualized objects, such as penises and vaginas, depicted in hundreds of drawings.

Those sexual activities also plagued her and made her feel contaminated with badness, a feeling she connected later in life with the imagined development of cancer, "the badness inside of me." The badness was related to a sense of guilt, for she felt that she had been equally responsible for the indulgence in sexual incestuous "games" and the fact that she had experienced them not just as pain but also with excitement and pleasure. After all, negative attention was better than no attention at all, as when her parents threw her in a closet and forgot her there for a day. The feeling of badness had been reinforced by her parents' image of her as bad. Therefore, when Eva first disclosed these sexual activities in her session, she had the panicky fear that I might permanently reject her as a "bad person," a strong transference reaction. My countertransference was in identification with the memory from my own childhood of my nonjudgmental and understanding father having been supportive of me and following up on and preventing a potentially sexually abusive situation without making me feel that I had been bad. I did therefore feel nonretaliatory when she acted out her feelings of badness by making so called "messes" for herself and others, including me, by example, not paying my bills, and smelling up my office by indescribably heavy perfumes. When she had worked on her self-image and her rage in treatment, she was able to "clean up her act" ("her messes"), and could, for instance, be more conscientious about paying her bills.

The neglect to which Eva was exposed in her early years evoked an aggression that stimulated the development of a sadistically cruel primitive superego. In the safe setting of my office, powerful oral-sadistic fantasies would surface—for example, transferential fantasies of cutting me up in pieces and spitting these pieces onto the walls and ceiling. Once, while indulging in these fantasies, making me, in my countertransference, feel uncomfortable, she "blacked out." For a few moments, my countertransference was a feeling of utter helplessness. Accepting my state of mind, I contemplated calling an ambulance but decided first to try to handle the situation on my own. Knowing that hearing is the sense that is the last to leave us, I told her that she felt too upset having these fantasies about me and therefore had "left" the situation. I added that I was sorry I had not been fully alert to how this experience was too frightening for her. Now my wish was to help her to come back to full conscious functioning again.

Having a sense that very basic experiences would be needed, I explained that I would take her by the hand and accompany her for a walk in the garden, where we would breath the air, listening to the bird songs, touch the tree trunks—fully experience the special world that is all around us. With her eyes turned upward so that her iris and pupils did not show, she came with me and within minutes came to full awareness. Returning to the treatment room, she could acknowledge her rage at her parents. She also recalled how in the past she would quickly turn the aggression onto herself, become neglectful of her own body, hurt herself severely. She looked upon herself as "the bad seed," who would ultimately be punished for her alleged crime of being born with the help of a Cesarean section, thereby "endangering my mother's life." Her self-punitive behavior expressed itself in her cutting and scratching her skin. She also felt, with great excitement, that at least then she was in charge of the physical abuse; she was no longer the passive victim as in the past. Feelings of satisfaction stemmed also from the reassurance she felt at still being alive when she looked at her blood and felt the pain the cuts caused her. It became a great victory for Eva, however, when she was able, as a result of treatment, to sublimate her aggressive drive and create "scratch drawings" instead of turning her aggression onto herself.

In one of these scratch drawings, there is an infant holding on to a syringe, the way ordinarily a baby would hold on to his mother. When her mother destroyed Eva's first transitional object, the mother's nightgown, Eva selected one of her mother's heroin syringes as something to hold on to for a feeling of safety. It seemed to be a conglomerate of what for Eva represented the concept of mothering: a fusion of her visual image of her mother and the baby bottle from which Eva was fed. Not until Eva, in her treatment, had worked out her complex relationship to her mother could she let go of the syringe. As a young woman close to 30 years of age, she conducted a burial ceremony of the syringe in my garden. After this symbolic act, thoughts of her mother's presence no longer bothered her.

Eva's anger was sometimes a defense against a lurking depression. When this was analyzed, Eva could recognize a deeply felt sadness about being seen as a reject. Many times she recalled incidents when her mother had given her the feeling that her mother needed to annihilate her. One of the earliest blows to her feeling of an identity of her own occurred when her mother exchanged Eva for one of her classmates for a family picture for a magazine article about her mother. Eva recalled how, at eight years of age, she had attempted to hang herself after learning about this deceit.

THE RESULT OF THE FIRST PHASE
OF TREATMENT AND WHAT PRECIPITATED
THE SECOND PHASE OF HER TREATMENT

The result of these therapeutic techniques after five years of analysis were extensive. Eva had developed meaningful friendships of a non-destructive character. She was functioning extremely well professionally. During the last two years she had given up acting on her aggression, endangering herself with destructive behavior such as suicide attempts, cutting herself, and drug and alcohol abuse. She had a more accurate sense of her body- and self-image and stopped referring to herself in the third person. Her voice no longer held the fluctuating quality of the girl–woman character. Her headaches and hallucinations were gone. Her impulse control had improved. At times, however, she could appear provocative, abrasive, and argumentative.

At this point, considering her improvements and that a reasonably long time had been given for their consolidation (two years), I thought it appropriate to introduce the idea of beginning gradually to reduce the number of sessions per week, with the ultimate goal of termination in a distant future. Eva seemed accepting of this plan.

Three months later, however, Eva reported to me that she had begun bleeding from her rectum. She said her condition had been diagnosed as inoperable carcinoma of the colon. A year later, she said her cancer had metastasized to the groin and the urethra and she had three to four years left to live. During the three and a half years that followed, after she claimed the initial diagnosis had been made, Eva reported periods of responding to chemotherapy and radiation but added that, in spite of everything, her cancer situation had worsened. She reported that lymphoma affecting neck, tongue, larynx, and eye was developing. Unknown to me, with Eva threatened by the possibility of loss of continuous psychoanalysis, Munchausen became the solution to secure care indefinitely.

THE SECOND PHASE OF EVA'S TREATMENT

During years of claiming she was a cancer patient, Eva faked her "cancer" so well that I, as well as the physicians treating her for her "symptoms," the so-called side effects of her cancer treatment, believed her cancer story. These treatments are documented; they took place in two reputable university hospitals. None of the professionals, however, were able to get any records regarding the diagnosis from the university hospital that was said to have made the original diagnosis of cancer. Eva explained this by saying that she was part of a research study group of cancer patients and that consequently all records were coded and therefore not identifiable by name.

Originally, when Eva told me she had cancer, I knew that heredity as well as milieu might have played a role in predisposing her for cancer. My countertransference was that of a state of deep sadness. I felt that life was never going to let up on her, would never cease to be the "scenes of hell" she had so vividly depicted in her drawings and words. My next response was to decide to research what could be important for me to know about cancer. I can see now that my decision, in addition to stemming from a sense of human compassion, was based on a powerful unconscious countertransference factor. Influenced by unconscious guilt, I leaped at the chance to do something that I could envision might be helpful. I first became aware of the source of my unconscious countertransference reaction at the time of the disclosure of Eva's having a factitious disease.

My conscious feelings of guilt led me to ask myself whether I had not perhaps caused her to develop cancer by prematurely introducing the idea of the termination of her treatment. Keeping in mind research findings (LeShan, 1977; Simonton, Mathews-Simonton, and Creighton, 1978), I asked myself whether Eva had perhaps been unable to cope with this idea of a future loss, and, as a consequence, her stress had lowered the function of her immune system, causing the outbreak of cancer. In Selye's (1979) hypotheses on stress, he stated that excessive stress impairs the immune system and renders the body incapable of combating abnormal, and sometimes malignant, cells. My speculations were numerous about how this illness possibly might have some connection with her own psychological factors. I realized that no answer could be given. Consoled by Groddeck's (1925) writings, I learned that to be ill has to mean something specific; it is impossible to find a general and universal meaning. We can only determine the specific meaning an illness has for each of us. Going on the assumption that Eva suffered from cancer, I decided to continue my psychoanalytic work with her and explore with her what she might be expressing by her illness, if anything at all.

I decided on a multidimensional therapeutic approach that I hoped might, in addition to her medical treatment, contribute to the remission of her cancer. Through workshops and readings, I learned that I had, in part, to modify my treatment techniques and to emphasize more modifiers (Blanck and Blanck, 1974) and parameters (Eissler, 1953) of a supportive character to make her psychodynamic treatment effective.

Of the most important parameters affecting her body- and self-image, one was the techniques that would diminish her fear and her feeling that she had no control over her body. Because of the dread of the severity of the cancer, this was a particularly prominent fear of hers related to the psychotic elements in her borderline character structure. In accordance with the techniques developed by Simonton, et al. (1978), I taught Eva how to relax, meditate, and visualize her cancer and the medical cancer treatments as being powerful in doing their job in arresting her cancer. Drawing No. 1 depicts her visualization of cancer as bugs on the beach (her favorite place) and the chemotherapy as powerful white birds consuming the bugs to eventual extinction. Note the ever-present love object Star(s) watching the process. Most important, her mother had taught her how to swim, how to preserve her body in an oceanic element.

The lack of family support and assistance was an immediate hardship for Eva. Efforts to engage on her behalf her family members still

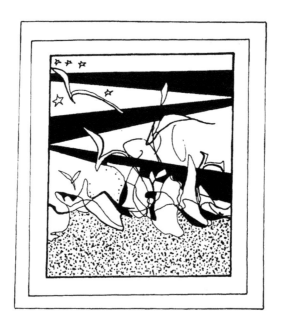

Drawing No. 1. *Visualization of Cancer Situation*

living were fruitless. Goodrich and Wise (1980) have emphasized the importance of the family in promoting healing of the cancer victim. I felt I would, whenever possible, try to supply some of the support a caring family ordinarily would give.

In Eva's transference reaction to me during this last period of psychoanalysis, sometimes I still represented the altogether idealized "good mother." However, she became increasingly able to express her anger toward me, at times reaching levels of intense fury. The defense mechanisms of splitting, dissociation, and fragmentation no longer came into play. In her transference fantasies about me as "the bad mother" she tested me out more extensively than ever before and accused me of a wish to reject her because of her cancer, her "badness."

The concept of cancer as a metaphor, with all its psychological implications, lent itself very well to Eva's need for a final opportunity to work through in her sessions, on a deeper level than ever before, her childhood traumas and her conflictual relationships with people of her past who had contributed to her distorted self-image. Under the influence of the repetition compulsion (Freud, 1914), Eva put herself through her present Hell, where her abusers were her parents, a powerfully introjected part of her, her imagined "cancer."

Living the role of a person with "cancer," Eva was torn between hope and despair over whether she was going to survive in her struggle to rid herself of her negative body self image. On Drawing No. 2, in black, white, and red, Eva has depicted this threesome, the

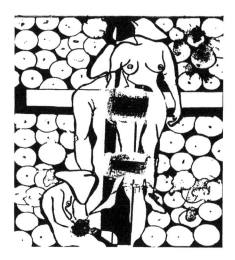

Drawing No. 2. *The Three Doomed People*

triangular setting of her parents and herself, being trapped and surrounded by cancer cells—a scene of three people about to be cruci-
fied for their sins. All of them are hurt in the genital area, a punishment
for their oral, anal, and genital sexual play. They are burnt out, doomed
and punished with cancer. At this time, she presented her "cancer"
as having metastasized to her groin, and she claimed the radiation
had burnt her skin so badly that she would have to undergo skin
graft. Even as Eva spoke of her parents' sexual abuse of her, she complained about intense cancer pains and spreading of the cancer (her
badness) into the pelvic area, so poignantly illustrated in Drawing
No. 3, in black, white, and red. Associating to the drawing, she underscored her body-image of herself as "bad" being related to her past
sexual excitement with her parents. After working through these early
experiences and feeling less guilty, she reported that her pains were
receding and her cancer was partially in remission.

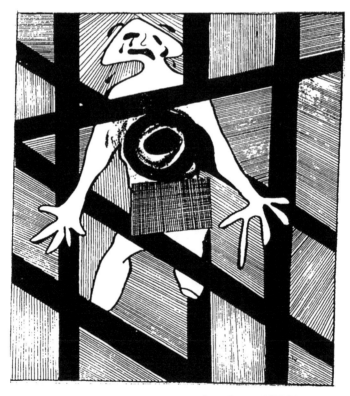

Drawing No. 3. *The Badness[the Cancer] Within*

The sexual play with her parents had not only a negative meaning but also a positive one. She had loved the fact that she could feel important to her parents. She expressed her guilt about having enjoyed the sexual excitement with her father in particular. She had always desired, as well as feared, the possibility of penetration. Her vagina caused her great conflict, however, she considered it the most vulnerable part of her body (Bernstein, 1990). Therefore, at times, she plugged it up with glue to preserve her body image. Her "cancer" now became "a baby," a rectal pregnancy fantasy in her transference to me as her oedipal father.

Eva had hated her parents' control over her. She indulged in fantasies about gaining omnipotent power over her abusers, what she called "penis-power." On Drawing No. 4 their power has been reversed; the power now being hers, she could do anything. Depending on which side of the drawing is up, it represents male and female power.

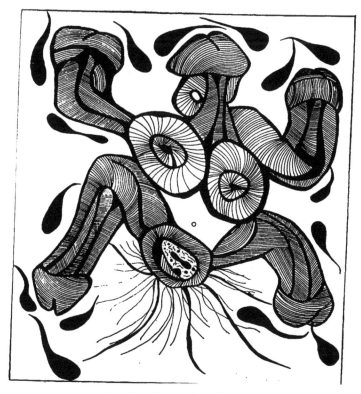

Drawing No. 4. *Penis-Power*

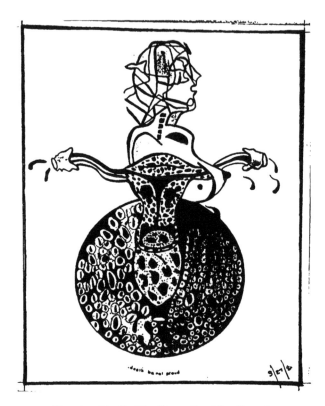

Drawing No. 5. *The Strength of the Female*

She was able gradually to gain a sense of her own strength as a female. In Drawing No. 5, the uterus and fallopian tubes symbolize her emerging regard for her own inner reproductive organs. She made use of this strength by being increasingly caring of herself. On the drawing, the bull's face in the middle symbolizes the strength she envisioned herself in need of to cope with her "cancer." Her "cancer" is contained in the circle, symbolizing the structure and the discipline one has to develop to hold oneself together, to preserve a good body image.

In the way she spoke about her cancer treatment, she continued to work through her past. The chemotherapy she envisioned herself getting, seems to have stood for her parents' abusive treatment of her when she was a child, as when her father would ejaculate in her mouth. As she had felt nauseous then, she vividly described feelings of nausea after receiving "her chemotherapy" (Drawing No. 6), which

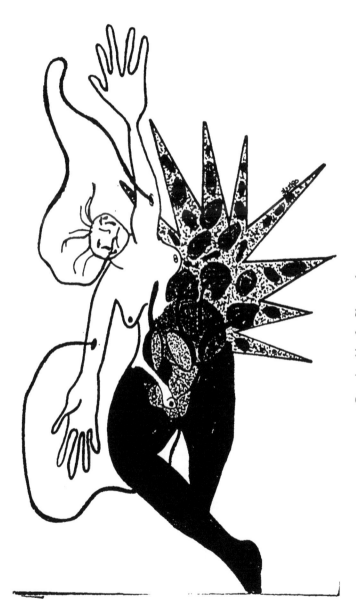

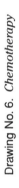

Drawing No. 6. *Chemotherapy*

lessened her ability to cope with "her pains." She commented, "I don't want them [the medical staff] to be mad at me like my parents were. I try to cooperate, to be a good patient so they will treat me well. The bottom part of me is black; that's where the cancer is. The chemotherapy is hitting the cancerous cells and POW they get hit and they try to run away. The treatment is hard but I put it in the Star; it stays contained in the Star." This concept made her feel safe and protected through the care of Star. She continued, "The Star is in the back of me, holding me together".

Continuing to associate to this drawing about the taxing cancer treatment, Eva associated her guilt-ridden memories to watching her father abuse her mother. Her chemotherapy made her feel as knocked out as she imagined her mother must have felt after such abusive treatment. It was hard for Eva to keep in mind that the treatment was not a way of being abused, or abusing oneself, but actually a medical treatment aimed at curing her. Her guilt about her oedipal fantasies, her wish to get rid of her mother, were worked on and resulted in her experiencing relief and led to a lessening of expressions of a primitive, sadistic superego.

After six and a half years in analysis, Eva reviewed with pride her accomplishments and expressed in particular her deeply felt satisfaction for having at last, in spite of all that had happened to her, managed to become a person with her own identity. She felt more truly differentiated from her mother, someone who could have a chance to be completely successful in counteracting cancer, someone who neither was a replica of her mother nor was responsible for her mother's problems and death. Eva claimed that she had been given an excellent prognosis, an 80% chance for complete remission of her "cancer."

Even with this gain, however, there was still unfinished business in Eva's puzzle of "piecing myself together," her body image: she had to deal more thoroughly with her relationship to her father. Eva had always felt responsible for the rapid deterioration of his health and functioning that had begun with her mother's death when Eva was 15.

Eva's father died when she was 30. Six weeks after she heard of his death, she showed a drastic change in her behavior; it reflected her way of coping with her loss as well as her efforts in working through more completely her complex relationship to him. In her mourning process, she took on her father's identity; that is, she replicated, to a large degree, his destructive behavior. She appeared immune to any attempt on my part to interpret her behavior in order for her to get control over her need to identify destructively with him. Her lack of response was due to her need to reenact fully her father's life style; the reenactments were so all-encompassing that they nearly cost her life on several occasions. Space permits only a few examples.

Soon after the death of Eva's mother, her father became paralyzed, almost unable to talk. Now, in coping with his death, Eva emulated his symptoms. In both cases, there was no apparent organic reason. It was as if Eva were, in part, giving up on life after the loss of a very important person, her father, just as he had done when hearing about the loss of someone important to him, his wife. On Drawing No. 7, she depicts herself as dead, and yet the position of the skeleton indicates some sense of aliveness. Completely identifying herself

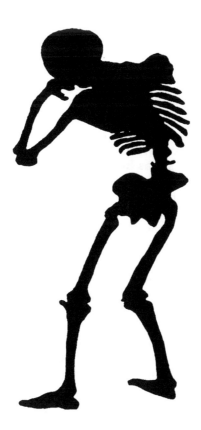

Drawing No. 7. *Sick to Death*

with her father, she thereby was denying his death and keeping him alive within her. Freud (1917) described that when somebody dies, for example, an ambivalently loved parent, the need to reproach and punish oneself in a hysterical fashion with the same illness that the person has had may occur. The self-reproaches against a loved object have been shifted away from it onto the mourner's own ego. When the work of mourning—that is, the decathexis of the libido toward the object—is completed, the ego becomes free again. Eva had to work on her relationship with her father before that freedom could be hers.

Her identification with her father took many forms. Eva developed symptoms indicating the possibility of brain damage exactly as her father's symptoms had mimicked brain damage. She also developed a fear of having a cancerous brain tumor, even when a brain scan showed no sign of it. Throughout his life, Eva's father had shown evidence of brain dysfunction, for example in epileptic psychomotor seizures following terrifying rages. Eva now underwent several incidents of being enraged and out of control. Once she had a seizure that resulted in a serious car accident. Her father had always been a reckless driver, and, during the months following the news of his death, she caused two car accidents. Before her father's death she had been a careful and competent driver. Her most serious accident, one that almost killed her, occurred, ironically enough, on the anniversary of the day her mother had set as Eva's new birthday after the plastic surgery on her face. On one occasion, Eva became unable to talk. She growled like a monster, the way her father had prior to his epileptic seizures, and she put on "a mean face" exactly as he used to do. For a few hours, she was totally inaccessible. On another occasion, becoming violent in my office, she broke a chair, the way she had described her father when he went berserk, breaking everything in his path.

In the midst of these agitated reactions to her father's death, she was able to express some amazement at the deep feeling of loss she experienced at the death of her hated father. Often, as she talked about him, she experienced him as being present as a "lump in my throat," associating to having been involved in fellatio with her father. Not long thereafter, she spoke about these sensations, a marked swelling appeared on the right side of her neck. She reported to me that the medical team had diagnosed her developing lymphoma, secondary to her chemotherapy. Her comment was, "My cancer is my father destroying me." Eva continued, "The cancer ran amuck with me, like my father used to do. The lump in my throat is like my father was still in there, choking me to death, pushing his penis into my mouth, dunking me in the feces water. I wish I could just spit him out, like they spat me out. I wish to spit out 'the cancer' and get rid of it. He caused the feeling of badness within me, but I am not really a bad person." This important statement shows the change in her self-image.

Eva had by now reached a phase of less resistance to my genetic and transference interpretations. She became more aware and acknowledged her intense and deep-rooted aggression, expressed in her oral-sadistic fantasies and in her frequent utterance, "Chew you up and spit you out," as well as in her excitement and fear. She realized that she had held back her oral-aggressive fantasies and had prevented them from fully becoming the focus of analytic work. Thus she could derive pleasure from silently dwelling on them. She was secretly fascinated by her frequent visits to the Brooklyn Aquarium. She observed the sharks and made a series of drawings of destructively interacting sharks, parents with their offspring. Interestingly, her body- and self-image were reflected in her purchasing an old, beat-up car, which was called "The Shark" because of its open front, which looked very much like the open mouth of a shark.

Accepting the aggression as hers, Eva's formerly cruel superego seemed gradually to become modified. She engaged herself in enjoyable activities and became capable of dealing with frustration without going out of control. Owing to her "cancer," she had a twofold loss: her former boyfriend (who had contacted her for the possibility of developing a relationship again, but then dropped her) and her job. Her job had meant everything to her and so had her boyfriend. But, she pulled herself together and tried to use her artistic talent to gain income from temporary jobs. As her professional trade mark, she took on the Swedish Dala-Horse, referring to me as Swedish and being 'a workhorse.' Eva's way of coping showed her strength from having developed a stronger sense of her body-ego and capacity to function well.

It, however, was as if Eva were driven to use the cancer concept to its ultimate limit, that is, as a symbol of "committing suicide" and then miraculously being resurrected (being redeemed). In spite of her physical appearance, in her mind she felt herself to be in remission from the cancer. She perceived herself as "cleansed from her sins" and felt rewarded with good health to enjoy for the rest of her life. In her self-proclaimed remission, she had finally rid herself of her "ghosts from the past."

Many events led to this final solution of her problems, "her cure." Eva had written her own will and made arrangements for the disposition of her remains. She left her assets to an already established organization for the support and care of children with cancer. She went to court to fight for her right to get the inheritance left by her father. The father's lawyer testified in court as to the reason why her father had wished his entire estate to go to Eva alone: her father wished to compensate her for the extensive abuses suffered at his hand, inflicted on her during childhood.

With the idea in mind of enjoying the remainder of her life, Eva informed me about her decision to end her medical treatment since, she said, it made her sicker than the cancer itself. In retrospect, one may think of this statement as a way of declaring that Munchausen had served out its role in her life. Her drawings no longer showed any signs of primary-process thinking; in fact, they took on the quality of life and joy and were now colorful. Drawing No. 8 she named "Springtime Is You," expressing how the therapeutic work had led her to hope and enjoyment of life. On the drawing, the women are surrounded

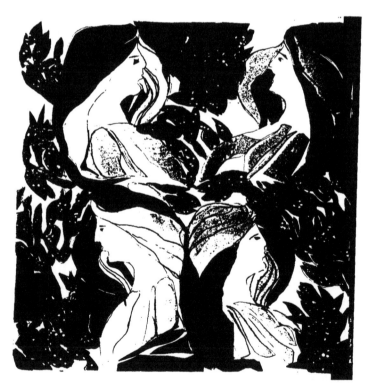

Drawing No. 8. *Springtime Is You*

by purple crocuses and sunshine. Note their positions in relation to each other: first there is the mirroring (Kohut, 1971) and then, below, the process of separation and individuation takes precedence (Mahler, Pine, and Bergman, 1975).

Even if Eva appeared spirited, as a cancer patient she looked extremely sick with her severe weight loss, inability to walk without a cane, difficulties holding her balance, tremors, bruise marks allegedly caused by a weakening of capillaries, and hair loss. (It was disclosed later that the latter two symptoms had been caused by her beating herself with cables and pulling out her own hair.) Because of her physical condition, my judgment was that she could no longer care for herself. Consequently, I suggested that she go for a thorough workup at the hospital in her community for the assessment of her chances to be eligible for a hospice service program, whereupon Eva became furious with me and stated that I did not care for her. She became hard to manage when she allowed herself to act out her anger. The oncologist who had seen her on occasion for consultation during the last three years followed a thorough diagnostic procedure in the hospital. The results revealed that Eva had no cancer and, in all likelihood, had never had it.

As her therapist, I was asked to convey to Eva the result of the medical workup. She became furious and insisted that she was a cancer victim, accusing us all of being out of our minds. In response to our request for release of information from the first hospital about her alleged cancer diagnosis, it became evident that the names of the oncology team were correct—they were the doctors involved in the cancer research program—but none of them had ever seen Eva. The truth was that Eva had never gone for any cancer diagnosis and treatment there. She had simulated the side-effects of chemotherapy and radiation. Being very well read on the subject of cancer and its treatment, she had done the simulation so convincingly that I, as well as the medical doctors who treated her for the side-effects of the so-called cancer treatment, never detected that her cancer was an invention of her mind. Eva was put for one week on Haldol and then discharged from the hospital.

I held off her psychoanalysis during the time our investigation lasted. I did not know how to assist her until her situation had been thoroughly assessed and I had had a chance to work through my own feelings about this highly unusual situation. Eva was furious; she experienced me as rejecting and distrustful of her. Using threats and attempts to disrupt my life, she tried to manipulate and intimidate me.

In my countertransference, I at first had felt numbed by the news that her cancer was a factitious disorder. Then I felt angry because I had been taken advantage of and fooled, though I was somewhat less upset knowing that so had the medical professionals in charge of her physical care. I resented all the time I had spent in a sincere effort to help to remedy a cancer situation that was not real. On the positive side, I felt pleased Eva was not suffering from cancer and that I had assisted her in successfully working through her body- and self-image as related to her complex past. I had gained knowledge about today's research about cancer. More important, in my own self-analysis, I gave myself a chance to gain more insight. I became aware that my childhood need to feel omnipotent was coverup for feelings of helplessness in the face of seeing my mother and other relatives die of cancer. My gratification had been to work with "the cancer-patient," Eva. I had unconsciously hoped this situation would be different in contrast to the one I had encountered as a child, when a cure for cancer was remote. The disclosure of Eva's factitious disorder had deprived me of a hope I must have harbored since childhood, the hope of being able to influence, to some degree, the progression of cancer and its end result, death.

I realized that with the sensitivity of a person suffering psychotic episodes, Eva had probably sensed my vulnerable spot and made use of it in the interest of her struggle to satisfy needs and obtain care and, finally, a psychological cure. Searles (1979) discusses the importance for the self-image of the psychotic patient to have had at least a chance to experience his own worth by finally enabling the mother (analogously the analyst) to become a whole and effective mother (analyst to him). In line with Searles's thinking, I believe that Eva benefited from seeing my pleasure in working with her. She had provided me with the opportunity for my increased self-knowledge, as well as to be of assistance to her. Supportive evidence for her ability to identify with me as "a good-enough mother" was that Eva replaced her murderous, sadistic fantasies about herself with some acceptance and a genuine appreciation of herself—an improved self-image.

I spoke to Eva a few more times about her situation and said that, if she wished to see me in psychoanalysis, we would naturally go back to the same treatment procedure, namely, the way we had worked before her "cancer"—a treatment relying entirely on verbal interaction. In addition, since she was not ill, she could now take on a job and pay regularly for her sessions. Eva did not accept this plan. In a few phone calls and correspondence, she spoke with genuine pleasure about the development of a relationship with a man. She continued to be a caring friend with parental qualities toward her best friend's son. Since analysis had been a special experience for her, she held on to the possibility of writing a book about herself, her legacy. Such a book would serve the purpose of giving hope to a person—a substance abuser with severe psychological impairments—that one can piece oneself together and function if the motivation is there. As part of that project, to be able to reach a wider audience with her message, she made three video tapes in which she talked about herself, her childhood, her creativity, and her "cancer." At our last meeting, we met to review the tapes. She said: "The circle is closed," referring to the place, the library, where our first contact had been. About 15 years have passed since then. Contacts with her have shown that there has been no reoccurrence of the factitious disorder.

DISCUSSION

The main pathology of Munchausen syndrome is an addiction to simulating illness. Eva, with her addictive personality, was able to give up her drug addiction when she became involved in her analysis and became addicted to me and her treatment. Only when she felt threatened by the prospect of the loss of me did her addictive personality express itself in the addiction to the idea of cancer in order to reinvolve me.

In pondering the sequence of Eva's addictions, I see Winnicott's (1953) theory about the transitional object as crucial to understanding her development. From early on, she had a continuous need to hold on to something for the sake of reducing her anxiety when confronted with loss. Her earliest transitional object was her mother's nightgown, subsequently destroyed by her mother. Thus Eva was deprived of the crucial opportunity to display her libidinal and aggressive drive energy on the transitional object while being reassured of its survival. Moreover, since her transitional object had been destroyed, it could not gradually and spontaneously be decathected either. Her mother's inability to adapt to her infant's needs and to provide opportunities for illusion and gradual disillusionment probably played a major role in Eva's pathology. She had been deprived of experiencing her transitional object as becoming naturally diffused. In Winnicott's conceptualization, this experience is crucial, for it encompasses the entire territory of outer reality as well as inner reality. Instead of the transitional objects being broadened into interests and

creativity, the partial lack of it led to Eva's development of an addictive character structure.

Hampered in her ego development, Eva cathected and secretly
kept what originally had been a transitional object, one of her mother's
syringes. It came to have more of the characteristics of "a psychotic
fetish" (Mahler and Furer, 1966), which in sharp contrast to Winnicott's
transitional object, does not facilitate object constancy. Characteristic of the psychotic fetish is that it draws almost all libido and aggression upon itself, as if the person's life depended on it. The person
clings to the burnt-out, deanimated, devitalized part-object as a
mother substitute. Eva's ego development had been neglected and
interfered with. It became thwarted in its capacity for object constancy and reality testing. Consequently, Eva developed a character
structure with the prominent regressive features of an addictive personality. Her drug addiction resulted from the fact that the transitional phenomena had basically remained unchallenged from early
childhood on and had thus predisposed her to hold on to the illusion
rather than to reality.

As you may recall, her attachment (addiction) to me came about
because Eva had listened to my presentation about the transitional
object. In her treatment, she was given an opportunity to receive
"good-enough mothering," with the restoration of the experience of
the transitional phenomena, self and object. The transitional object
ultimately enables the person to journey from what Winnicott (1953)
called "the purely subjective to objectivity." In this way, the transitional object seems to antedate the establishment of reality testing.
In analysis, Eva went through all the necessary steps toward attaining the capacity for reality testing and the development of a well-
adjusted, mature adult's ego functioning.

From our knowledge of Eva's infancy, it was clear that there had
been few opportunities for bonding and establishing, through touch,
a sense of her body. Ashley Montagu (1971) has described the necessity of tactile experience in human development. Anna Freud (1965)
underscored what Erikson (1950) was among the first to acknowledge, namely, the importance of "the incorporative mood" during the
oral phase, when the sense organs and the skin are receptive and
increasingly hungry for proper stimulation. Anna Freud (1965)
wrote:

> At the beginning of life, being stroked, cuddled, and soothed
> by touch libidinizes the various parts of the child's body,
> helps to build up a healthy body image and body ego,

increase its cathexis with narcissistic libido, and simultaneously promotes the development of object love by cementing the bond between child and mother. There is no doubt that, at this period, the surface of the skin in its role as erotogenic zone fulfills a multiple function in the child's growth [p. 199].

To assist Eva in gaining a physical sense of her own being, I understood her need for a modicum of physical touch (Kupfermann and Smaldino, 1987). Winnicott (1989) warned against not responding to the need for touch in a patient who is in a psychotic state. A failure to respond means that the unintegrated self falls forever. When in deep distress, Eva used to repeat, "Put on the lines." She needed me to stroke her back with my fingers apart. When associating to this need, Eva said she remembered the crib bars onto which she used to push herself as a child to get a sense of the existence of her body. Later this memory was transferred to her experience of the soothing quality of striped patterns in my office and then to follow the differently colored lines in hospitals that guide patients to different departments for care.

The eight years of treatment strengthened her sense of body- and self-image. A true sense of self began to be solidified to the point that she was able to invent creatively a "cancer" when she felt threatened by a loss she was not ready to fully accept. As a cancer patient, she received the additional concrete care she needed. I believe that my not knowing the factitious character of her illness was a crucial factor in Eva's improvement. If I had been aware of it, I would not have been able to be in true and full empathy with her situation, to respond to her need for a modicum gratification, and consequently no effective corrective experience could have been provided. At the end of the treatment, she could relinquish the concept of cancer and feel entitled to enjoy improved mental health after eight years of difficult analytic work. A follow-up has shown that Eva has functioned fairly well with the support of a few deeply important friendships and group activities. As mentioned, there has been no evidence of the recurrence of Munchausen syndrome, since the termination of her analysis 15 years ago.

In view of the poor prognosis regarding Munchausen Syndrome, which many clinicians have reported (e.g., Bursten,1965; Zastrov, 1989), one may ask, does the reason for the difference in outcome between Eva and other cases of factitious disorder lie in the fact that Eva received a very special type of psychoanalytic attention and intervention? I believe that, as clinicians, we may be able to prevent the reoccurrence of factitious disorder if we respond in insightful ways to our patients' needs. The corrective social and emotional experience should be provided during a transitional period when the therapeutic aim is to give optimal empathic attention, care, validation, and understanding for the purpose of mending and compensating for earlier deficits. In contrast to other clinicians (Crabtree, 1967), I believe that, as a result of psychoanalytic efforts to afford the patient insight into the dynamics of the pathology, the patient can give up the need for this devastating and destructive syndrome, the factitious disorder.

We need to be especially cautious in the way we expose our patients to the fact that they are feigning illness, as well as in the way we assist them therapeutically to deal with this fact. Most patients described in the literature leave the medical setting where they have been treated, only to reappear in another similar situation in an endless, futile, repetitive search for satisfaction of their need to be attended to. Some unable to cope with the exposure have been known to lapse into psychosis. When Eva was faced with our knowledge of her deception, she did not become devastated and wish to disappear. She became furious but saved face by telling others a story about the complete remission of her cancer. In contrast to other patients, she no longer needed to use factitious disorder as a way of temporarily fulfilling her needs for attention and care. Owing to intensive analytic intervention, the factitious disorder had served out its purpose.

In summary, my conjecture is that the development of factitious disorder seems in this case to have been rooted in inadequate parenting during infancy and childhood, which caused distortion of the body- and self-image. In this state of vulnerability, Eva was predisposed to develop a factitious syndrome later in life under stressful conditions. The adult patient's experience of a corrective emotional experience and "good-enough mothering" assisted her in developing a solid sense of her body ego. In addition, psychoanalysis—the working through of the patient's traumas as well as clarifications and analysis of resistance and transference—enabled Eva to fully renounce the factitious syndrome addiction as a way of coping with life. In that sense, Eva's case is unique compared with those of other patients described in the literature who remained addicted to the use of factitious disorder as a coping mechanism. A case such as Eva's testifies to the fact that patients with factitious disorder can be successfully treated with psychoanalysis provided that the psychoanalyst is willing to be flexible enough to include the use of various parameters and modifiers. The patient's self-image and body-image can be worked on to restore the perception of self and reality.

REFERENCES

Alexander, F. (1954), Some quantitative aspects of pychoanalytic technique. *J. Amer. Psychoanal. Assn.*, 2:685–701.

———— (1958), Unexplored areas of psychoanalytic theory and treatment Part II. In: *Selected Papers.* New York: Basic Books, 1961, pp. 319–335.

———— (1960), Psychoanalysis and psychotherapy. In: *Selected Papers.* New York: Basic Books, 1961, 310–318.

American Psychiatric Association (1994), *Diagnostic and Statistical Manual of Mental Disorders, DSM-IV*, Washington, DC: American Psychiatric Assn.

Asher, R. (1951), Munchausen syndrome, *Lancet*, 1:339–341.

Bernstein, D. (1990), Female genital anxieties, conflicts and typical mastery modes. *Internat. J. Psycho-Anal.*, 71:151–165.

Blanck, G. & Blanck, R. (1974), *Ego Psychology, Theory and Practice.* New York: Columbia University Press.

Bursten, B. (1965), On Munchausen's syndrome. *Arch. Gen. Psychiat.*, 13:261–268.

Crabtree, J. H., Jr. (1967), A psychotherapeutic encounter with a self-mutilating patient. *Psychiat.*, 30:91–100.

Eissler, K. R. (1953), The effect of the structure of the ego on psychoanalytic technique. *J. Amer. Psychoanal. Assn.*, 1:104–143.

Erikson, E. H. (1950), *Childhood and Society.* New York: Norton.

Federn, P. (1943a), Psychoanalysis of psychoses. I. Errors and how to avoid them. *Psychiat. Quart.*, 17:319.

———— (1943b), Psychoanalysis of psychoses. II. Transference. *Psychiat. Quart.*, 17:246–257.

———— (1947), Principles of psychotherapy in latent schizophrenia. *Amer. J. Psychother.*, 1:129–144.

Freud, A. (1965), *Normality and Pathology in Childhood.* New York: International Universities Press.

Freud, S. (1914), Remembering, repeating and working through. *Standard Edition*, 12:147–156. London: Hogarth Press, 1958.

———— (1917), Mourning and melancholia. *Standard Edition*, 14:237–258. London: Hogarth Press, 1957.

Goodrich, C. H. & Wise, H. (1980), Family healing strategies with cancer. Presented at workshop on Cancer and the Family: The Healing Context, New York City.

Greenacre, P. (1958), The relation of the impostor to the artist. *The Psychoanalytic Study of the Child*, 13:521–540. New York: International Universities Press.

Grinker, R. R. (1961), Imposture as a form of mastery. *Arch. Gen. Psychiat.*, 5:449–452.

Groddeck, G. (1925), The meaning of illness. In: *The Meaning of Illness*, ed. L Schacht. New York: International Universities Press, 1977, pp. 197–202.

Gunderson, J. G. & Singer, M. T. (1975), Defining borderline patients: An overview. *Amer. J. Psychiat.* 132:110.

Kaplan, H. I. & Sadock, B. J., ed. (1975), *Comprehensive Textbook of Psychiatry, Vol. 2*. Baltimore, MD: Williams & Wilkins.

Kohut, H. (1971), *The Analysis of the Self*. New York: International Universities Press.

Kupfermann, K. (1996), The ilmportance of lines. *Amer. J. Art Ther.*, 34:62–74.

—— & Smaldino, C. (1987), The vitalizing and the revitalizing experience of reliability: The place of touch in psychotherapy. *Clin. Soc. Work J.*, 15:223–235.

Le Shan, L. (1977), *You Can Fight for Your Life*. New York: Jove.

Mahler, M. S. & Furer, M. (1966), Development of symbiosis, symbiotic psychosis, and the nature of separation anxiety. Remarks on Weiland's paper. *Internat. J. Psycho-Anal.*, 47:559–560.

—— & Pine, F. & Bergman, A. (1975), *The Psychological Birth of the Human Infant*. New York: Basic Books.

McDougall, J. (1989), *Theaters of the Body*. New York: Norton.

Miller, A. (1981), *Prisoners of Childhood*. New York: Basic Books,

Montagu, A. (1971), *Touching*. New York: Columbia University Press.

Nadelson T. (1979), The Munchausen spectrum: Borderline character features. *Gen. Hosp. Psychiat.*, 1:11–17.

Pollock, G. (1970), Anniversary reactions, trauma and mourning. *Psychoanal. Quart.*, 39:347–371.

Searles, H. I. (1979), *Countertransference and Related Subjects*. New York: International Universities Press.

Sechehaye, M. A. (1951), *Symbolic Realization*. New York: International Universities Press.

Selye, H. (1979), Stress, cancer and the mind. In: *Cancer, Stress, and Death*, ed. J. Tache, H. Selye & S. B. Day. New York: Plenum, pp. 11–19.

Simonton, O. C., Mathews-Simonton, S. & Creighton, J. L. (1978), *Getting Well Again*. New York: Bantam Books.

Sontag, S. (1979), *Illness as Metaphor*. New York: Random House.

Spiro, H. R. (1968), Chronic factitious illness. *Arch. Gen. Psychiat.*, 18:569–579.

Winnicott, D. W. (1953), Transitional objects and transitional phenomena. *Internat. J. Psycho-Anal.*, 34:89–97.

—— (1960), True and false self. In: *The Maturational Processes and the Facilitating Environment*. New York: International Universities Press, 1965, 140–152.

—— (1989), *Psychoanalytic Explorations.* Cambridge, MA: Harvard University Press.

Zastrov, F. (1989), Vorgetauschte Krankenheiten, Insbesondere das Munchausen-Symdrom, [Simulated illnesses, especially Munchausen syndrome] *Versicherungsmedizin*, 1:41:191–192.

7

DISSOCIATION AND PHYSICAL DIFFERENCE

The Case of the Transformed "Short" Person

Barbara K. Eisold

Small, pretty, and obviously bright, Stacey at 18 had definite charisma. The essence of her charm lay in a contagiously cheerful mood, coupled with the capacity to respond quickly to others. I met her early in my career, when she came to the hospital clinic where I then worked as a psychologist. She was seeking help for a pronounced stutter.

Stacey belonged to a family of people whom she described as "short." In fact, they were afflicted with a sex-linked, genetic anomaly called antrogolospia,[1] the most telling effect of which is stunted growth. Thus in Stacey's household, which included her paternal grandparents, her father, two younger sisters, and a half-brother, only the grandfather and the half-brother were of normal height. Because they were "short," none of the women, even the grandmother, had ventured much into the world, at least during Stacey's lifetime. Indeed, her father had kept them virtually locked up at home, in this way hoping to protect them from the pain that he had endured as a "short" person in the world at large.

In contrast to Stacey and her sisters, an older half-sister, also "short," had not been raised in this household and thus had been free to create a life for herself that included not only education and employment, but eventually a husband and children. This half-sister, Mitzi, visited Stacey often and played a very important role in Stacey's life. Less attractive than Stacey by far and hardly without problems of her own, Mitzi was nevertheless Stacey's closest friend and her model for the good things life had to offer, physical handicap and all. It was Mitzi who knew about the clinic at the hospital and she who sent Stacey there to get help with her stutter. In fact, the trip to the clinic was among the first Stacey made, once she gathered the courage to go out into the street alone.

Stacey herself was the first child born of her father's union with an adolescent girl, whom he had brought home pregnant to join his family. For a brief period immediately following Stacey's birth, her mother was content. But this relatively happy state ended as more children were born and drugs appeared on the scene, introduced by the new man in her mother's life. Stacey could remember how this man had bullied her mother to take the drugs, how her mother quickly became addicted and developed the habit of screaming tearfully when drugs were unavailable, while Stacey and her sisters clung to one another in fear. When Stacey was four, her mother moved in with this second man and took her children with her. Eventually Stacey's mother had many men from whom she bore a total of 13 children, most were taken away and put into foster care. This, however, was not the case with Stacey and her sisters. They remained in their mother's care for another two years until eventually they were stolen by the new woman their father had installed at home. Childless herself, this "stepmother" had grown attached to the little girls when they visited their father; on one such visit, with Stacey's encouragement, she refused to send them back. Too addicted to care, Stacey's mother never tried to repossess them.

Meanwhile, Stacey's father, an intelligent, but wily and suspicious man, was supporting his family by various illegal means. During his more prosperous years, he was a bookie. With the proceeds, he purchased a white Cadillac in which he proudly drove his children to the expensive parochial school he had enrolled them in. In addition, he bought piano lessons for Stacey, who was by far his favorite child and the one he hoped would make a name for him in show business. Stacey's father was impressed by celebrity and very much wanted to have a star in his own family.

Things went on like this until Stacey was eight or nine, when, apparently, hard times hit and her father could no longer afford either the fancy car or the school tuition. Formal schooling was totally abandoned at this point, and the children were kept at home, where television and newspapers comprised all the outside stimulation they were allowed. Financially the family survived on the various public assistance checks collected by their grandfather and whatever Stacey's father himself could earn by whatever means.

I cannot begin to describe the hovel in which this family lived. A visiting nurse, sent by us to assess the family's needs, had the following to say about what she saw there:

> VN observed entire setting to be depressing and deplorable. Building appears hazardous to health and safety. Walls in outside hall have large holes, leading to the street. Halls are dark. Windows are broken. Family resides in first floor apt. in 6 rooms. D (sister) opened door for me wearing her hat, coat, gloves. I noted cracks in ceiling; constant water flows through cracks. Family had two pails to catch water. Apt so cold that ice had formed around the pails. D informed me that father was asleep (at noon). E (other sister) refused to come and speak to me. And I did not go to where she was because she was with family dog, half german shepherd, half doberman! I do not feel that lack of motivation is financial because family continues to pay rent. VN cannot return to family due to lack of safety.

Depression, which was pervasive among all members of this family always, grew over the years.

Given her history, it is hardly surprising that Stacey hated most things about herself. She hated being short; she hated the color of her skin. She experienced both of these physical attributes as shameful humiliations that made her feel even more diminished in size than the barely 3'7" of her actual height. And she hated the surroundings in which she lived and the poverty of opportunity available to her.

The intensity with which Stacey experienced shame cannot be underestimated. Along with an equally intense need for stimulation, it eventually led to the development of a relatively felicitous means of escape: Stacey learned to escape in fantasy. Regularly, from age 10 until the time she first came to see me, she sat at home, alone, in front of a broken t.v., imagining antennae emerging from her head. There she transformed herself, in fantasy, into "Jennifer," a tall woman of American Indian origin, a lawyer, around whom she created an imaginary television drama, a "loved version of her life" (Allison, quoted in Jetter, 1995, p. 56) to take the place of the version of her life that she was living. Somewhere in Stacey's past there actually had been a Native Indian relative, and she was proud of this. In this new version of her life, she incorporated this pride and made Jennifer tall and light skinned as well. Above all, Jennifer was intelligent, a woman whose mission in life was to defend the downtrodden and exploited. Normal height was crucial to the sense of personal agency Stacey experienced in this fantasy. She envied normal height above all and held steadfastly to the belief that one day she herself would grow, despite the fact that a doctor whom she had visited once (after looking him up in the yellow pages and going by taxi to his office with money she had begged from her grandfather) had told her this could not be.

Along with normal height, Jennifer's Native American origin was also very important in Stacey's eyes. Not only did it achieve a wished-for change in skin color, but also it allowed Stacey an alternative to a lineage peopled entirely by other imprisoned souls. Native Americans may be a minority group, she thought, but slaves they have never been. Freedom seemed implicit to Stacey in their original style of life.

To feed her fantasy, Stacey watched televsion and read the newspapers hoarded by her grandfather in piles around the house. Although in her fantasy Jennifer had a boyfriend, Stacey was not much interested in elaborating this romance. Instead she used news stories to develop cases in her head for Jennifer to argue in court. This routine taught her something about logical reasoning and allowed her to play with the thrill of winning. By imagining success and tasting in fantasy what it felt like to be a respected member of society, she was able to feel positively about herself. This positive sense of self stood in juxtaposition to the negative feelings she also carried inside.

Stacey also used her fantasy life to experiment with identity, as defined by race and class. This was a subject that interested her immensely, in part because it was a source of constant dissension at home. Her irritable, somewhat paranoid father thought that all white people were mean and criminal by "nature." Stacey passionately disagreed and feared, in fact, that blacks might be the ones who were more "naturally" unpleasant. Out of her conflicted interest in this subject, she created for Jennifer a set of half-siblings, each from a different ethnic background. Jennifer had various, not very well-delineated relationships with these brothers and sisters, but in the last analysis they had to be accepted, regardless of their ethnic origin and skin color, because they were "family" and family members were valuable to her. In this ingenious way Stacey contended with many issues raised for her by differences of all sorts.

Outside of fantasy, meanwhile, she learned as much as she could from watching the way her grandfather took charge. Unlike her father, he stayed at home, read the newspaper, talked to his grandchildren, and doled out the meager financial resources of the family. He went to the supermarket himself and made sure that there was enough to eat. In her dreams it was always he who questioned her anger and advised her to control it. With him she also attended to the comfort of her siblings; since their early lives together, she had always been the one to care for them. Although much in need of relief from the sad desperation of her life, Stacey's day-to-day existence, in fact, was remarkably reality bound.

Before I continue this story, before I describe the course traversed by Stacey and me over the nine years we saw one another, I want to address some questions about what it was within Stacey that guided her to the creation of her fantasy and, once created, what its dimensions were. These questions seem particularly salient now because of the rekindling of interest among psychoanalysts, especially those writing from a relational perspective, in the phenomenon of dissociation as a "normal" defense (Lampl-de groot, 1981; Bromberg, 1996); and in the observation that "normal" dissociation is accompanied by the existence, in all of us, of multiple self-states that appear in response to specific relationships (Davies, 1996a,b), developed with different people in different contexts. In this regard, Stacey's is a particularly interesting case, for the Jennifer-self she created went on being alongside other aspects of herself that she loved far less. The Jennifer-self, however, came *fully* into being only when Stacey put herself physically in a certain place, in the room at home in front of the broken t.v. In retrospect, then, Stacey seems an excellent example of a person who could consciously tolerate the internal existence of at least two rather robust self-states, one of which was carefully put out of mind, "dissociated," in circumstances in which the other came to the fore.

It is important to note here that Stacey's ability to create an alternative self in this way is not unusual. Others among the handicapped have done the same (Gleitman and Roth, 1978), as have people victimized in other ways (Herman, 1992). Novelists and playwrights also have been known to become the characters they create for short periods of time. If Stacey is unique in any way, it is perhaps that her fantasy emerged from a background of such utter deprivation. Indeed, how do we explain this young woman's ability to move from a stark, unstimulating reality, in which her growing self was subjected to much more negative than positive affirmation, to a reality in which a sustained experience of self-affirmation was achieved? What personal qualities seem to be required to construct the latter reality, and out of which experiences in her own life did they emerge? Her case may shed some light on the way in which normally dissociated self-states come into and go out of existence in us all.

PERSONAL QUALITIES

Stacey was physically attractive and had a pleasing disposition. In addition, she was unusually intelligent and had a gift for what E. J. Anthony (1987) calls "representational competence" (p. 22), the capacity to put thoughts into words. According to him, this kind of creativity can give a person the illusion of power. Finally, temperamentally Stacey was both energetic and strong. Thus, Stacey was genetically well endowed and, as is often true of those who survive desperation (Warner and Smith, 1992), others were attracted to her. This had been the case from her earliest days.

EXPERIENCE

Stacey had had a number of experiences, both positive and negative, which together seem to have determined the creation of her fantasy world.

Attention as the Favored Child

Not only did Stacey have a consistent support system, which tends to promote psychoimmunity (Anthony, 1987, p. 7), but for various extended periods in her life she had been the best loved child in her family. First, when Stacey was an infant, her mother had loved her best; then briefly her father's new girlfriend had; and finally her father had, during the period in which he chose her to bring celebrity to his family. "A man who has been the indisputable favorite of his mother," Freud (1925) has written, "keeps for life the feeling of a conqueror, that confidence of success that often induces real success" (p. 26). Presumably this truism holds for women as well. Brief as these periods were, Stacey knew what it felt like to be highly valued and the center of attention, "a jewel," as she put it "for everyone to see." Almost in spite of herself, she felt compelled to make this feeling a continuing part of her reality.

Shame

Stacey endured extreme experiences of shame in reponse to her circumstances. The pain of her response was obvious in the lowered gaze and hunched-over body posture she assumed as she talked about them. Experiences of shame and humiliation had first appeared early in Stacey's life and had continued to grow.[2]

Opportunity for Instruction in Frustration Tolerance

Because it was she who, early in life, had been the one to negotiate with her mother for food and care for herself and her sisters, she had learned to set impulsiveness aside, to assess others, and to keep trying; in fact, she had nurtured a kind of determination in this regard and was surprisingly self-disciplined in its pursuit. This specific resilience was apparent to me at first in the way she contended with homework assignments at school. For example, when she first came to the clinic, she had only the most rudimentary math skills; she was also unable to create a written paragraph. In spite of the pain these deficiencies caused her, she persisted, and in surprisingly little time, had mastered sufficient academic skills to pass the test to obtain a high school-equivalency diploma. When asked to explain the well-spring of her motivation, she said that it was a matter of life and death to her to end her dependence on her father and learn to depend on herself. She was sick to death of his despotic ways.

The Ideal of Being a Show Business Personality

Stacey came from a family in which there was a lively interest in show business, in which the stars of screen and stage, often seen on television, were discussed at great length. Their success was held up to her by her father as an alternative to the poverty and degradation of their daily lives. Stacey experienced this alternative as extremely compelling. It fit well with her intense need to be the center of attention.

Encouragement in the Creation of False Selves

In Stacey's family, pretense and bravado were positively valued; her father was always putting on airs to "meet the man," so to speak, or to "play the dozens" (Labov, 1978). Stacey herself was surprisingly practiced at pretending. Without conflict, she knowingly used this ability to secure for herself things she needed. Indeed, no ideal of a single, unified self existed anywhere in Stacey's family milieu; the contrary, in fact, was the case. Thus, in creating the Jennifer fantasy, Stacey had no internal resistances to overcome; no one told her that her fantasy was "crazy"; she did not therefore have to hide it from others. Stacey created Jennifer consciously, as a respectable way to gain relief from her life. In her words, "I let Jennifer come when I don't have to be me. I give all my troubles to her and her family. It's a relief because I get rid of my problems for a little while. I don't have to remember what it's like being small, living where I do, not having friends, not having all the things that I read about other kids having." Jennifer was an alternative self-state deliberately created by Stacey for relief and recreation.

No theory can yet explain the ways in which multiple self-states develop. In reviewing this concept, Jody Messler Davies (1996b) suggests that "multiplicity of ego states" represents "dynamically interacting representations of self in relation to the internalized significant others in childhood" (pp. 559–560). I have said that Stacey internalized some positive early experiences of herself in interaction with others, as the favorite child, as the organized, self-disciplined one. Together these positive experiences of self seemed to have emerged, in amalgamated form, in the representation of self-in-relation-to-others called Jennifer. Once created, Jennifer could then be used by Stacey to go beyond her original amalgamation. Through Jennifer, Stacey's remembered positive experiences could grow and change and be put to use to counteract other, more negative self-states, internalized experiences in relation to others, of shame, powerlessness, and rage.[3]

THERAPEUTIC CONTACT

As her therapist, I found work with Stacey compelling. Her intelligence, her liveliness and honesty, above all, her proclivity for metaphor and therefore for analytically oriented thinking, captivated me for some time. During the nine years of our relationship, we met twice a week for the first five, once a week thereafter. In her presence, I often had definite sensations. Often I felt gigantic, even sitting down. When we stood, I was inevitably aware of how much good-humored buzzing (smiling, humming, phrase-uttering) she did and how much this seemed to fill the space created by the difference in height between us. Later, as black and white differences came more to the fore, I became increasingly uncomfortable with my own presumptions as a white woman and with the way in which these seemed to locate my expectations of the world. I began to question myself about these presumptions more deeply than I had before. In fact, I had never worked with someone whose plight was as desperate as Stacey's in regard to the very basics of *physical*, no less psychological, survival. For example, there was, at one point, a gas leak in her building, while she was out, that knocked her sisters unconscious and killed her grandfather. Later, her father was shot in the eye and her half-brother killed during random shootouts between strangers; such incidents occurred regularly on her block. The backdrop against which Stacey and I worked, addressing fantasy and the unconscious, was full of very real perils of its own. Her dreams often reflected these dangers. Once, for example, she dreamt that she "walked into a store. Men came in and held up the store. I started running and they shot me." Another time: "I'm running down the street and being chased by a little boy with a toy. The moment he hits me, the toy turns into a hammer and he hits me and I fall unconscious in a pool of blood." We proceeded, nevertheless, interpreting not only the manifest content, but the less conscious meaning of these dreams, the sense of doom she experienced just below the surface. Indeed, her treatment was based to a great extent on these dreams, most of which I wrote down. They are the material from which I am writing this paper.

For the sake of clarity and relevance to the subject of this book, I have artificially organized Stacey's treatment into theme sequences, each theme relating to a different aspect of her body. She had very specific feelings about her height, her color, and her sexuality. Her relationships, with me and with other important figures in her life, were implicit within each set of feelings.

Stacey was mortified by her height. Poignantly she described the ways in which children she met treated her as though she were their age. "They pester me with questions," she said. "I so hate myself for being short." The stutter, in fact, seemed to come into existence in part out of the hope that she might be able, magically, to exchange it for normal height. "I would so much rather have a terrible stutter than be short," she said. "Every Sunday I go to church and pray to grow taller. I'd settle for four feet. God doesn't answer. I always figure He'll pick his own time."

When we first began seeing each other, she blamed her height for rejection of many kinds, especially for the rejection she experienced from the young male speech pathologist to whom she had been assigned at the hospital and on whom she had developed a crush that pained her. A fear of being unattractive as a female, shut out by other women from the terrain she imagined they occupied in their pursuit of men, for reasons that were not so clear, but that seemed to be related to the inadequacy of her physical self, surfaced in numerous dreams during this period. Here is one of those dreams:

> I went up to the hospital to see Mitzi [half-sister] and she was all dressed up. She was her usual self, staring at me and everybody else [Mitzi had inherited their father's stare, which scared Stacey] and she told me I could tag along. She was going someplace in the hospital. We went to a big room with two windows and I was looking through the windows. Yvonne [Mitzi's half-sister] looked nice. She had bangs and earrings and a green dress. You were there too in a black dress. You were standing in a group of men. Even Mitzi was there. I felt so sad. I was looking at everyone. When I woke up I was mad at Mitzi.

Negative feelings about her height started to recede very soon after we began working together. Within the first six months, during which she also made a great deal of progress toward obtaining her high school diploma, she was able to relinquish the long-held belief that one day she would grow. She gradually stopped going to church to pray for this. The Jennifer fantasies also began to recede at this juncture. Secretly, in fact, she came to like her size: "I am getting to like short more than tall," she told me at this point. This new conviction fit in with the belief that she was, as she said, a "jewel for all to see." Although she always believed that "tall people command respect," it began to occur to her that short people might also.

A more insidious kind of self-doubt seemed to take over at this point: she began to think of herself as seriously "deformed." She looked in the mirror at her arms and legs and saw them as "crooked" or misshapen. When men paid attention to her (as many did), she could not believe in the sincerity of their admiration. "Is it my size they are attracted to? Would I be a trophy, an oddity to them?"

She also did not have positive feelings about her sexuality. She had watched her mother be pushed around by various men, and this had frightened her. In addition, she had been given no information about sex when she was a child. Thus, when menstrual blood first appeared (when she was 12), she thought it was a sign of cancer, of which she was convinced she would die. This misinformation, which was finally corrected by her father's girlfriend at the time, left its mark on her already uncertain sense of the health of her own inner organs. Indeed, in retrospect, as I reread my notes, the idea of her deformity seemed to extend beyond her limbs to her sexuality and to become a shield of embarrassment that kept her from examining her feelings about her body in greater depth. In retrospect, I am not only sorry, but I do not know why I did not insist that we investigate this area more deeply.

Not surprisingly, contained within Stacey's feelings about her sexuality were her most intense ties to her parents; these feelings, in turn, were tied to her ambivalence about aggression. Sex with men scared her because it implied not only that her humiliating "deformity" would be revealed, but also that she would be forced into passive surrender; she would become bonded to a person on whom she would have to depend, the way her mother had on various men. This dependence horrified her. It was similar to what she perceived as her long dependence on her father.

Stacey's feelings about her father were more complex than those about her mother. He appeared occasionally in her dreams in veiled sexual relationship with her, dreams she reported with the utmost embarrassment and shame. As her model of masculinity, he repelled her. He bullied her and her siblings every day and wore an expression on his face that was appallingly unattractive. Although her will toward independence from him was the motive for all her actions, the energy required to sustain it is testament to the difficulty she had in separating from him. Propelled into action by the intensity of her feelings on this subject, one day, soon after she began with me, she impulsively hit her father back as he meted out the slaps he regularly aimed at her. A fight erupted and, to her surprise, she emerged victorious: she had punched him so hard that he withdrew in terror. This was a turning point of huge proportions for Stacey. After that, although her father threatened her, he no longer expected that she would do as he said. A more immediate side effect was evident in her school work: her reading scores advanced two grades!

Despite her ability to overcome her own passivity in regard to her father and fight him back, her fear of and adversion to men continued. For a time, dreams about having sex with her father were replaced with some explicitly homosexual dreams. In some of these dreams, whiteness and her relationship with me seemed implicit. Here are two of those dreams:

> I come in and am sitting on a long flat couch. You are there and so is Bianca [a light-skinned acquaintance]. She says, "Come, Barbara, let's show her how its done." You get up and come together. I am not shocked, not surprised. It's like looking at a ballet, Alvin Ailey, people coming together beautifully. After you were finished you said, "That's how its done" and smiled at me. I smiled back.

> I see myself on a ship. The wind is blowing very strong and I'm totally in control. I meet this girl, white, good looking. We come into a deep and meaningful relationship. She teaches me about me, and I'm not afraid of it. I understand myself between the times I am with her. There are no demands, no ties. I am free and honest. But other people in the dream are taunting us. Then the relationship becomes embarrassing and repulsive.

To some extent we explored the sexual aspects of her feelings for me in regard to their meaning as a way to get closer to me and to the qualities—the freedom, respect, self-knowledge—she so deeply wished for. But when it came to sex, Stacey was very inhibited. She forbade herself any deep exploration of the subject, either in her body or in her mind, and, sorry to say, I did not push her. In her relationship to me, instead, skin color and its implications came to play an increasingly important part as we proceeded. This was apparent in dreams about competition with me and achievement in general.

Stacey's feelings about skin color were perhaps the best barometer of the changes she experienced in self-esteem during the years we met. At first she was convinced that no black woman could be beautiful. She picked apart black women she knew, feature by feature. She hated the looks of Mitzi, her half-sister, whose resemblance to their father frightened her. She connected their similar looks (including their blackness) with their nastiness and, even though she did not look like them, worried that, if she were nasty to anyone, she would "get into a pattern of nastiness like them" and get "ugly" in other ways too.

Gradually, however, these feelings began to give way to others. She would report, "I have days when I feel black and want to wear an Afro and make the power sign to the black brothers on the block. But deep in my heart I can't hate whitey and I wonder about that." Her family milieu required at least a minimum of skepticism about white people. Thus, implicit in her relationship with me, was much ambivalence about my whiteness. In the beginning, I was more attractive because I was white than I might have been had I been black. But, as time advanced and she got closer to achieving her goals (which included earning a college diploma and getting a good job), whiteness took on qualities that frightened her; and I, as the white person she knew best, became less and less attractive. Her dreams were loaded with imagery in which racial feelings were apparent. Here are some examples:

> I'm at what looks like the North Pole. Its snowing, blizzarding. I'm walking and falling in the snow. I get up and am trying to find you. Finally I find you and you say, "See Stacey, it's not so hard." But it is!

> I died and went to heaven and this nice, sweet man came to take me to my destination place. I said I wasn't going. Then Father Time came and asked to check my time. They found it wasn't my time so they had to take me back. But they had cremated my body. They had to find me one. There were only white ones. I was very picky. I settled for this person who was successful, brilliant, and rich. When they put me in it I didn't like it and wanted to get out. But they told me I had to stay in it. It was so boring! I had to do the same thing every day, so they told me they were going to take my memory away. I wouldn't remember anything. As my memory was going, I was screaming, "No,no, not yet!"

As we talked about these dreams, it became clear that the white world was connected in her mind with achievement (money, power), but also wtih coldness, isolation, boredom, repetitition, and obliteration of her past. Each of these issues had to be discussed.

By this time, well into her treatment, the retreat into fantasy had all but disappeared. Jennifer had been gradually abandoned as Stacey had less and less time for her and was herself feeling more satisfaction in the "real" world. It seemed that Stacey had been unable to preserve or elaborate on the proclivity to use fantasy in this way, and, perhaps partly as a result, she was feeling bereft of some of the high points of her previous existence. She may have blamed my whiteness, my achievement-organized values for her loss. Dreams of all sorts in relation to me appeared at this point. In some we were friends; in others, competitors. In some, I was beckoning her to a fate that required submission to me. In some, our paths were separated and she was going off to a life of desperation. Her dependence on me had became an issue for her, one on which we worked for some time. Meanwhile she had graduated from college and won a prize (for high achievement against great odds) and had been accepted at a graduate school in another city. She turned this offer down in order to remain near her sisters and to work in an administrative capacity at a university.

The final period of our time together centered on Stacey's feelings about herself in the world of work. She read a book called *Drylongso* (Gwaltney, 1980) about the attitudes of black people toward whites and was feeling intensely that she was somehow not like other black people in her attitudes. During this time, however, she was habitually late to work and, consequently had been accused by her fellow workers of being an example of a person who lived by "colored peoples' time." This accusation infuriated her. Needless to say, she stopped coming late, but the wish to end her appointments with me seemed to accelerate. In retrospect, I can see that she thought her feelings for me kept her from being able to identify fully with the fate of black people. Be that as it may, soon after she graduated from college she announced that she felt that "pieces of me are breaking away and I have to stand up for myself. It's scary, but I have to. I'm sprouting my wings. Time is my enemy. When I'm afraid, time just stops. I don't plan anything or do anything about my schedule or my social life. I just fill up my life with appointments with you and other people. I need more of a life than that."

As I explored with her what she meant when she said that "pieces" of herself were breaking away, it seemed that she felt more unified inside. And so she became, I believe.

Last year, after a break of 15 years or more, I called Stacey to ask permission to write about her. I learned that she had just applied, and been accepted, for a course of professional training in a field that had always been of interest to her; she had spent the last 10 years working in one city office after another, usually, I think, as a secretary. Sadly, she has never established a primary relationship with anyone. Although she lives alone, she is in constant communication with her sisters and with the now grown children of Mitzi. As for fantasy, when I mentioned Jennifer, she did not remember much about who Jennifer was! She still reads a good deal and talks to herself when she has problems, she said, but there is not a fantasy world to which she retreats. Now in her mid-40s, she said her life has been hard, but not without rewards.

CONCLUSION

In summary, in these pages I have described Stacey, a "short" black woman, who located her self-hatred in her physical characteristics, which she detested for years. Locked up by her father for much of her early life, she regularly put her considerable gifts to use by transforming herself, in fantasy, into Jennifer, a self-respecting woman of normal height and normal opportunity. Stacey then used this parallel self to practice the skills of living. In this way, she experienced the world as she imagined other, more privileged people might.

Stacey is a woman who possesses the capacity to create, and then use, a parallel self. As others before me have observed (Herman, 1992; Warner and Smith, 1992), this capacity is a life-preserving one. Those who have it have at their disposal a powerful adaptive resource. This is perhaps especially the case when, as was true of Stacey, the parallel self-state, first created as a means of escape from particular daily events, becomes a consciously invoked vehicle used for *self-enhancing* self-preservation. Stacey came to use Jennifer to locate her own interests and gifts in ways that she could then enlarge on and expand. In sharp contrast to alternate self-states that appear to be disconnected from one another and cannot be consciously recalled, recorded markers of time and space were defining aspects of Stacey's parallel self-state, built in to the "person" Jennifer became. Thus Stacey was able to use all of what Jennifer learned.

What is the fate of the ability to create in this way, once the creating person is removed from the conditions in which it first appears? Why, in some people, does this ability seem to become permanently affirmed, become a part of self that is pleasurably exercised again and again in, for example, the creation of fiction, whereas in others it gets pushed aside?. Here, I think of Hannah Green (1964), who recorded her own retreat into fantasy and her analysis of it with Frieda Fromm-Reichmann in her novel *I Never Promised You A Rose Garden* and then went on to write many other books. Do the circumstances in which the original fantasy creation appears badly color the capacity to create itself, in some people, so that they cannot make use of it, once its life saving aspects are no longer necessary to them? Is it that other abilities, beyond the basic ability to create, the abililty to discipline the talent, for example, to rewrite again and again, are required, if the original talent itself is to bear fruit? Finally, how much responsibility does the therapist bear for the encouragement of such talent, and how should this be done? I raise this question because, beyond minimal encouragement to "write some of your life history down," I did not directly attempt to encourage Stacey's development as a creator of fiction. Encouragement, I think, has a large impact on budding abilities, perhaps especially when the therapist does the encouraging (see, for example, Bader, 1997). Although historically many analysts have thought encouragement of this sort unconscionable in analytic work (see, Aron's, 1996, discussion of Etchegoyen, p. 95), in retrospect I wonder what kind of disservice to Stacey it might have been to have been inactive in this regard.

As much as I rue not having explored and encouraged her creative talent more deeply, I regret that I did not work harder with Stacey on another, perhaps related, aspect of her creativity, her sexuality. Unlike men, women in our culture, as Ethel Spector Person (1980) has pointed out, can live relatively "normal" lives with almost no sexual experience, even masturbation, even in fantasy. Stacey, I surmise, has become one of those without; beyond one short-lived, intense romantic fantasy (her crush on her speech therapist), which ended when she decided it gave him more power over her than she liked, Stacey had no elaborated romantic fantasy at all during the time I knew her. Her homosexual dreams embarrassed her to such a degree that they too were eventually shelved and sexual attachment to women eschewed as a subject she allowed herself to think about. Finally, in our most recent conversation, my tentative queries on this subject were answered in the negative. I regret not having pursued discussion of this area with her more intensely. Were she to see me now, I hope we might do better.

NOTES

[1]I can find no reference to this disorder in the sources I have consulted. I do, however, remember looking it up, some years ago, when Stacey first told me about it, and finding a reference to it somewhere. Whether I have misspelled it in the years since then, or it is no longer mentioned in the books I have consulted (which are relatively "popular" medical guides, a large number of them, in fact, found in local libraries and book stores), I do not know. For the sake of this chapter, it seems sufficient to say that Stacey suffered from a genetic disorder that affected her height but otherwise did not seem to be deforming.

²Shame, according to Alan Schore (1991), first emerges in relationship to the mother as "an inhibitor of hyper-aroused states, in the early separation-individuation phase . . . specifically from 12 to 18 months." It reflects "a sudden shift from sympathetic-dominant to parasympathetic-dominant autonomic nervous system activity. Crucially important to "the resolution of the rapprochment crisis and the genesis of the ego ideal" (pp. 187–188), it continues to grow to greater and lesser degrees, depending on the child's environment.

In Stacey's case, the opportunity for growth had been large and the concommitant wish to escape it large as well. Shameful feelings pressed her hard from within to find a respectable escape.

³There are great differences between multiple self *states* and multiple personality disorder, or dissociative identity disorder (DIS), as this is now called (American Psychiatric Association, 1994). A great deal of controversy has recently developed around this subject and seems to center on the question of whether MPD or DIS exists at all and if so, how to diagnose it. In differentiating between multiple self-states and DIS, Davies (1996a) is again helpful: "True multiple personality disorder . . . is, in fact, a foreclosure of multiplicity: [the latter seems to be] a linear series of separate lives, sequentially lived, in which *awareness* of their dynamic interplay collapses into a scotomatous narrowing of consciousness" (p. 566, italics added).

According to psychiatrist Colon Ross (1995), this narrowing occurs because people who suffer from DIS have inserted "an amnesia barrier" between themselves and their "newly created identity" so that the traumatic abuse they have suffered (often the instigator of DIS, in the first place) can appear not to have happened to them (p. 67).

Thus, it is reasonable to suppose that DIS is an escape mechanism that evolves in some individuals when they have endured overwhelming trauma, trauma that, probably for many reasons, is not, or cannot be, preserved in memory with the markers of time and place necessary for coherent, integrated biography (Olds and Cooper, 1997).

Stacey did not seem to have experienced trauma to this degree. On the contrary, the traumatic aspects of her life seemed to make her all the more anxious to keep ordinary markers of time and place intact, in order to mitigate the potential threat they posed of keeping her from living a decent life.

REFERENCES

American Psychiatric Association (1994), *Diagnostic and Statistical Manual* 4th ed. Washington, DC: American Psychiatric Association.
Anthony, E. J. (1987), Risk, vulnerability, and resilience: An overview. In: *The Invulnerable Child*, ed. E. J. Anthony & B. J. Cohler. New York: Guilford, pp. 3–48.
Aron, L. (1996), *A Meeting of Minds*. Hillsdale, NJ: The Analytic Press.
Bader, M. J. (1997), Altruistic love in psychoanalysis: Opportunities and resistance. *Psychoanal. Dial.*, 6:741–764.

Bromberg, P. M. (1996), Standing in the spaces: The multiplicity of self and the psychoanalytic relationship. *Contemp. Psychoanal.*, 32:509–535.

Davies, J. M. (1996a), Dissociation, repression and reality testing in the countertransference: The controversy over memory and false memory in the psychoanalytic treatment of adult survivors of childhood sexual abuse. *Psychoanal. Dial.*, 6:189–218.

——— (1996 b), Linking the "pre-analytic" with the postclassical: Integration, dissociation, and the multiplicity of unconscious process. *Contemp. Psychoanal.*, 32:553–576.

Freud, S. (1926), Inhibitions, symptoms and anxiety. *Standard Edition*, 20:1–70. London: Hogarth Press, 1959.

Gleitman, J. & Roth, W. (1978), *The Unexpected Minority.* New York: Harcourt Brace Jovanovich.

Gwaltney, J. L. (1980), *Drylongso.* New York: Random House.

Green, H. (1964), *I Never Promised You a Rose Garden.* New York: Holt, Rinehart, Winston.

Herman, J. L. (1992), *Trauma and Recovery.* New York: Basic Books.

Jetter, A. (1995), The Roseanne of literature. *New York Times, Magazine Section*, Dec. 17, pp. 54–57.

Labov, W. (1971), The logic of nonstandard English. In: *The Language of Poverty*, ed. F. Williams. Chicago: Markum, pp. 153–189.

Lampl-de Groot, J. (1981), Notes on multiple personality. *Psychoanal. Quart.* 50:614–624.

Olds, D. & Cooper, A. (1997), Dialogue with other sciences: Opportunities for mutual gain. *Internat. J. Psycho-Anal.*, 78:219–225.

Person, E. S. (1980), Sexuality as the mainstay of identity. In: *Women, Sex, and Sexuality*, ed. C. R. Stimpson & E. S. Person. Chicago: Chicago University Press, pp. 36–61.

Ross, C. A. (1995), The validity and reliability of dissociative identity disorder. In: *Dissociative Identity Disorder*, ed. L. Cohen, J. Berzoff & M. Elin. Northvale, NJ: Aronson, pp. 65–84.

Schore, A. N. (1991), Early superego development: The emergence of shame and narcissistic affect regulation in the practicing period. *Pschoanal. Contemp. Thought*, 14:187–250.

Warner, E. E. & Smith, R. S. (1992), *Overcoming the Odds.* Ithaca, NY: Cornell University Press.

8

BREAST CANCER
IN THE ANALYST

Body Lessons

Barbara Pizer

> A woman's breasts bear the paradoxical burden of being esthetic organs. They are modified sweat glands that secrete what is essentially enriched sweat, a lactational charge without which the human race, until very recently, could not have survived. At the same time breasts in Western culture have long been considered the paired centerpieces of female erotic beauty, a woman's 'natural jewels,' in the words of the culture critic Anne Hollander, and the things that make men "stupid" as the humorist Dave Barry has put it. Imagine if the pancreas had to be pretty while releasing insulin. Or, just for fun, imagine if fashion and female taste dictated the display of a man's reproductive organs through a bit of pelvic decolletage [Angier, 1997, p. 4].

When the Editors asked if I would provide a chapter for this book, I felt flattered and excited by the invitation. At the same time, I was fairly sure that they were not aware of my abiding interest in the mind–body relationship, and so my immediate question was, "Why me?" They told me that they considered a paper I had written about illness

I gratefully acknowledge my husband, Stuart, my daughter, Andrea, and Dr. T, each of whom contributed lovingly to the subject and substance of this chapter.

191

in the analyst (Pizer, 1997) to be a valuable contribution to their subject. So it was *my body* I was being asked implicitly to write about— my body in relation to my patients' *bodies*, during (and after) my illness. But in the context of a chapter for this book, "illness" becomes a euphemism for Breast Cancer; that is, my earlier exploration of an analyst's illness as an impingement on the treatment situation needed here to be unpacked in terms of a more explicit examination of my breast. (Yikes!) The editors were inviting me to talk in more detail about an organ that patients and therapists don't usually refer to in relation to each other—aside from the more experience-distant phantasms of Kleinian metapsychology. I felt asked to draw attention to my breasts. How fraught this is for a woman analyst. To my knowledge, few analysts, (Ehrenberg, 1995, is a notable exception) have written about their patients' explicit references to their breasts as objects of notice and interest. It's my impression that patients don't readily speak about the esthetic presence of their therapists' breasts. And while they may voice their dread of losing their analyst/breast, they do not ordinarily express the threat of losing their analyst's breast.

Although my earlier paper takes up the issue of how and when I spoke about my illness and the loss of my breast, its primary focus is on the analyst's disclosures—not only in illness, but in a broader and more general context. I wrote the piece during my summer break in 1995, just one year after receiving the startling diagnosis of breast cancer. The writing process forced me to revisit the eclipsed vacation of the previous year. It was motivated by three personal urgencies.

First, having retreated in the 80s from my characteristically open, interactional, and experimental perspective with patients (as I recoiled from the string of revelations concerning respected analytic guides and idols who abused the relational elements of analysis), I found myself gradually returning to my more naturally inclined clinical stance of active engagement. But now, in my return, I wanted to find and set down, if not a "technique," a standard or framework outside of the clinical moment to which an analyst might refer as she considers how she feels urged to use herself in a therapeutic interaction. My own particular investment in carefully conceptualizing such issues as self-disclosure is born of the conviction that the mental discipline inherent in using a systematic approach (despite its inevitable shortcomings) serves the function of "checks and balances" on the necessarily intuitive and authentic responsiveness of the analyst immersed in the current of a clinical moment. And I believe that, as the analyst further introduces the relational use of body cues (her own or her patient's) into the clinical discourse, disclosures need to be as grounded as possible in self-awareness as well as an orienting conceptual framework.

Second, I felt the need to chronicle for myself, as well as begin to share with colleagues, some of my recent experience of working with patients while dealing with a life-threatening, body-altering illness. I was eager to contribute to the opening of the subject of what is, and what is not, speakable in the clinical situation; to draw attention to the analyst's owning and respecting what she herself can or cannot bear to say before defaulting to thoughts about what she thinks may or may not be useful for her patients to hear.

And, third, perhaps most deeply motivating, I wanted to write a memorial for my mother, whose death I had, until then, been unable to grieve fully. In matters of the body and the heart, my mother had been unusually reserved and nondisclosing. Ironically, it was not until Alzheimer's, with all its accompanying terrors, began to loosen her fine mind that she was able to speak with me about the details of her growing up and how she had experienced herself back then as well as now. In a small window of time, my mother and I were deeply in touch with one another, allowing me to appreciate more realistically both who she was and who she could not be for me in my own development. Although they were tantalizingly brief, I believe these few years of closeness did make it easier for me to embrace my own independence, to let her go—in some ways sealing many of my convictions about the value of the relational school in psychoanalysis.

So, even though my focus in this chapter is on relational perspectives on the body in psychoanalysis rather than self-disclosure, it has become obvious to me—as when I was asked to write about the feelings in my body and how the loss of my breast affected my feelings about myself, my patients' bodies, and their feelings about mine— that there is, indeed, an overlap of subjects.

I begin here where my earlier paper began, in the midst of those particular conditions that prevail "When the Analyst is Ill" (Pizer, 1997). Now, two years later, I can illustrate, through personal anecdote and clinical vignette, the changing relationships between me and my body, and the existing or potential mind–body relationship between myself and others. After a brief exploration of body as metaphor for mind, cancer as metaphor for death, I integrate these phenomena, through a description of a few of the ways in which I believe my heightened body awareness contributes to the development of my analytic self and, it is to be hoped, the selves of my analytic partners.

LIFE EVENTS AND THE PERSON OF THE ANALYST: INESCAPABLE IMPACTS ON THE ANALYTIC PROCESS

In my earlier article (Pizer, 1997), I described the personal circumstances under which, as an analyst, I judged the clinical necessity for inescapable self-disclosure to my patients. Specifically, in the last days of May 1994, four weeks prior to my annual vacation month, a routine mammogram revealed a startling abnormality. With little notice, I would begin my vacation a few weeks earlier to undergo a lumpectomy on June 15 and, subsequent to the pathology report, a mastectomy in July. I would return to work at the end, rather than at the beginning, of August. Chemotherapy began in September of that year and was administered every three weeks for six months. I arranged to have my chemo on Friday afternoons so that the worst of the side effects would abate by Monday, when I would be back at work. I rearranged my patient schedule to accommodate one to two hours in the middle of each weekday for rest and meditation. Other than a radical change of hairstyle (very short; I never lost it all) and four unanticipated days out of the office due to a need for a blood transfusion, there were no major disruptions of my schedule. I cannot say the same for the process and content of the work itself. Perhaps my patients would call the term disruption an understatement. I told them all I had breast cancer.

I experienced this self-disclosure as inescapable. I define inescapable self-disclosure as the analyst's action resulting from the presence in the treatment situation of a circumstantial event whose disruptive properties *in the mind of the analyst* can be handled only by verbal acknowledgment. More simply stated, it is the "elephant in the room" phenomenon.

The circumstantial event may originate in the life of the analyst (e.g., a fire or an illness, or the death of a loved one) or in the patient, as in the case of Donald (S. Pizer, 1992), in which the therapist felt it necessary to say that he was distracted by the effort to tolerate his patient's body odor (an instance of the body achnowledged in the analytic session).

The elements of time and choice distinguish inescapable self-disclosure from inadvertent and deliberate self-disclosure. In contrast to inadvertent self-disclosure, inescapable self-disclosure allows the analyst time to consider what he or she feels must inevitably be said. And, in contrast to deliberate self-disclosure, in inescapable self-disclosure the analyst's subjective choice of what and how much must be said is dictated by a particular obtrusive circumstance rather than by the intrinsic clinical process. To emphasize, the omnipresent threat of disruption is most often the thundercloud contained within an inescapable disclosure. In other words, along with the analyst's awareness of the necessity for some kind of disclosure is the concomitant awareness and dread of a subsequent eruption in the analytic interaction.

I emphatically believe that the degree and manner of a self-disclosure by any analyst is, and must always be, inextricably linked to that analyst's conscious and unconscious dynamics.[1] Participation through self-exposure, to whatever degree and whatever the content, is necessarily determined not only by the analyst's technical framework but also by her personal boundaries, beliefs, and sense of comfort. For example, Abend (1982) describes how, on his return to work after a serious illness, he overrode his determination not to disclose. Responding to persistent inquiries, he did disclose his illness to several patients. Abend then reports his subsequent second thoughts about these disclosures: retrospectively he regarded them as being unnecessary distractions from the transference implications of his patients' inquiries (see also Dewald, 1982). Many analysts locate their comfort in, and advocate, keeping their private selves at a distance from the analytic discourse.

Yet another position was bravely taken and bravely reported by Amy Morrison (1997), a clinical social worker well known in the therapeutic and analytic community around Boston. She continued to see her patients as her own health declined unto death from breast cancer. She described how she carefully, selectively, tactfully, and responsibly discussed the reality of her illness with *some* of her patients. Not every therapist with breast cancer would make the personal choice to disclose her condition to her patients. *Nor should she.* Among the many private issues one may or may not choose to share with a patient, cancer is an intensely personal matter. And a matter of this magnitude—with a course both invisible and invasive, with an outcome at best unpredictable and at worst leading to death—may certainly plunge the person of the analyst into a state of uncertainty or anxiety, even terror. While the analyst's awareness of uncertainty or anxiety will most likely be communicated to her patients, these raw states—as states in themselves—are problematic when either denied or directly "bled" out into the room. The analyst must find some words to explain and contain these affects, although not necessarily in concrete informational form. For both persons, the stark exposure of the analyst's anxiety surges—specifically about her cancer—can be a mutually destabilizing force that undermines the analytic process in

a variety of ways (e.g., the patient may flee, deny his senses, or attempt to take care of his analyst). Thus, each analyst must remain
attentive and connected to her own sense of how stable she can remain in the face of her uncertainties, how grounded and prepared
she is to deal with whatever surprises of affect or inquiry may arise.
My own choice to disclose my illness to patients grows out of who I
am as a person and who I am as a practicing clinician.

My Awareness of Self in Self-Disclosing

At the most conscious level, I felt a sense of responsibility to disclose—to give my patients maximal opportunity to process and plan
in the face of an unwanted, unpredictable situation; to think about a
referral, a consultation, an interruption; to express a variety of feelings at a time when I felt whole, strong, calm, and surprisingly capable. (This management style is characteristic of my emergency
mode.) I hasten to add that this sense of responsibility, this sense of
wanting to let my patients in on the beginning in order to maximize
their choices of action, does not originate in an abstract principle of
how one "ought to behave." I have an aversion to out-of-control surprises. When I was a young child, my sister and I were walking home
with my mother late one winter night when suddenly she compelled
us to run ahead of her. "Run ahead children, *run ahead!*" My mother
was unbelievably private about her person and inexpressive in general. It was not usual for her to raise her voice; we had never seen her
cry. Now, without warning or explanation, she was pushing us away
from the comforting presence of her body, shoving us forward into
the dark. And then, through the darkness I heard these intense, gut-
tural, wracking sounds and an inexplicable splatter. I felt certain that
my mother was being cut apart and bleeding. Rooted to the spot on
the sidewalk to which we had been commanded—too far away from
my mother—I stamped my feet and wailed through the blackness:
"Mommy's dying, Mommy's dying!" "Barbara," said my elder sister,
who managed upsets with disdain, "Mother is throwing up." (Following this event, our mother took us home and happily informed us
over cocoa and cookies that we were going to have a new baby.)

Despite the stresses and shocks of growing up, I am by nature a
hopeful person. When the toxicity of chemo did indeed cause cells to
die and I did indeed feel as though my life were ebbing away, I nevertheless did not expect to die at this particular time. Further, I did not
experience myself as a person who is preoccupied with death. I am

more afraid of not fully living in the moment than I am of dying. (I used to say I am much more afraid of throwing-up than of dying, but chemo has cured me of that fear!) There are those who have told me that they have benefited from my "courage"—although "courage" is not my felt experience. If courage is the operative word, then I resonate with it in terms of what for me may be the tributaries of courage: faith and discipline—happily augmented by loving support, all of which were available to me before the event of cancer. I believe that throughout my illness I could say to myself that I have never felt so sick and so well at the same time.

The more neurotic components of my awareness involved shame, embarrassment, and guilt. (Therapists and mothers betray their contracts when they draw attention to themselves.) Although I would certainly not deny needs for sympathy (see Renik, 1993), I sense that my guilt was the stronger affect. This may have operated in favor of the work; that is to say, when I received sympathy, I was—along with my gratitude—hyperalert to what might lie beneath or alongside of it. I was anxious, perhaps overanxious, to do the analytic job. I recognized all too well that whatever else my patients and I would be able to make of my inescapable self-disclosure, cancer was—and is—an invasion into our interaction.

At the same time, issues of life and death, change, loss, grief lie at the center of human experience and growth; and I took hope in the belief that my patients and I could put this inescapable event to analytic use. Today, I would include the body in that critical list. Life, change, loss, grief, and death begin and end in the body—the visible and palpable container of these phenomena. Life, change, loss, and grief are not disembodied abstractions (although our fashion icons, with their derealized shapes and poses, and our more specific professional culture, with its speech practices of "psychologese," may seem—or seek—to belie this). After all, it is the *body* that actually lives or dies or changes through excitement, exercise, growth, aging, illness, or decline. Loss and grief, when some*body* is missed, are housed in our body and often take over the house. In Lacanian terms, our body experience locates us in the register of the Real, which our words and our dialogues can never entirely grasp. Perhaps it is because the body, one's corporeal house of spirit and desire, is so powerful, so dangerous, that we tend to inhibit access to its messages. The admission of cancer into analytic discourse has sharpened my awareness of a particular irony: we are somehow bred to steer away from critically important discussions about the processes of dying, especially when they involve the inevitable deterioration (developmentally "normal," as well as pathological) and ultimate loss of one's bodily states and functions.

The circumstantial unfolding of more open conversation between me and my patients has led me to wonder about how we, as analysts, participate in three interlocking taboos on discourse: taboos concerning matters of the body, sensuality, and death.[2] Of course, the intimate environment of the consulting room, along with the power inequities inherent in the analytic setup, requires the analyst's mindfulness of how and how much her visceral responses and experiences are offered into dialogue. Nevertheless, it is worthwhile to continue to think about the ways in which we hinder or facilitate our patients' revelations about the body and related matters. How many analysts, like McLaughlin (1987, 1991, 1995), focus beyond the verbal interchange to include the messages conveyed by bodily gestures and states? And how many analytic therapists, like Jane Burka (1996), explicitly invite patients to consider the shape and weight of their therapist's body as a source of unconscious fantasy and transference? Do we automatically assume that conversation about clothing (ours or the patient's) is a diversion from the task at hand? Do we allow ourselves to be aware that we may dress in certain ways for particular patients and use this information as data for personal reflection and countertransference analysis? Do we feel more comfortable *behind* the couch? What is the cost and benefit of a "poker face" in a particular clinical instance? Do we take note of how it is that most of us unwittingly adhere to the unwritten rule against display of family pictures (visible evidence of loving attachment), so common in physician's offices? Legitimate reasons for this practice notwithstanding, we do need to consider how we contribute to promoting the myth—or wish—that we have sprung from the head of Zeus, fully formed, detached from earthly processes like birth and death.

I cannot tell to what extent my invitation to patients to consider with me the impact of a life-threatening, body-compromising illness influenced them to disclose related issues of their own. Interestingly, some patients expressed more concern about having to deal with the potential loss of my hair from chemo than with the surgery itself. The issue of their fear of my hair loss—whether they preferred to see me in a wig or with a scarf wrapped around my head—became a speakable topic of discussion. On one hand, hair loss may be easier to talk about than breast loss; on the other hand, it comes closer to the changes and losses we all experience, but hesitate to talk about, in the aging process.[3] Today, with many of my women patients (and one male patient), we consider together the grief and loss experienced in the gradual sagging and drying up of tissue and skin, the shock of seeing one's aging face reflected in a shop window—an image so discrepant with one's internal sense of self.

I believe that these inevitable, concrete body experiences of change, loss, and felt betrayal are critical issues to be recognized and addressed in the clinical setting. Not surprisingly, we tend to feel shy about inviting them into discourse. It is worth noting that the social taboo on body talk that refers to actual functions experienced in and by the body finds an outlet in the myriad ways we engage in "body talk" as *metaphor for mind*. Surprise, for example, may be expressed as, "She threw me for a loop," or disdain as, "He holds me at arm's length," or distrust as, "Something smells fishy," or felt intimacy as "I'm touched." Then there are those metaphors for mind accepted in polite company perhaps because they aptly illustrate matters *in the mind*. From more innocent metaphors like "father hunger" and "love starved," we move to such expressions as "verbal diarrhea" and "mind fuck."

Then there are those real bodily events occurring in life that can become, over time, what I call *signal metaphors,* metaphors that bridge physical and psychic reality. Take my aversion to "out-of-control surprises," for example. For me, they hook up to a body event named "throw-up." Of course, aversive to us all, "throw-up" in my mind understandably became a metaphor that releases a primary fear of abandonment as well as shame over the spilling out of inner contents. For others, more than for me, the loss of limb or organ evokes the notion of "mutilation" as a metaphor more all-encompassing than the terrible reality itself. I have found that, in my practice, physically intact people who have endured childhoods of psychic invasion and impingement talk about their fear of death in imagery of bloody collision or crash—they picture their last moments in terms of bodies punctured, lacerated or mashed. Conversely, I note another group of people, who grew up fitting themselves into an assigned parental role, whose death fears share a common metaphor: an almost phobic terror of being "buried alive."

Consistent with the unexamined acceptance of bodily images as metaphors of mind, cancer still remains a metaphor for shamefulness and death (see Sontag, 1978), a word to be whispered or avoided. When my cancer was first diagnosed, a sympathetic relative called to inquire—amid embarrassed pauses—about my "condition"; another called to tell me how sorry she was to hear about "my problem." "I don't *have* a *problem*," I retorted in rebellion, "I have *breast cancer*."

In time, most patients were able to share with me their genuine

concern for me *and* for themselves. "What if you die before I'm done?"
"If you die, I'll never be able to do this again"; we could *talk* about
these things. Or perhaps I should say we could allow *some* aspects of
concern to surface into dialogue. A number of patients initially kept
my self-disclosure to themselves: "If people find out, it will ruin your
practice!" In doing so, these patients denied themselves the comfort
they might have received from friends. Indeed, some patients (I can
never know how many) denied themselves the opportunity to fully
share *with me* all their responses to my self-disclosure as long as they
considered me "too sick" to tolerate the depth of their fears about
the cancer or their disappointments over how I handled our freighted
relational space.

One analysand, who recently reminisced with me during a visit
two years after termination, offered this example. Although we had
both worked hard to explore the myriad ways in which my illness
had invaded and scarred the final phase of her successful analysis,
we both had been left with a sense of something unspoken, or unspeakable. And now, to my surprise, she found the words I would
never have imagined! For her, in this period of *her* leave taking, she
felt deprived of the person she had come to know before the cancer.
Together we had grown her up, and now she found me insufficiently
sharing my own bodily concerns or sufferings—she felt that I kept
too tightly in control; she felt suddenly "infantilized," "shut out" of a
more adult mutuality of exchange. I remember that, as I began chemotherapy treatments, I had indeed sensed her urgent need for more
contact with my experience, more responsiveness to her wish to offer "help"; and I remember the wince of guilt that reverberated through
my analyst-self when at last I said to her that, if she so keenly wanted
to do something for me, I would be grateful if she could find me some
eye-catching earrings (to divert attention from my short and thinning
hair style). And now she reports that particular connection between
us to have been one of the most relieving and comforting experiences
in our final year. In her experience of my cancer, this competent and
loving woman had felt essentially "helpless," "useless." In her words,
"For the first time in this marvelous space we had created, I now felt
somewhat silenced."

Without a doubt, it seems to me, cancer is an unavoidable blight
on dialogue.[4] Both in and out of the consulting room we have to come
to terms with that and do the best we can to listen and remain open.
I have learned that, for some patients, my illness was not merely a
matter of whether I would die sooner than other therapists. Some
patients harbored a deep fear that I was already terminally contami-

nated by a rampant proliferation of nasty internal activity. I remember certain ineffable experiences among my colleagues as well. During professional gatherings, there were those who would ordinarily come up to me and chat—and now they cut a wide berth around where I stood. One woman colleague—to this day—will not relate to me beyond a glancing, courteous smile. I wonder if I make more of this than I should or if I offended her in some other way; I run through the possibilities in my head; but I also cannot bring myself to approach her and inquire. It is indeed as if I had contaminated myself! Another woman has, after considerable time, come to tell me explicitly, "I just *could not* talk to you; I was much too upset about your illness."

A HISTORY OF MY BREAST

In the final paragraphs of Natalie Angier's (1977) review of Yalom's *A History of the Breast,* she writes:

> Only in recent years have women begun to claim their breasts as their own, as they did in the 1960's and 70's by dispensing with bras altogether, or by declaring, as some women do now, that breast-feeding can be a sensual pleasure. Women can also find a distinctive humor in breasts, one that has nothing to do with the kind of adolescent humor found in Playboy cartoons. . . .
>
> This exhilarating burst of female takes on the breast underscores what is so lacking in the historical material: women's voices and women's vision. Ms. Yalom rues the fact that despite her best efforts, she found very little in the record to indicate how women have felt about their breasts: whether they took pleasure in them, the extent to which they chose to display their breasts, or if they had any say in the debate over wet-nursing. Hence, much of the documented epic of the breast is a voyeuristic one, told from the perspective of those who lack the organs yet still claim the ultimate authority on the subject. Let's hope that women keep talking on the subject. Let's hope that women keep talking if only to say, as Marilyn Yalom does in paraphrasing Freud, "Sometimes a breast is just a breast" [p.4].

In discussing the writing of this chapter with me, Fran Anderson asked that I consider (1) how had I felt changed by my mastectomy?

(2) how had it affected my view of patients? and (3) whether it had left me feeling somehow "flawed"?

Initially, I thought I might escape "the worst": the surgeon believed that a lumpectomy would serve to remove the cancer. I remember the distinct experience of relief when she first reported that "the margins looked clean!" But, by the end of the week, the pathology report reflected otherwise. Lymph node involvement bumped me up to "Stage II" cancer, and the cells appeared invasive. The surgeon offered to go in again, to excise more tissue . . . and if that didn't do it . . . we could proceed with a . . . blankety blank. . . .

Mastectomy! I could hardly bear the word. To me, "mastectomy" conjured up the lopping off of an entire organ, just like that!—much as an axe might, with a single chop, hack off a vital branch of tree. Then what shape would I be in? The image that came to mind was much like what a young child would draw of the human figure with a squared-off blank space where genitals should be. But moving upward along the body and to the left, where once there was my breast, I pictured a spidery scar, webbing out from the center of the blank— a sucked-in, closed-up hole.

Subsequent consultations provided more realistic and less terrifying information. The breast surgeon and the oncologist agreed that a total mastectomy was ultimately the most likely outcome and the wisest choice to make now. I did have the option of electing immediate reconstruction, a procedure that could be piggy-backed along with a mastectomy. When the breast surgeon had carved out an eye-shaped area around, and including, my nipple, and scooped out all of the breast tissue, the plastic surgeon would come in to take her place and do his work.

I discussed the issue of mastectomy alone versus reconstruction with my husband and my daughter. Stuart felt uneasy about prolonged anesthesia. The choice involved either a four- or an eight-hour procedure. "Of course it's up to you," he said, "but know that what I care about is having *you* alive." My daughter wanted to know what I would do if it were *only* up to me. Impossible question. Thoughts about the incredible strictures on "vanity" in the household of my growing up were suddenly broken by a recollection that struck me as so funny that it seemed to hasten my decision. My immigrant parents used to refer to people who were volatile or "mentally ill" as "unbalanced." Mrs. Gruenhut (translates Mrs. Green Hat), for example, a refugee wife who would come to sell us soaps and perfumes and chocolates and once (to the great giggles of my sister and me) had locked herself in our upstairs bathroom, was "unbalanced." I did not wish to appear "unbalanced"; nor did I wish to insert a prosthesis, like some kind of green hat, into my brassiere each day, a ritual reminder that I was, after all, "unbalanced."[5]

Perhaps because I did opt for reconstruction (and because my daughter told me that, when she saw me being wheeled into my room from Recovery, her first immediate relief came when she noticed the outline of what looked like two breasts under the sheet), I feel my body "flaws" in much the same way as I felt them before the mastectomy. I often wish I had inherited my mother's or my grandmother's "flawless" legs, somebody else's hips. But the terrors of "mutilation" that haunted my first fantasies of breast removal are gone.

That I feel "balanced" doesn't mean that I did not experience a loss. As Love (1993) writes, "What's constructed is *not* a real breast. When it's well done, it will *look* real, but it will never have the full sensation as a breast does. It's more like a prosthesis attached to your chest!" (p. 350).

In the weeks before the surgery, I spoke to Stuart about the upcoming loss. "Stuart," I said, "we need to say goodbye to this breast." Stuart held me, looked at my naked body, and spoke. "Breast," he said, focusing there and addressing it directly, "it should come as no surprise to you that I will miss you. . . . You and I have been friends for a long time."

So I would take issue with Yalom's statement (quoted in Angier, 1997) that "sometimes a breast is just a breast." In my experience, a breast—if we stop to think about it—is never just the thing itself. Although it need not adhere merely to standard societal associations, the body of the breast is a rich, communicative resource of individual metaphor and meaning.

THE BREAST AS METAPHOR:
A CLINICAL EXAMPLE AND A LETTER TO MY DAUGHTER

The following clinical vignette was first described in my 1997 paper to illustrate "inadvertent self-disclosure." It constituted the first inadvertent instance in which I referred to my breast in relation to a patient as more—or other—than just the location of a cancer.

Inadvertent self-disclosure, an inevitable outcome of the analyst's active engagement with a patient, may or may not contain within it elements from the analyst's life experience. The responsible analyst, with appropriate caution, and respect for the power inherent in any self-disclosure on her part, must be prepared for this eventuality. Inadvertent self-disclosure requires, above all else, the analyst's skill in utilizing the potential of the shared contents of her experience in the service of the analytic process.

Dr. T is the eldest daughter of a large, well-to-do family dominated by a narcissistic, neurasthenic, alcoholically unpredictable mother who delegated Dr. T as a caretaker of her siblings, as well as of the mother herself in her various moods of exaltation or despair. Promised rewards of special luncheons out or shopping expeditions were more often than not rescinded because mother would claim a headache or some "fatigue" of unknown origin. Even before my illness, Dr. T and I were not surprised by her incredible vigilance over my states of being. We knew that, for her, any distractions or discomforts on my part would be perceived as signals to negate her needs and to tend to mine. Dr. T has required much of me over the years. But one of her most impressive characteristics is the unflinching and persistent way in which she has required as much of herself. She does not spare herself. On days that she would rather do anything else than come to analysis to face our work, she drags herself in to pursue it. Throughout the stormiest of times she has never let me lose sight of her integrity. Over the years, my admiration for this woman's relentless quest for herself has deepened into love.

On this Monday morning she came into the office and, rather than taking up where we had left off on the Thursday before, she sat down in an uncharacteristic manner, assuming a body position that I have come to associate with her sense of unarticulated outrage. Although she didn't say so, I suspected that she somehow knew I'd had my chemo on the previous Friday. She asked me how I was, and I answered, "Pretty good, thanks." There followed a long silence. Then, sitting back, she spoke in an unusually soft and solicitous tone: "I am not going to sit here and tell you what's going on inside of me. How can I? I bring in ordinary, run-of-the-mill issues, and you bring cancer. I'm not" she said softly, "going to tell you how I am in pain." At that, I discovered myself leaning forward in my chair and heard myself saying, in a tone also uncharacteristically low but fairly spitting out the words, "I have lost a breast. Now do you want to take my milk away from me too?"

The acknowledgments that followed opened the way to our better understanding (through our experience in the interaction) of how each of us responded to her distrust of women (now speakable between us) as well as the hostility that accompanies her expectation of abandonment. In my efforts to provide a safe place, in which Dr. T might open and deepen an exploration of her desires, I had neglected a crucial aspect of her person. At last she upped the ante in such a way that I could no longer avoid talking back to her rage. It would be nice to be able to report that we were both cured, that I no longer slip into the "correct mother" role, and that she is now at home in her desires and aggression. But although in our time to come she may not remember this moment (she may hold another moment), for me it is an important marker—a moment in which we broke through a critical resistance.

Not until thinking about writing this chapter did I realize—even though the arduous, exhausting process of chemo overshadowed the original traumas of surgery—how deeply my metaphor of breast had implanted itself in consciousness. During the three-and-a-half-hour chemo sessions, Stuart and I together would fantasize and plan a Wellness Party to be given at the end of our ordeal. We wanted to celebrate and thank the many people who had so generously provided caring support. When the time came, on a cool, soft evening in May with our dogwoods and azaleas in full bloom, and we said our thank-you's to the large gathering of relatives and friends, I read this letter to my daughter: I include it here as an illustration of how, having begun to find the words to think, feel and talk about my breast as metaphor (originating *in my body* rather than as an intellectual abstraction), I could now *connect* the *word* to inner and outer events. My "breast" became a complex signal metaphor. And so, in the wake of a profound body experience, heightened body awareness, and an intensified articulation of body based issues, my own past and present experiences—as here expressed to my daughter—have become increasingly registered, recategorized and revisited subjectively in the connecting form of body memories.

Andrea

"Andrea, you and I have come so far in time and space and spirit since that first miraculous event when I felt the vibration of your cry inside of me moments before you broke into the world. That was in the 'olden days,' when godliness took second place to cleanliness, even in Texas hospitals. Although I insisted on a natural childbirth (then 'unheard of' for 'white women' of my station), I had you in the O.R., strapped down for fear I might infect you with my touch. Imagine!

"But once in my room, no one paid much attention to us. A sterile white-capped nurse with a rolling tray of babies, just dropped you in my lap and promptly moved on with her wailing, hungry cargo. And this is really true Andrea. I had little idea what to do, and found myself in tears. An elderly black cleaning woman who was mopping the halls heard my distress. She came in and smiled, and with such confidence and care, showed me how to breast-feed.

"In later years and harder times, I could have used such patient and unpressured tutelage. I often wish I'd known much more about myself and how to better be with you. But with my efforts and your forgiveness, it seems that we have found our way to an adult relationship, and an attachment deeper than the bond of blood and milk. And then, last year, events occurred that brought me to yet another miracle. I say miracle again, not because it was unreal at all—on the contrary!—but because what happened was both the last thing I expected or that, as a mother, I had ever wanted to expect; and that I learned to take it in.

"You were such a holding presence for me, Andrea, caring for me throughout two surgeries—so that when, I, your mother, lost a breast, you, my daughter, lovingly and with such exquisite nurture and great humor, nursed me through."

                                                                                    May 20, 1995

CONNECTING THE BODY AND MIND

While I do not hold with the extreme psychosomaticist view that I caused my cancer, I do believe that intensification of stress compromises the immune system, and, more broadly, I believe that the mind–body connection, so simply manifested in the lifting of one's arm when the mind asks it to do so, is also manifested in more complex and subtle ways, ways that our discipline is far from fully understanding. Some examples: the ways in which competitive athletes sharpen their performance through the use of preparatory imaging practices; or the way a hypnotizable patient can manage surgery without anesthesia; or the way a person's body recognizes the moment to die when loved ones at that person's bedside finally shift within themselves and let go. We tend to think of these phenomena as more mysterious than the interplays of mind and body and symptoms we are used to witnessing in our daily practices, yet I believe that, beyond what we have dreamt of in our own psychology, there are everyday occurrences that remind us that psyche, soma, and spirit are interrelated component aspects of one unity. My chemotherapy experience is a mind—body tale in itself. Stuart (who never translates anxiety or distress into stomach upset) accompanied me to each procedure. While I was hooked up to the IV, Stuart hooked himself up to me via a "Y" jack and one of the dual headphones we had attached to our tape recorder. We listened together, taking in the same music and meditation tapes. Later, at home, Stuart, in true couvade fashion, would experience sensations of postchemo nausea.

I was in the midst of undergoing tests for breast cancer when my sister called from Ohio to say that Mother, who had been moved to a Care Center there, was dying. Unable to leave before completing these tests, I asked my sister to tell Mother to hang on until I could get there at the weekend. Knowing her, I felt certain that she could, and would, hang on for me. What I had not counted on, however, was my loving daughter's immediate flight from graduate school to Ohio to wish her grandmother goodbye. To my way of looking at it, Mother mistook her for me and died quietly a few hours later.[6] Once again, I was struck by the connection between the body and (even a demented) mind.

In the next few months, I could not make room for the visceral memories of maternal comfort during my early childhood illnesses, nor for the loss of such containing comfort in the present. Mother died in May. I find it remarkable that, at the end of *July*, as I emerged from anesthesia after the long surgery was finally over, I made this first (unconscious) statement to my husband and daughter: "Did you know that Mother died?" (I imagine I was only just beginning to feel safe enough to take in the loss . . . of mother/breast.)

Following the wishes of both of my parents, their bodies were donated to medical schools. The image of their dismantled cadavers was actually less disturbing to me than the notion that their bodies would be dispersed and I would have no *place* to *find* them. So I requested the ultimate receipt of their ashes. My office is attached to a small sunroom where I often stand between appointments. I look down into a garden that now includes two Japanese dwarf maple trees. Beneath each tree, the fertile soil is mixed with a ring of a parent's ashes. Dad's tree actually reaches out toward Mother's, which stands straight and tall. These trees embody the two of them for me and my husband, Stuart, as well as for my children—a source of connection and comfort, a location, a transformational image of the cycle of life and death.

If we consider patients' inquiries into our family ties, what are the downsides of analytic anonymity? "Families" and "parents" in the psychoanalytic framework most often conjure up the problematics in developmental history. While this may be ever true, it may not be the whole truth. My trees stand for that perspective from which parents serve us as elders, reminding us of our inherited traditions, some of which we may have rejected, transformed, or embraced.

Furthermore, I am convinced that the majority of people who come to our consulting rooms make their final choice of a therapist on the basis of some more personal aspect of the therapist's "stock" than on theoretical roots or institutional affiliations. Years ago, a person in our field came for a consultation to consider therapy and analysis with me. She had three questions: Was I Jewish? Did I have children?, and Had I witnessed death? I answered them all, and, happily for us both, we set out to work. Another person, also in the mental health field, said she chose to work with me because I looked to her like a person who, at my age, still embodied a sense of passion and sexuality. Recently, she reminded me of this, adding that her experience of me continues thus, unaltered by my mastectomy.

BODY LESSONS

In the midst of my illness, a patient blurted out, "You're so *lucky* you have cancer!" She went on, "You know how to talk about it. It comes in *a word* that people understand. They can believe it, they can sympathize and give support, and feel good about that. What can I say about what goes on inside myself?" She sighed. "There's no 'reality' I can name, like cancer. Why should people feel sorry for me? I can't even feel sorry for myself!" I considered this a courageous statement. I could well understand her view. Another patient's sentiment, one more commonly expressed: "My God, you must be seething over this! You must be asking yourself over and over, again, 'Why me?'"

I found this empathic assumption the most difficult one to respond to with the appreciation it deserved, while still maintaining my integrity. What was the matter with me? Was I denying the full weight of my feelings? I think not. I am readily furious when my back goes out, enraged at betrayal by a trusted friend, and palpably saddened by the physical ravages of the aging process (particularly since it was not until my 40s that I truly experienced coming into my own life—feeling finally old enough to be young). But, for me, "Why me?" signifies not rage, but surprise over something that I cannot yet justify or comprehend. It is a question that ultimately has an answer. Cancer is too large for such a query. "Why me?" makes me too important in nature's scheme of things. Why *not* me? Or why not anybody?

That is not to say that I am devoid of fear. Far from it! I am subject to near phobic fear of what I cannot know and only sense. Meditation and visualization practices continue to teach me how to remain present, accepting; to ease into the unknown—body, mind, and spirit— learning as I go along. Isn't that what we, in our best analytic selves, are meant to do? To ease into being with wherever we are in relation to what we hear, both from ourselves and from the people with whom we sit?

Experiencing cancer has also sharpened my awareness of my own processes, teaching me when to move into the center of pain and nausea, and when to detach and contain it, treating each sensation as an ordinary object in the wide array of objects within my domain— a kind of disciplined meditative control that is, paradoxically, accomplished only by letting go. By extension, I apply this dialectic to include the people with whom I sit in therapy. There are moments when I move with them into the center of their felt experience, and moments when I detach, in order to contain it for us like an ordinary object in the wide array of objects within our shared domain.

I find that practiced observation of such processes has contributed to a heightened sensitivity to states and moods that are nonverbally expressed. I see a gradient in which the posture of terror differs from anxiety; the manner in which muscles go flaccid in a rigid skeleton distinguishes dissociation from the more relaxed states of dreamy distraction.

Clearly, a mindful integration of mind–body experience in analytic practice requires further study. The technical issues to be explored include questions about how we learn, let alone teach, the ability to distinguish between what we keep private and to ourselves and what is in danger of becoming a withholding secret that distorts the analytic process and progress. What, precisely, are the ways in which we differentiate tact, propriety, and open sharing from seductive, enmeshing, or power promoting dialogues?

I conclude with a recent dream from Dr. T's analysis. For many days she had sustained a serious infection, an illness so threatening that she felt forced, for the first time in all our years together, to cancel a session. On the following Monday, just a week before I would take three weeks off to write this chapter, she reported having had this "horrible dream":

"I am lying in bed with Molly [her daughter] and the dog. You are sitting on the bed, holding my hand. You are very pale. . . . Your skin looks awful. I ask over and over if you are in pain. 'No' you say, 'I'm not in pain. I'm dying, but I'm not in pain.' I lie there thinking to myself, 'How *can* she, how can she *do* this to me?'"

I see this as an early termination dream. Her rage over what had happened to me and what had happened to herself—a rage over repeated, unbearable separations that had kept her out of touch with tenderness—had bridged to a now speakable grief, which indicates to me that she is on the verge of emerging from the middle phase of her analysis. We can recognize in the dream imagery her conjuring of themes that constitute our actual experiences together, including my illness and what had happened (and might still happen) to my body, in order to construct a symbolic rendering of an early termination dream. The dream, given shape from the material at hand in our shared intersubjective experience, seems to me to represent Dr. T's anticipation of my abandonment of her through her arrival at her own readiness to terminate in the foreseeable future. The dream composes a describable presence (life, change, death), to prepare for absence (loss, grief)—symbolizing in vivid corporeal form how one may carry absence inside without emptiness. Such a central symbol would be described by some analytic colleagues as the *navel* of the dream.

It has been aptly said that "life is a terminal disease, and no body survives." We are lucky if we have some freedom to choose how we cope with what is given and what is taken away. I believe that our essential work and play, in and out of our consulting rooms, is to find our way to facilitate those connections that make person-al sense of inexplicable experience. Often the connections that we make or facilitate are formed as they are in meditations or dreams—comprehensible only in retrospect. For example, had Frances Anderson and Lewis Aron asked me at the outset to trace the relationships among breast cancer, loss, and reconstruction as they influenced my connections to parents, patients, immediate family, and the planting of trees, I can't imagine ever having begun this task.

NOTES

[1]Renik (1995) emphasizes that "an analyst's personality is constantly revealed, *in one form or another*, through his or her analytic activities" (p. 469). See also Aron (1992).

[2]Important contributions to this subject are offered by Davies (1994), Aron (1996), Gerson (1996), and Crastnopol (1997).

[3]I cannot help musing here on collected clinical experience of hair loss registered in the unconscious as dream images representing powerlessness or enfeeblement; or, where the unconscious sprouts at the surface of conscious action, the frequency with which (particularly) women mark profound life transitions, changes in status for good or ill, by suddenly adopting a new haircut.

[4]In my practice, one patient interrupted contact until after chemotherapy, another terminated prematurely without accepting a referral.

[5]I elected a procedure called "myocutaneous flap" in which "a flap of skin, muscle, and fat [was] taken from . . . [my] back (latissimus). . . ." In this miraculous procedure, "[t]he tissue is removed except for its feeding artery and vein, which remains attached, almost like a leash. . . . The site from which the tissue was removed is sewn closed. The new little island of skin and muscle is then tunneled under the skin into the mastectomy wound. Since the blood vessels aren't cut, the blood remains" (Love, 1993, p. 363).

Later, a nipple may be carved—lifted up and constructed, origami fashion—from the sufficiently thick flap of skin taken from my back.

[6]Another one of my sisters, unaware of my request, might say that it was her whispered permission—"It's okay, Mother, you can let go now"—that eased Mother on her way. But the point is the same.

REFERENCES

Abend, S. M. (1992), Serious illness in the analyst: Countertransference considerations. *J. Amer. Psychoanal. Assn.*, 30:365–379.

Angier, N. (1997), Goddesses, harlots and other male fantasies. *New York Times*, p. 4, Feb. 23.

Aron, L. (1992), Interpretation as expression of the analyst's subjectivity. *Psychoanal. Dial.*, 2:475—507.

——— (1996), *A Meeting of Minds*. Hillsdale, NJ: The Analytic Press.

Burka, J. B. (1996), The therapist's body in reality and fantasy. In: *The Therapist as a Person*, ed. B. Gerson. Hillsdale, NJ: The Analytic Press.

Crastnopol, M. (1997), Incognito or not? The patient's subjective experience of the analyst's private life. *Psychoanal. Dial.*, 7:257–280.

Davies, J. M. (1994), Love in the afternoon. A relational reconsideration of desire and dread in the countertransference. *Psychoanal. Dial.*, 4:153–170.

Dewald, P. A. (1982), Serious illness in the analyst: Transference, countertransference, and reality responses. *J. Amer. Psychoanal. Assn.*, 30:347–363.

Ehrenberg, D. (1995), Self-disclosure: Therapeutic tool or indulgence? *Contemp. Psychoanal.*, 31:213–228.

Gerson, B. O.,ed. (1996), *The Therapist as a Person*. Hillsdale, NJ: The Analytic Press.

Love, S. M. (with K. Lindsey) (1993), *Dr. Susan Love's Breast Book*. Reading, MA: Addison Wesley.

McLaughlin, J. (1987), The play of transference: Some reflections of enactment in the psychoanalytic situation. *J. Amer. Psychoanal. Assn.,* 35:557–582.

———— (1991), Clinical and theoretical aspects of enactment. *J. Amer. Psychoanal. Assn.,* 39:595–614.

———— (1995), Touching limits in the analytic dyad. *Psychoanal. Quart.,* 64:433–465.

Morrison, A. (1997), Ten years of doing psychotherapy while living with a life threatening illness: Self-disclosure and other ramifications. *Psychoanal. Dial.,* 7:225–241.

Pizer, B. (1997), When the analyst is ill: Dimensions of self-disclosure. *Psychoanal. Quart.,* 66:450–469.

Pizer, S. (1992), The negotiation of paradox in the analytic process. *Psychoanal. Dial.,* 2:215–240.

Renik, O. (1993), Countertransference enactment and the psychoanalytic process. In: *Psychic Structure and Psychic Change,* ed. M. Horowitz, O. Kernberg & E. Weinshel. Madison, CT: International Universities Press, pp. 137–160.

———— (1995), The ideal of the anonymous analyst and the problem of self-disclosure. *Psychoanal. Quart.,* 64:466–495.

Sontag S. (1989), *Illness as Metaphor and AIDS and Its Metaphors.* New York: Anchor Books.

PART IV

*The Place
of Bodily Experience
in the Psychoanalytic Process*

9

LISTENING TO THE BODY

Somatic Representations
of Dissociated Memory

Karen Hopenwasser

The emerging study of consciousness is an interdisciplinary effort that poses significant challenges to traditional psychoanalytic theory of the mind. It is also, however, an area of study that promises to enhance our psychoanalytic and psychotherapeutic work. The centerpiece of this chapter is a lengthy case presentation. The clinical material is woven into a review of current neurobiological theory, in an effort to explain the relationship between dissociation, memory, and somatic symptoms. This relationship is explored within the context of a shift from the philosophy of mind–body duality to what can be called a post-Cartesian neurophilosophy. The current attack on the authenticity of memory has failed to consider extensive knowl-

I am grateful to those who have made suggestions and helped me to integrate the complex material presented in this chapter: Jenny Heinz, Marlene Hunter, Richard Kluft, Andrew Levin, and Rosemary Masters; to those who have given me unfailing support in my clinical work, including Lynn Pearl, Carol Levine, Donald Brown; to the other members of my dissociative disorders study group: Jack Dunietz, Arlene Levine, Kathleen Hynes, Norman Kaplan; and, of course, to my patients, who often could not locate the words and have given me permission to tell their stories.

edge outside the limited scope of laboratory cognitive psychology. Arguments about notions like true versus false memory do not address more compelling questions, such as what is consciousness? how do we know what we know? This is a question that has been addressed in the psychoanalytic literature by only a few authors.[1] But this is a question we must pose if we are going to explore how information is held within or expressed through the body.

How does the study of consciousness relate to somatic memory? I imagine the men and women who have floated in space, tethered to the machine of transport that carried them beyond the atmosphere. For most, the awareness that one could be lost in space, disconnected yet awake within the universe, sends a chill through the body. It is this chill through the body that holds my focus here: physical sensation is a source of information historically devalued and often clinically trivialized. When physicians cannot find the etiology of somatic symptoms, they often dismiss the patient as "hysterical." When analysts view somatic symptoms as hysterical, however, they often limit their interpretations to metaphor. Clinically we need to understand the body as an agent of metaphor.

Consciousness can be viewed from two quite distinct positions: from the bottom up, that is, neurons, neural networks, and electrochemical transmissions, or from the top down, that is, spirituality, philosophy, and cognitive psychology. Among the philosophers who have taken the leap from top down to bottom up is Patricia Churchland (1986; Churchland and Sejnowski, 1992), who predicts that our understanding will ultimately reduce the mind to a computational brain. Some neuroscientists also put forth a reductionist view of the material basis of the mind. Molecular biologist Francis Crick (1994) postulates that consciousness is dependent on oscillating connections between the thalamus and certain cortical layers. Gerald Edelman (1987, 1992) has put forth a theory of neuronal group selection, that is, that consciousness has emerged through the evolution of neuronal connectivity. There are many new voices participating in this dialogue, including those who believe that consciousness is an irreducible entity, like a physical property, that cannot be reduced to neurobiological parts (Chalmers, 1996).

The intersection of bottom up/top down theory is the grey zone of clinical practice. The data reviewed from neurological and neurobiological studies are just a glimpse through this grey zone. But these data can help us to validate our increasing appreciation of somatically expressed perception and recall.

CARTESIAN DUALISM

While the debate rages with regard to a neuronal basis for conscious-ness, researchers are showing that the mind can be mapped in the brain and are subsequently shifting the frame to the post-Cartesian theater.

Our work with patients who exhibit dissociative disorders en-tices us to think about both philosophy and biology. Within the psy-choanalytic frame the dualist roots of psychoanalytic theories can create a therapeutic stumbling block, highlighted in this population. A brief review of the history of dualist philosophy will clarify the im-portance of the post-Cartesian theater.

Before Descartes, as far back as Plato, we see the origins of a philosophical dichotomy between mind and body. Plato, attempting to "prove" the immortality of the soul in the Phaedo, established the presumption that there is a component of our self that is separate from our body. In the *Thaetetus* and the *Symposium*, his lively dia-logue on love, he essentially said that knowledge obtained through the sensorium (through bodily perception) is not "true knowledge" (Plato, N. D.). Here we have some of the first evidence of the Western bias against imagination.[2] This devaluation of sensory perception as knowledge helped to shape an overvaluation of the rational or "sci-entific mind" as opposed to the artistic, "imaginative mind." While the study of imagination is relevant to debates about the authenticity of memory, it is beyond the scope of this chapter. Suffice it to say now that it is not until Kant that we have an elaboration of how the imagination serves to synthesize sense perception with semantic concepts into mental representations (Johnson, 1987). If we then look to literature we can explore the relationship between memory, imagi-nation, body and self. Julia Kristeva (1993) explains, "Proust uses time as his intermediary *in the search* [*a la Recherche*] for an embodied imagination: that is to say, for a space where words and their dark, unconscious manifestations contribute to the weaving of the world's unbroken flesh, of which I is a part" (p. 5).

In his search for scientific truth, Descartes (1637) proclaimed *cogito ergo sum*, I think therefore I am. In his *Discourse on Method*, he described that the mind stuff and the body stuff were of essence sepa-rate (*res cogitans* and *res extensa*). He speculated that the pineal gland, a small structure centrally located in the brain, served as a valve through which the spirit or soul could retrieve information from the brain. Except for a notable few (Eccles, 1989; Penrose, 1989, 1994), most researchers and theoreticians, and many philosophers, have produced arguments counter to Cartesian dualism.

One of the first extensive descriptions of the post Cartesian model can be found in Daniel Dennett's (1991) treatise, *Consciousness Explained*. His Multiple Drafts theory of consciousness attempts to synthesize several disciplines: mathematics, philosophy, biology, cognitive psychology. He states, "All varieties of thought or mental activity—are accomplished in the brain by parallel, multitrack processes of interpretation and elaboration of sensory inputs. Information entering the nervous system is under continuous 'editorial revision' " (p. 111).

It is the advancement in neurophysiological cartography that allows us to reformulate our understanding of awareness. Neuroanatomical and neurophysiological studies support the multitrack pathways concept. And it should be possible to support this reformulation further through our observation of dissociative phenomena in a clinical sample. Ultimately it should be possible to understand how multiple pathways of information retrieval connect together and, inversely, how multiple pathways of information retrieval may be biologically disconnected.

Toward the end of *Consciousness Explained*, Dennett arrives logically at a brief discussion of what he considers one of the

> terrible experiments of nature. . . Multiple Personality Disorder. . . . The idea of MPD strikes many people as too outlandish and metaphysically bizarre to believe. . . I suspect that some of these people have made a simple arithmetical mistake: they have failed to notice that two or three or seventeen selves per body is really not more metaphysically extravagant than one self per body. . . [p. 419].

RELATION BETWEEN MEMORY AND CONSCIOUSNESS

In the classic medical text of Plum and Posner, *The Diagnosis of Stupor and Coma* (1972), consciousness is defined as

> awareness of self and environment. . . there are two aspects of consciousness, and different types and distributions of brain disease affect them differently. One is the content of consciousness, the sum of mental functions. The other is arousal, which behaviourally at least, is closely linked to the appearance of wakefulness [p. 2].

Those who work daily with people who suffer from posttraumatic problems know that it is the very relationship between the content of consciousness and the concept of arousal that demands explanation. Neurobiologically we can understand the difference between awake (a higher brainstem function) and aware (necessitating cortical function). What we remember about our awareness is contingent on the wakefulness of our senses and their connections to the cortex. The link between our senses and our consciousness is the body. As Diane Ackerman (1990) says, "[o]ur senses define the edge of consciousness" (p. xv). Sensory perception is the motor of subjectivity. Yet what we remember and when we remember it remain something of a mystery. How much memory is necessary to maintain awareness? How much memory is necessary to maintain identity? In Korsakov's syndrome, a consequence of chronic alcohol abuse, the destruction of the mammillary bodies and connecting tracts may make all new learning impossible. In severe cases, this may lead to a need constantly to reconstruct one's sense of self. In Alzheimer's, the progressive loss of mental functioning will ultimately shrink conscious awareness entirely, perhaps secondary to the loss of mass, the volume of complex cholinergic neural networks that disappear with massive degeneration.

As the neuroscientist C. M. Fair (1992) states, "we might have to conclude that the substrate of 'consciousness' is memory" (p. 161).

While the substrate of consciousness may be memory, memory seems not to be restricted to consciousness. Therefore questions we need to ask are:

1) Can we understand certain physical sensations as memory, even if there are no simultaneous semantic associations?

2) How and why do physical sensations trigger retrieval of previously stored mental representations?

3) Can an exploration of how the brain stores and retrieves memory clarify the inconsistency of remembering?

4) If we abandon dualism and consider some physical sensations to be memory, then are somatic memories a substrate of consciousness?

CLINICAL CASES

Well over a decade ago, in the midst of a session with a patient, I realized that her symptoms could be understood as somatic memories.[3] She was a 28-year-old woman who had attempted suicide following the termination of a previous treatment. Some of her chief complaints on entering psychotherapy initially were panic attacks since early adolescence and the sense of being "just a pair of eyes." During the course of her psychotherapy she had become increasingly obsessed with her male therapist until he finally ended the treatment. Several weeks after termination, she took a near-lethal overdose of tricyclic antidepressants. She was stabilized in an intensive care unit, was transferred to a psychiatric hospital, and began outpatient treatment with me in anticipation of discharge. The first weeks, even months, of treatment focused on her continued suicidal ideation as well as homicidal ideation toward the previous therapist. I struggled to understand why this extremely bright, capable woman had slipped into such a desperate state. I also struggled to know whether I needed to warn the previous therapist about her homicidal fantasies.

During the initial months of treatment she had frequent panic attacks. She remained depressed and had active suicidal ideation. She had moved to a new apartment shortly before the suicide attempt and now found herself isolated in an unfamiliar neighborhood. She returned to work, however, and worked without impairment. She acknowledged that the move had been related to an "awareness" that the previous therapist had recently moved into that neighborhood. Although she did not say that she wished to be near him, she recognized that her move and his neighborhood appeared to be connected. In one of the first sessions, she said, "I'm afraid, I don't feel like myself. Everything feels different. Up in [town]—how could I be there? I must have been in a dream to move there."

As her history unfolded, she revealed lifelong anxiety, panic attacks, and a profound sense of humiliation. Both she and her brother had been subjected to relentless criticism from their mother. Extreme reprimand followed any loss of control of body function, such as diarrhea on the way home from school.

She described her father as shy and awkward, but a fierce disciplinarian. Each Saturday morning he would take the children to the basement and drill them in military-style exercises. Frequently the children would be punished by being whipped with a belt on their bare bottoms. Her father was the child of a deaf father and a nearly deaf mother and, openly ashamed of his family of origin, he minimized contact between my patient and her paternal grandparents, who communicated primarily through signing. (Recall her initial complaint in therapy, that is, "I am just a pair of eyes.")

In relationships with men she was particularly drawn toward men who "revolted" her. She reported the recurrent experience of being with men and entering into a frightful state, certain that they would suddenly become violent toward her. Although she recalled the incidents of corporal punishment by her father, she never made any sense of these fears until the following emerged.

About nine months after the start of our work she told me a dream she had years before that she remembered in the hospital.

> She is about 3 years old, in her aunt's house, on a mink farm. Her father is leaving after a fight with her mother. She is thinking, "What about me, what about me?" Her brother is in the kitchen with cowboy hat and guns. Brother says to mother, "Look at A, something is wrong with her." Mother says, "It's OK, he's not leaving." Mother goes to put coat on her— can't stand it, can't stand to have mother touch her.

Upon awakening she has the following thought: "There is something I am too afraid to think."

Her first association is to a memory, uncertain at what age, when she cut her foot on a stone at a lakefront beach. Her father is carrying her. She is screaming, and she recalls feeling ashamed—she did not want anyone to see him holding her. This association comes up dozens of times over the next years of treatment. She dreams abundantly, with much recall of dream images and easy access to extensive free associations during sessions. As she emerges from her depression and sense of loss, she draws a portrait of a family crippled by humiliation.

About 12 months into the analysis, she tells me the memory of a "fat Sunday school teacher with hairy arms" who frightened her. She has no recall of his harming her and remembers her parents being unable to understand why she would not return to the Sunday school class. She has several associations to this memory: the only men she has felt sexually attracted to were "fat"; her maternal grandfather was "fat with hairy arms." Looking at a map for the lake of her lakefront beach memory, she began to think about her maternal grandparents growing up in a town with a name including the word stone (she had cut her foot on a stone). She then states, "I remember not liking my grandfather." Her grandfather died when she was eight years old. She has previously told me of the memory of her maternal grandfather's taking her to school with mother in the car. She often cried, and on one occasion he said to her, "Your tears are gonna freeze on your face." She recalls thinking, "He's in the front seat. I can only see the back of his head. He's not able to look me in the eyes; there is something about eyes."

For many months she continues to function without acute symp-
tomatology. She is no longer suicidal. She dates men and, if they wish
to have sexual contact, she complies, although she needs to have a
few drinks before she is able to have sex. We focus on and try to
explore her inability to say no to a man. She presents recurrent dreams
about her basement and the stairs leading down to the basement.
Her associations are to her father and often to an incident when he
kills a sick bird in the basement.

Then, at about month 18, she reports the following experience:

> I'm in bed, not quite awake, not quite asleep. Some-
> thing is gonna come at me, it's just out of my vision.

Over a period of months she has recurrent nighttime episodes. Sometimes they seem like night terrors; she awakens, heart pounding, unable to move. Sometimes they are dreamlike but not quite during sleep.
In some of these episodes she feels pinned down, that she is choking;
she is aware of pain in her genitals; someone is pinching her; she is
aware of pain in her rectum.

Concurrently all is going well at work, and she moves from one
job to a better position, higher salary, and more responsibility. She is
planning a visit home to her parents. Then she comes in with the
following:

> Last night, I felt paralyzed. I was on my stomach—as
> if someone were over me—I'm being hurt. I'm on my
> pillow; it's slid out from under my head. I'm kissed
> on the cheek—it feels as if it's not a dream.

It was becoming clearer to me that these episodes at night were dissociated flashbacks that during the daytime were often not remembered or were remembered without the intense terror reported in
association with them. Since her intensive treatment had been so rich
with dream material, I could wonder about the quality of these "not
quite asleep" dreams and contrast them with her abundantly recalled
dreams.

At approximately the beginning of the second year of treatment,
we are in a session discussing her difficulty saying no to men. She
reports the fantasy that, if she says no, she will be in danger. She then
reports the following nighttime episode:

> I'm laying on my stomach. He's over me. I have a
> feeling it's my grandfather; it's just a feeling. He's

> touching me all over—it's not sexual—it's cruel. He's
> pinching me. I was definitely a child, but I felt sexual
> excitement. I have a feeling it's coming, on my back, a
> big person coming down. I'm waiting for the pain. I'm
> clawing at his hands, to get him to stop.

She continues to have elaborate dreams, many containing explicit sexual content, frequently focused on fear of rape, containing visual images of male genitalia, and occasionally manifestly about her father. In these dreams she expresses both a sense of obligation and the desire to have physical contact with him. In her nighttime episodes of dissociation, however, she rarely has a visual image. Much more frequently she relates a touch sensation, either apprehension or actual pain, in her body. Most of the time she describes a clawing sensation and an awareness of trying to bite someone's fingers. Frequently she describes pain in her rectum.

Years ago my patient and I exercised a freedom to explore these associations and respect the emergence of memories, however blurred, about her parents and grandfather. Although her memories of her grandfather were never absolutely clear, we could maintain an open, curious stance as the information cascaded before us. As is often the case, the possibility that these feeling states might have been associated with actual experience allowed her to contain her daytime anxiety, decreased her fear of "going crazy," and increased her self-esteem. She never felt it necessary to know for sure in order to grow and heal. The very possibility of asking the forbidden question was reparative for her.

After years of psychoanalytic treatment, this patient's daily symptoms diminished to a minimal level. However, her core fearfulness of men persisted to the extent of inhibiting a sustained, intimate relationship. A few years ago we introduced the use of Eye Movement Desensitization and Reprocessing (EMDR, Shapiro, 1995) to tackle the basic physiologic terror of sexual intimacy. Not only did she begin to have sexual experiences in a nondissociated state, but she has been in a serious, increasingly intimate relationship for more than a year. Later in this chapter I elaborate about the role of EMDR as a vehicle for weaving a bridge between affect and cognition in psychoanalytic treatment.

A number of years ago, prompted by a patient in the hospital, I more systematically began to study the neurobiological relationship between somatic sensations and memory. This patient was a 25-year-old woman who had been in the hospital for about four weeks, following a suicide attempt. She gave a history of being the subject of chronic violence during her childhood and had clear recollections of having been chained to chairs, beaten with hairbrushes, locked in closets, burned on her arms, sexually abused, tied up and neglected for long periods of time. She had a history of addiction to crack but had been drug free for several weeks when I first met her. She had been previously diagnosed as multiple personality (now called Dissociative Identity Disorder). She spontaneously slipped into trance states and manifested parts (sometimes called alters) during her sessions.

Since relapsing addiction to crack is a primary obstacle to any recovery, I tried to explore her drug abuse with her. She claimed that it was only one part of herself that sought use of crack. I suggested that the crack-using part needed to participate in the treatment. She went into a trance and swiftly developed rhinorrhea, lacrimation, pilomotor activity on her arms (gooseflesh), and diaphoresis. If we had been in the emergency room I would surely have admitted her to the detoxification unit. But within moments of her switching back into other parts, the physicial signs of withdrawal ceased.

In yet another patient with a dissociative identity disorder, the following somatic manifestations of memory emerged. She acknowledged that she was aware of parts that seemed to be particularly mistrustful about taking the prescribed medication. At my request to work with those parts, within moments she transformed from a physically robust, articulate woman into a state of deformation. She manifested a left facial droop, with subsequent uncontrolled salivary drooling and slurred speech. Both hands appeared cramped into a position of contracture. In this state she was able to tell me about memories from her middle-childhood years in a convent, where, she alleges, she was given drugs, physically restrained, and sexually abused.

TRAUMA AND SOMATIC MEMORY

In these three cases we see physical sensations that either trigger the memory of experience or actually represent the experience (i.e., in an abreactive sense). The abreaction is perhaps best understood from the extensive research on posttraumatic stress disorders. There is a substantial literature on the psychobiology of PTSD (van der Kolk, 1987, 1994; Pitman, 1989; Pitman and Orr, 1990; Yehuda et al., 1991; Charney et al., 1993; Murburg, 1993; Friedman, Charney, and Deutch, 1995; van der Kolk, McFarlane, and Weisaeth, 1995) and a growing literature on the psychophysiology of dissociation (Putnam, 1984, 1988; Coons, 1988; Miller, 1989; Putnam, Zahn, and Post, 1990; Spiegel, 1991; Brown, 1994; Krystal et al., 1995). Flashbacks and nightmares can be understood as eidetic (photographic) memory dislocated in time. These experiences correlate with activation of certain neuronal pathways, particularly the noradrenergic tracts between the locus coeruleus (LC), the hippocampus, and the amygdala. Bessel van der Kolk (1987) has suggested "that LC-mediated autonomic arousal activates these potentiated pathways when conscious control over limbic system activity is diminished, as it is under stress and during sleep" (p. 70). Van der Kolk (1994) describes studies that suggest that intense stimulation of the amygdala may interfere with hippocampal function, leading to registration of sensorimotor perception (affective or somatic memory) without symbolic or semantic coding. Recent research on the connections between higher cortical pathways and these limbic system networks may, however, help us to understand how the sudden retrieval of symbolically encoded information that is triggered by somatic stimuli can occur in the absence of excessive stress or sleep states. In particular, we are coming to appreciate the role of the pre-frontal cortex, frontal lobes, anterior cingulate gyrus, and other parahippocampal structures in integrating information (memory). A particularly exciting area of research involves the use of positron emission tomography (PET) to look at brain activity during mental processing. One study in particular (Rauch et al., 1996) looked at the experience of flashbacks following script driven imagery. While activity increased in right limbic, paralimbic areas and visual cortex, activity was remarkably decreased in the left inferior frontal (Broca's area) and medial temporal cortex, where one would find the words to describe these experiences.

To understand the emergence of awareness through body sensation, we first need to review some basic concepts about memory. Memory begins with perception. Sensory perception peripherally is relayed to the sensory cortex, where there is process of registration, followed by consolidation into both short-term and long-term memory. Although there are specific anatomical locations in the brain correlating with these processes, both cortical and subcortical, the processes are best understood as feedback loops between anatomical structures. A simplified model for understanding the actual recall of information would be to imagine that stimuli activate neural network pathways, and it is the actual firing of pathways that leads to the recreation of "representations" in the cortex.

Long-term memory can be classified in two broad categories: 1) procedural memory or implicit, that is, learned, skills, like riding a bicycle and 2) declarative memory or explicit, that is, learned, facts. We are here specifically looking at the relationship between declarative memory—information that may be retrievable in visual or semantic representations—and sensation in the body.

The diencephalon (thalamic structures) in the upper brainstem is a main convergence zone of information from the brain and body. Its function is crucial to the state of wakefulness. The neuropsychologist James Newman (1996) emphasizes that this convergent zone is key to consciousness and names it ERTAS: the extended reticular thalamic activating system.

The hippocampus, an "old-brain" structure (evolutionarily predating the appearance of the mammalian neocortex) is part of the limbic system and is essential to the registration of memories. It functions primarily as a structure that facilitates memory and has many connections to other structures: the neocortex, the amygdala, and brainstem structures that carry input about basal body states. Somehow in the complex relatonship between thalamic structures, amygdala, and hippocampus we have the enigmatic regulation of cortical "awareness" of somatic experience.

NEURAL NETWORKS

Neuroanatomists and neurophysiologists studying neural networks understand that these are circuits or loops of information (Anderson and Rosenfeld, 1988). Connections between structures are both afferent (coming toward) and efferent (moving away from). Fair (1992) proposes two stages of hippocampal function: "the recycling of sense-data (cortex-hippocampus-cortex)" in short-term memory and "consolidation, [during which] return fibers from the hippocampal system may release trophic factors that result in long-lasting, site-specific changes in the postsynaptic membrane of the cortical units to which they project" (pp. 4–5) This mechanism, most commonly suggested for the creation of long-term memory on a cellular level, is long-term potentiation (LTP), a phenomenon in which electrical stimulation of a synapse causes a strengthened postsynaptic response, even when repeated stimuli are weaker (Lynch and Baudry, 1984; Gabriel, Sparenborg and Stolar, 1986).

Molecular biologists have identified within the hippocampus various receptor types and their particular sensitivities to circulating neurotransmitters. Particularly relevant in posttraumatic stress disorder are receptors with high sensitivity to the glucocorticoids, such as ACTH (adrenocorticotropic hormone). Since ACTH release is increased under stress, there is likely an increased firing of hypothalamic-cortical pathways, leading to increased facilitation of long term memory. It also appears, however, that there exists the possibility of down regulation, whereby overstimulation may be diminished through decreased sensitivity. The activation of these pathways is also contingent upon activation of hippocampal-brainstem connections, that is, input from basal body motivational systems.

In dissociative states the thalamus appears to play a crucial role. It "serves as a sensory gate or filter that directly and indirectly modulates the access of sensory information to the cortex, amygdala and hippocampus" (Krystal et al., 1995, p. 245). Studies looking at the excitatory (excitotoxic) neurotransmitter glutamate and specific receptors such as NMDA (N-methyl-D-aspartate) are giving us a theoretical basis for understanding the neurobiology of dissociation.

Fair (1992) outlines the way in which primary sensory input is processed in the neocortex as generic or generalized memory, primarily through a corticocortical relay system. Long-term potentiation, leading to long-term memory through various feedback loops between sensory cortex, association cortices, and limbic system, leads to consolidation of specific information. The associational connections over time are subject to modification and consequently substitutions in memory. In addition, associative changes can cause blocking of pathways, a "corresponding memory may become . . .strongly resistant to reactivation via the usual cortical routes. (It may still be accessible by way of affect-related retrieval. . . [through] subcortico-cortical circuitry. . .)" (p. 56). This statement means simply that a feeling state can trigger a memory and that the memory may or may not be closely associated with clear content. The study of both the blockage of pathways in the associational cortices and the reactivation of pathways through subcortical (limbic system-brain stem) pathways may be the substrate of scientific inquiry that can help us to clarify the concept of delayed recall ("recovered memory"). There are over 100 billion neurons in the brain, and each neuron has about 10^4 synapses. The number of possible routes of connection is astronomical. The possibility of triggering recall is omnipresent.

This is not to suggest that affect-mediated retrieval is the only mechanism of delayed recall. In the case of Mrs. O'C presented by Oliver Sacks (1970), we see the emergence of previously inaccessible memories from the first five years of life as a result of a stroke induced temporal lobe epilepsy. In this case, the involvement of limbic system-temporal lobe pathways produced auditory hallucinations in the form of long-forgotten Irish songs, associated with profound nostalgia, "an overwhelming sense of being-a-child again, in her long-forgotten home, in the arms and presence of her mother" who had died when she was five years old" (p. 136).

Much of our understanding of how information from the body is processed in the brain comes from studying patients who have cerebral illness or injury that interferes specifically with that processing. Somatosensory memory has been studied and documented in people who experience the phantom-limb phenomenon (Katz and Melzack, 1990; Katz, 1992). Phantom limb is characterized by either the persistence or the recurrence of pain in a limb previously amputated.

> The affective or emotional tone that accompanies the experience of a pain memory appears not to be a re-activation of a stored representation, but is thought to be generated on a moment-by-moment basis. . . .The separate somatosensory and cognitive components that appear to underlie the unified experience of a pain memory are consistent with recent evidence of multiple, dissociable memory systems which specialize in processing specific kinds of information (Katz and Melzack, 1990, p. 333).[4]

The neurologist Antonio Damasio (1994) has been studying patients with anosognosia, a condition in which the individual fails to recognize information from the body. The most common example is a hemiplegic patient who does not recognize that the left side of his or her body is paralyzed. The injury is to the right brain; a mirror-image injury on the left side of the brain would not cause this loss of "awareness." Damasio has also recognized that some patients with anosognosia have an impaired ability to reason and make decisions as well as a defect in processing emotions. The study of these patients has contributed to his belief that there is in the brain a particular area (the anterior cingulate cortex) where emotion, attention, and memory are integrated.

There is no consensus as yet that any such integrative activity can be localized anatomically. Damasio himself states, "A composite, ongoing representation of current body states is distributed over a large number of structures in both subcortical and cortical locations" (p. 154). He has developed a theory, which he calls "the somatic-marker hypothesis," that may be very helpful in understanding somatic memory. His theory is dependent on the following concepts:

1) There are, within the brain, "dispositional representations" and these representations are clusters of synapses enabling the reconstruction of a memory. These dispositional representations exist in potential states once information has been processed initially. One could think of these representations as gates that must be decoded before they will excite adjacent neurons, thereby facilitating recall.

2) There are "as-if" activity patterns, where information is triggered not by the actual change in body state but by a symbolic representation (used in the psychological, not neurological sense) of a somatic state.

3) "Convergence zones located in the prefrontal cortices are . . . the repository of dispositional representations for the appropriately categorized and unique contingencies of our life experience" (p. 192).

In summary, he is saying that, somewhere in the ventromedial (bottom and central) portion of the prefrontal cortices (the front of the frontal lobes), pathways from the somatosensory aspects of the neocortex (holding the potential for recovery of certain information about one's mind) are converging with pathways from the limbic system and brainstem (holding the potential for recovery of information about the body). This convergence, whether anatomically located or diffusely distributed, is most certainly crucial to the emergence of consciousness.

The neurologist V. Ramachandran is also researching this phenomenon of anosognosia (Shreeve, 1995). He has suggested that the right parietal lobe is crucial in the detection of an anomaly—something not working according to script. When a stroke damages this area, neglect of the anomaly occurs. He has also noticed that rapid eye movement can stimulate this part of the parietal cortex and trigger awareness of the anomaly. He compares the effect of induced rapid eye movement to REM sleep, when dreaming brings dissociated perceptions into awareness. Clinicians utilizing the technique of EMDR for posttraumatic symptoms also note the triggering of awareness as well as desensitization (Shapiro, 1995). While it remains to be studied, one possible explanation of EMDR's efficacy is that alternating bilateral stimulation to the brain through sensory perception has an impact on gating properties in neural networks, allowing for an enhanced integration of thalamic, limbic system, and cortical function. Some unpublished studies using electroencephalography suggest that EMDR resynchronizes hemispheric activity that has uncoupled from pacemaker cells (Bergmann, 1995). As a result of the downregulation of a chronically sensitized system, individuals are able to integrate higher cortical function more fully. Once noradrenergic firing is diminished, self-perception is actually altered and people are able to self-reinforce cognitively more mature explanations of traumatic experience.

MECHANISMS OF AFFECT
AND SOMATIC MEDIATED RETRIEVAL

Finally, we look specifically at affect-mediated retrieval of memory and its relation to sensations within the body.

Both Damasio (1994) and Fair (1992) have established theories about a correspondence between higher cortical memory function and lower, brainstem activity. Fair calls these "brainstem tags" (p. 133). While there is a limited number of basic drives and affect states, there is an unlimited number of higher cortical associations. Consequently, a great many loops of information (memories) may be tagged to the same emotional state. The implication of this idea is quite complex. It suggests an anatomical explanation for how information retrieval can be influenced by powerful emotional states that are not temporally related. The association of emotional states with higher cortical function (vision, language, symbolic representation) gives us some sense of personal continuity. When the cortico-subcortico-brainstem loops are somehow intermittently blocked there is a disruption of this sense of continuity. Hence the subjective experience of discontinuous conscious states, that is, dissociation.

Nonsymptomatic dissociation occurs all the time, when implicit memory is disconnected from self-awareness, for example, having a conversation while driving a car. Symptomatic dissociation occurs when self-awareness is disconnected from declarative memory, for example, fugue states and traumatic black outs.

One final clinical example that specifically suggests some sort of consciousness manifest through the body is two cases presented by Damasio and Tranel (cited in Fair, 1992, Appendix). They tested two patients who suffered from prosopagnosia, the inability to recognize familiar faces. They showed these patients pictures of faces, both familiar and unfamiliar. Visually the patients were unable to distinguish between familiar and unfamiliar faces. However, measurement of galvanic skin conductance revealed significant changes when they looked at what should have been the familiar faces. Both patients had lesions in the white matter of the occipitotemporal cortex, which suggests that some brainstem-limbic system-cortical loops were activated, stimulating these brainstem "tags" and leading to arousal. Key neuronal pathways in the cortex, however, were damaged and there-fore "conscious" mental recognition of the faces was impossible.

LOST IN THE SYNAPSE

Let us now return to my three clinical cases. In the first patient, the emergence of pain in her body during dissociative episodes at night was the first indication of somatically held information somehow dis-connected from declarative memory. Her persistent skepticism and her own value of authenticity inhibited willful imaginative elabora-tion. But how valid were her associations, particularly ones such as, "I have a feeling its my grandfather; it's just a feeling"? She seems to be like Damasio's (1994) patients with prosopagnosia: one part of the brain registers retrieval of stored perception, while another series of associations seem to be blocked. The verbal process of psychoanaly-sis facilitated a complex series of associations, like meandering through a maze that is vaguely familiar. We did not need to validate the details of content in order to validate the somatic memory.

In the patient who developed symptoms of a narcotic withdrawal syndrome, we were witnessing a different process. The memory was more like the phantom-limb state, presented entirely as a physiologi-cally reproduced state. We need to know more about the relationship between cortical mental representations and the triggering of brain stem stimulation and autonomic nervous system response.

While there is ongoing research on the neurophysiology of dis-sociation, there is much that remains mysterious. In patients who have dissociative disorders, what is the neurochemical mechanism by which transmitters such as glutamate may block or unblock asso-ciations? Should the black hole of dissociation be renamed "lost in the synapse"? Why is switching so often accompanied by headache? Is psychotherapy a process of down regulation, whereby pathways previously shut as a result of flooding (over stimulation) are now gradually open to electrochemical stimulation? Does the psychothera-peutic concept of "making it safe" simply mean deactivating certain memory/information loops between cortex, limbic system, and brain stem? Or does it mean activating new loops, so that the information can be "stored" at a higher level of organization? Is that how affect is mediated by cognitive development?

In a sense, aren't alters simply collections of memories in search of a self? Like the patient with Korsakov's syndrome who needs con-stantly to reconstruct himself through confabulation, isn't the patient with dissociative identity disorder a self with multiple constructions at various levels of cognitive development? Whereas patients with Korsakov's confabulate because no new information is ever stored and they are not aware of this lack, patients with dissociative identity disorder maintain enough sense of self that confabulation is usually not so necessary. They sometimes know that they do not remember.

There are times in our clinical work, however, that we do listen to lies. Perhaps some of the misinformation, as well as the absolute denial of trauma we sometimes hear, is a form of confabulation, the construction of the non-traumatized self. I am reminded of the words of the poet Adrienne Rich (1978):

> No one ever told us we had to study our lives,
> make of our lives a study, as if learning natural history
> or music, that we should begin
> with the simple exercises first
> slowly go on trying
> the hard ones, practicing till strength
> and accuracy became one with the daring
> to leap into transcendence, take the chance
> of breaking down in the wild arpeggio
> or faulting the full sentence of the fugue.
> —And in fact we can't live like that: we take on
> everything at once before we've even begun
> to read or mark time, we're forced to begin
> in the midst of the hardest movement,
> the one already sounding as we are born.

It is the clinician who sits with the patient "in the midst of the hardest movement." It is the clinician who listens to the mental representation of both symbolic and physical experience. And it is the clinician who must learn to listen to the body as well.

We are at a stage of understanding where we can suggest that affect-mediated and somatic-mediated retrieval of memory has validity, but we do not know if it is reliable. One hypothesis to test is that the eidetic nature of traumatic memory increases the reliability of specific recall. Another hypothesis is that, if discontinuous conscious states lead to temporal dislocation, then layers of associations become like transparencies superimposed on one another. It is more likely that memories are blurred into each other than that they are wholly unauthentic. Yet another hypothesis to explore pertains to our understanding of affect states. In patients who have a symptom picture of dissociation, are cycling moods actually episodes of memory retrieval, that is, affective abreactions in the absence of semantic memory. How many patients with a diagnosis of rapid cycling mood disorder are actually patients with dissociative disorders?

In conclusion, if consciousness is a complex integration of information processing dependent on memory, and information is retrievable through both cortical function and basal body state, then the body seems to have the capacity to "hold" information, as in a potential state, even if the associational pathways to mental representation are somehow blocked. In people who have no structural neurological damage,[5] such as patients with chronic posttraumatic symptoms, changes in basal body states and intense affective states can then trigger areas of cortical potentiation (dispositional representations). In some cases, associated pathways will allow for the linkage of semantic information with these body states. In other cases, associated pathways remain blocked, and the memories are represented entirely in either somatic sensations or affect states. It is particularly in cases where associated cortical pathways remain inaccessible that we must respect the risk of suggestibility in traumatized individuals. We must, however, also respect the integrity of somatic memories and validate the recall of experience without semantic clarification.

NOTES

[1]See the work of Khan (1971), Bromberg (1991), and Kennedy (1996).

[2]For an excellent discussion of the influence of Eastern philosophy and meditation practice on our understanding of the mind/body unity see Varela, Thompson, and Rosch (1992).

[3]Although a definition of somatic memories is ultimately an endpoint of this discussion, it would be useful to clarify a distinction between the terms psychosomatic and somatic memory. Psychosomatic implies a channeling of mental affect, such as anxiety, into the body and is actually consistent with dualism, that is, the displacement of mental phenomena into body experience. Somatic memory implies the very processing (potential storage) of experience (information) simultaneously within the body and mind, mediated through the brain, which is the intersection of the mind and body. This information can be symbolic, or, as discussed by Davies and Frawley (1994), "can exist outside the usual domain of recalled experience, unavailable to self-reflective processes and analytic examination" (p. 45).

[4]The concept of modular brain systems is exquisitely described by Squire (1987).

[5]There are studies suggesting that severe emotional trauma may have some "structural" effect on the brain, such as decreased volume of hippoc-

ampal cells (Bremner et al., 1995; Stein et al., 1997). However, we do not know if there exists a direct cause and effect between these observations, nor do we know the significance of these changes.

REFERENCES

Ackerman, D. (1990), *A Natural History of the Senses*. New York: Vintage Press.
Anderson, J. & Rosenfeld, E. (1988), *Neurocomputing*. Cambridge, MA: MIT Press.
Bergmann, U. (1995), Speculations on the neurobiology of EMDR. Unpublished manuscript.
Bremner, J., Randall, P., Scott, T., Bronen, R., Seibyl, J., Southwick, S., Delaney, R., McCarthy, G., Charney, D. & Innis, R. (1995), MRI-based measurement of hippocampal volume in patients with combat-related posttraumatic stress disorder. *Amer. J. Psychiat.*, 152:973–981.
Bromberg, P. (1991), On knowing one's patient inside out: The aesthetics of unconscious communication. *Psychoanal. Dial.* 1:399–422.
Brown, P. (1994), Toward a psychobiological model of dissociation and post-traumatic stress disorder. In: *Dissociation*, ed. S. Lynn & J. Rhue. New York: Guilford.
Chalmers, D. (1996), *The Conscious Mind*. New York: Oxford University Press.
Charney, D., Deutch, A., Krystal, J., Southwick, S. & Davis, M.(1993), Psychobiologic mechanisms of the post-traumatic stress disorder. *Arch. Gen. Psychiat.*, 50:294–305.
Churchland, P. (1986), *Neurophilosophy*. Cambridge, MA: MIT Press.
———— & Sejnowski, T. (1992), *The Computational Brain*. Cambridge, MA: MIT Press.
Coons, P. (1988), Psychophysiological aspects of multiple personality disorder: A review. *Dissociation*, 1:47–53.
Crick, F. (1994), *The Astonishing Hypothesis*. New York: Charles Scribner's Sons.
Damasio, A. (1994), *Descartes' Error*. New York: Grosset/Putnam.
Davies J., & Frawley, M. (1994), *Treating the Adult Survivor of Sexual Abuse*. New York: Basic Books.
Dennett, D. (1991), *Consciousness Explained*. Boston: Little, Brown.
Descartes, R. (1637), *Discourse on Method*, London: Penguin Classics, 1968.
Eccles, J. (1989), *Evolution of the Brain*. London: Routledge.
Edelman, G. (1987), *Neural Darwinism*. New York: Basic Books.
———— (1992), *Bright Air, Brilliant Fire*. New York: Basic Books.
Fair, C. (1992), *Cortical Memory Functions*. Boston: Birkhauser.
Friedman, M., Charney, D. & Deutch, Y., ed. (1995), *Neurobiological and Clinical Consequences of Stress*. Philadelphia, PA: Lippincott-Raven.
Gabriel, M., Sparenborg, S. & Stolar, N. (1986), The neurobiology of memory. In: *Mind and Brain*, ed. J. LeDoux & W. Hirst. New York: Cambridge University Press.

Giller, E., ed. (1990), *Biological Assessment and Treatment of PTSD*. Washington, DC: American Psychiatric Press.

Johnson, M. (1987), *The Body in the Mind*. Chicago: University of Chicago Press.

Katz, J. (1992), Psychophysical correlates of phantom limb experience. *J. Neurol. Neurosurg. Psychiat.*, 55:811–821.

——— & Melzack, R. (1990), Pain "memories" in phantom limbs: Review and clinical observations. *Pain*, 43:319–336.

Kennedy, R. (1996), Aspects of consciousness: one voice or many? *Psychoanal. Dial.*, 6:73–96.

Khan, M. (1971), "To hear with eyes": Clinical notes on body as subject and object. In: *The Privacy of the Self*. New York: International Universities Press, 1974, pp. 234–250.

Kristeva, J.(1993), *Proust and the Sense of Time*. New York: Columbia University Press.

Krystal, J., Bennett, A., Bremner, J., Southwick, S. & Charney, D. (1995), Toward a cognitive neuroscience of dissociation and altered memory functions in post-traumatic stress disorder. In: *Neurobiological and Clinical Consequences of Stress*, eds. M. Friedman, D. Charney & A. Deutch. Philadelphia, PA: Lippincott-Raven, pp. 239–269.

Lynch, G. & Baudry, M. (1984), The biochemistry of memory: A new and specific hypothesis. *Science*, 224:1057–63.

Miller, S. (1989), Optical differences in cases of multiple personality disorder. *J. Nerv. Mental Dis.*, 177:480–486.

Murburg, M., ed. (1993), *Catecholamine Function in Posttraumatic Stress Disorder*. Washington, DC: American Psychiatric Press.

Newman, J. (1996), Putting the puzzle together. Part I: Toward a general theory of the neural correlates of consciousness, *J. Consciousness Studies*, 4:47–66.

——— (1996), Putting the puzzle together. Part II: Toward a general theory of the neural correlates of consciousness, *J. Consciousness Studies*, 4:100–21.

Penrose, R. (1989), *The Emporer's New Mind*. New York: Penguin.

——— (1994), *Shadows of the Mind*. New York: Oxford.

Pitman, R. (1989), Posttraumatic stress disorder, hormones and memory. *Biol. Psychiat.*, 26:221–223.

——— & Orr, S. (1990), The black hole of trauma. *Biol. Psychiat.*, 27:469–471.

Plato (n.d.), *Plato, The Collected Dialogues*. New York: Charles Scribner & Sons, 1871.

Plum, F. & Posner, J. (1972), *The Diagnosis of Stupor and Coma*. Philadelphia, PA: Davis.

Putnam, F. (1984), The psychophysiologic investigation of multiple personality disorder. *Psychiat. Clin. No. Amer.*, 7:31–39.

——— (1988), The switch process in multiple personality disorder and other state-change disorders. *Dissociation*, 1:24–32.

——— Zahn, T. & Post, R. (1990), Differential autonomic nervous system activity in multiple personality disorder. *Psychiat. Res.*, 31:251–260.

Rauch, S., van der Kolk, B., Fisler, R., Alpert, N., Scott, O., Savage, C., Fischman, A., Jenike, M. T. & Pitman, R. (1996), A symptom provocation study of posttraumatic stress disorder using positron emission tomography and script-driven imagery. *Arch. Gen. Psychiat.*, 53:380–387.

Rich, A. (1978), Transcendental etude. In: *The Dream of a Common Language.* New York: Norton.

Sacks, O. (1970), *The Man Who Mistook His Wife for a Hat.* New York: Simon & Schuster.

Shapiro, F. (1995), *Eye Movement Desensitization and Reprocessing.* New York: Guilford.

Shreeve, J. (1995), The brain that misplaced its body. *Discover*, May, pp. 82–87.

Spiegel, D. (1991), Neurophysiological correlates of hypnosis and dissociation. *J. Neuropsychiat.*, 3:440–444.

Squire, L. (1987), *Memory and Brain.* Oxford: Oxford University Press.

Stein, M., Hanna, C., Koverola, C., Torchia, M. & McClarity, B., Structural brain changes in PTSD, *Annals of the New York Academy of Sciences*, 821:76–82.

van der Kolk, B. (1987), *Psychological Trauma.* Washington, DC: American Psychiatric Press.

——— (1994), The body keeps the score. *Harvard Rev. of Psychiat.* 1:253–65.

——— McFarlane, A., & Weisaeth, L., ed. (1995), *Traumatic Stress.* New York: Guilford.

Varela F., Thompson E. & Rosch E. (1992), *The Embodied Mind.* Cambridge, MA: MIT Press.

Yehuda, R., Giller, E., Southwick, S., Lowy, M. & Mason, J. (1991), Hypothalamic-pituitary-adrenal dysfunction in posttraumatic stress disorder. *Biol. Psychiat.*, 30:1031–1048.

10

"MAMA, WHY DON'T YOUR FEET TOUCH THE GROUND?"

Staying with the Body
And the Healing Moment
In Psychoanalysis

Tamsin Looker

Several years into her analysis, my patient Iris said to me, "Our work will be done when I have had enough time with you, when I have been as comfortable in my body as one can be in an old sweatshirt." When I asked her to tell me how that might feel, she said, "I would be able to be fully in my body, in your presence, and able to move freely around your room and touch and see things from my real self without fear. I would be able to give up the fear that comes with constantly overthinking and evaluating whether I really have or deserve your availability. I would be able to take for granted that it is fine with you that I can take you for granted." This vision marked a nodal point in Iris's growth in her treatment, and has served as a beacon for changes to come. I am grateful to Iris for her imagery. We analysts need more descriptions of mutative events (Spence, 1996), of healing moments and states of wellness, in our literature.

The kind of well-being Iris hopes to achieve is not easily come

I would like to thank Drs. Carolyn Clement, Fran Anderson, Zeborah Schachtel, Susan Coates, Susan Kraemer, Felicia Rozek and Ron Balamuth for their helpful comments on earlier drafts of this chapter.

by, either in the natural course of development or through the efforts of psychoanalytic treatment. Indeed, many people are unable to produce such images of psychosomatic unity and health. Those who have suffered gross neglect, or physical or sexual abuse, are afflicted with dramatic dissociative symptoms well documented in the clinical literature (Putnam, 1989; Davies and Frawley 1994; van Der Kolk, 1994). In my clinical experience, however, the problem of psychosomatic disharmony is much more widespread, perhaps ubiquitous. Nearly all my patients suffer from some degree of disconnection from their bodies and, therefore, from their truest feelings and core sense of self. Patients complain of not being able to breathe naturally or to feel entitled to take up space or to move about the world propelled by authentic feelings and needs. They suffer from a deep conviction that they cannot occupy their bodies while maintaining mutually safe and intimate contact with the people they need most. I believe that these dissociative conditions are often the cumulative developmental sequelae of various forms of parent–child misattunement.[1]

In this chapter I explore the rift between psyche and soma as a problem rooted in the child's relationship to the mother's body. Through clinical examples, I show how the mother's disconnection from her own body can promote dissociation of psyche and soma in her child. I also explore the idea that if psychoanalytic work is to facilitate the bridging of psyche and soma in the patient, the analyst must keep her own body present in the treatment room. The analyst's attention to her own and her patient's body-based experiences, and to connections and disconnections between psyche and soma, are critical to the analytic holding environment. During enactments of troubled relational patterns, analyst and patient will share or take turns feeling all kinds of disturbing experiences of psychosomatic disunity. These states of disconnection are powerful diagnostic tools that guide us to the places that need to be healed. I demonstrate through clinical examples that it is the analyst's struggle to remain embodied consciously throughout these enactments that makes the patient feel, quite literally, held and, consequently, safe enough to experiment with new relational patterns.

I want to convey my appreciation of analytic space, not as a playground for abstract ideas, but as a place where the actual body and the imagined body coexist and interplay. In this interplay, bridges between body, thought, and affect are built, and feelings of being alive are enhanced. In this interplay, the analyst is fully used and taken in. If healing moments are to occur in treatment, the analyst must be able to surrender to body-based experience and to the flow of bodily imagery before giving in to the inevitable press to abstract and verbalize. Such surrender can feel very risky to both patient and analyst. It can lead to moments of boundary loss and to violent imagery that register in the body and, therefore, feel real. At other times this immersion can create an intimacy that can feel too good to be true. I offer no specific techniques for staying with bodily experience in clinical work. It is enormously difficult for most of us to do, not only in treatment but in any aspect of life. Rather, through clinical vignettes, I aim to convey the significance and power of bodily presence and bodily absence in the treatment setting.

RECLAIMING THE BODY FOR PSYCHOANALYSIS

When Freud removed his hand from his patient's forehead and invited her to free associate, he empowered her mind but abandoned her experiencing body.[2] He abandoned the body that remembers and carries meaning, and that, above all, seeks to connect her to others for the sake of connection. With the development of the structural theory, the primacy of the Oedipus complex and the call for abstinence, the actual body was eclipsed by the fantasized body and the intrapsychic fate of the sexual and aggressive drives. The touch taboo and the fixed postures of patient and analyst that we have inherited from the classical model inhibit not only what we do and say with our patients, but also *even what we are able to imagine and feel*.[3] We have been taught to be quick to reflect interpretively, to impose rational order on bodily experience. We foreclose our opportunity to learn from the body and to connect it to both affect and abstract thought.

The dichotomization of mind and body is much older and more pervasive than psychoanalysis. The tendency to split mind and body appears to be universally human. Ernest Cassirer (1944), the anthropologist, suggested that as a species we have evolved into symbolmongers: the symbolic functioning that makes us human can take on its own reality and leaves us cut off from our more biological and emotional selves.

Similarly, Ernst Schachtel (1957) described the loss of infantile psychosomatic unity as a culturally shaped and repressive developmental event, which is largely responsible for infantile amnesia. When, in the third year of life, memory in the service of recognition and naming of objects takes precedence over experiencing, a unique and autobiographical self gives way to the conventionalized memory that

accompanies language. Then the senses of smell and touch recede
and the distant senses of sight and hearing take primacy. This shift
away from immediate bodily experience, he believed, constitutes a
rupture in the continuity of self that cannot be overestimated. More
recently, Daniel Stern (1985) has restated Schachtel's thesis: "There
are enormous gains and enormous losses with the advent of language.
With entrance into the cultural membership is the loss of the force
and the wholeness of original experience" (p. 178). He explains that,
since language demands a categorization of information and cannot
express many nuances of affect, it forecloses certain kinds of communication between child and parent. Frustration with this gap in understanding motivates the child to learn more and more a communally
based language, which, in turn, decreases his or her ability to communicate subjective experience.

The difficulties and limitations of language-based interactions
between patient and analyst are similar to those between parent and
child. We and our patients are involved in teaching each other or
coconstructing a common language. When that language excludes
sensorimotor, kinesthetic, proprioceptive, and imagistic experience,
we drift away from the more personal, the subjective, and the affective.

Much in the psychoanalytic literature supports a nonlinear,
nonhierarchical, nondichotomous relationship between body-based
and language-based experience. These experiences can be seen as
parallel, different, complementary, and, in health, fluidly linked. Noy's
(1969) ideas on the relationship between primary and secondary process and Fosshage's (1997) views on waking and dreaming mentation
support the idea of a complementary relationship. They both contend that we do not grow out of, nor should we be cured of, intuition,
sensorimotor or imagistic intelligence, primary process, or dreaming
mentation. Bucci (1985) and Epstein (1994) suggest that these processes operate according to a logic and foster adaptation and growth,
just as language-based processes do, throughout the lifespan. They
emphasize that these processes are often closer to affect, to a core
sense of self, and to a sense of agency than are the more language-
based processes. They are, indeed, closer to the body. They are the
processes on which we rely for "self-righting" (Fosshage, 1997) and
for the bridging of body and mind.[4]

Winnicott, because he was not only an analyst but a pediatrician
who worked directly with mother–child pairs, was no stranger to touch
or to the bodies of both mother and child.[5] In all his writings, the
body is present, staying well-connected to the mind through his po-

etic, rather than scientific, use of language. His concept of premature ego development prefigures the kind of mind–body dissociation I will explore in the clinical material to follow. Winnicott (1949) said that, when a mother cannot hold her child, the child begins to take care of herself with her own mind. Such precocious caretaking of both the self and the mother brings with it a feeling of being less alive in one's own body. In subsequent clinical examples, I expand on the importance of psychosomatic awareness and integration in the caretaker and in the analyst as a prerequisite for a capacity to hold.

It is hard for us psychoanalysts to think about and work with the fact that the body is not a metaphor. The body is a wonderful source of metaphor, but it is also something to be reckoned with on its own terms. I learned this when I worked with toddlers and their parents together in a therapeutic nursery.[6] There we tried to repair disturbed interactions by working directly with body-based attachment behaviors, as well as with talk and play. This hands-on clinical experience impressed me indelibly with the fact that, when an analyst focuses directly on the body, she has unique access to the most severe mind–body splits associated with terrors related to ego annihilation and abandonment, as well as to the more subtle dissociative consequences of parent–child misattunement. Extreme examples of attachment disturbances abound already in the literature. The following is an example of the sort of subtle, mild attachment problem that might have been experienced in childhood by any of our patients.

ATTACHMENT AND THE BODY: EMERGENCE OF DISSOCIATIVE PROCESSES IN A MOTHER–DAUGHTER PAIR

Deedee is an 18-month-old girl who is coping with her mother's mild to moderate depression.[7] This mother–toddler pair spends a reasonable amount of time together in close contact and a reasonable amount of time pursuing separate activities. They also seem to negotiate separations and other changes in closeness without too much trouble and would probably not fit into any of Ainsworth and colleagues' (1978) disturbed attachment groups. A close look, however, reveals that when mother and child are in close physical contact, they almost never have simultaneous mutual eye contact or even direct body angulation. There is a subtle but purposeful disconnection between what is happening in their bodies and how they share and validate their experiences through an affective visual exchange. Deedee is learning to dissociate in order to cope with the fact that her mother's face is a foggy mirror or a frightening window. Without clear communication and validation about what they are doing and what they feel about what they are doing, they cannot negotiate shared affect or closeness and separation during this critical phase of rapprochement as well as it might appear at first.

When you look closely, you see that Deedee moves her body more stiffly and less steadily than do many of her peers. She falls more often. She cannot be fully in her body while using her antennae to monitor her mother's moods. She is overdeveloping her capacity for empathy and not paying attention to her own insides. This is Winnicott's (1949) premature ego development in progress. Unable to rely on her mother's body and her mother's boundaries, she must work overtime, both cognitively and defensively. She is taking care of herself with her mind.

Lichtenberg (1989) suggests that, when a child's cognitive development is not well-enough grounded in a body relationship with her mother, there is a hollowness about it. This disconnection is evident in Deedee's body and is heard in her language. The periphery of her body, her musculature, and her movements are stiff as she tries to keep certain things out and certain things in. Her language is taking off like a rocket, sometimes in an almost manic way. Her language is almost entirely social, adapted to her view of her mother's needs, and not well-enough connected to her personal self and to her body self. It fills in sad holes. Sometimes her language seems almost to hold her body together and hold it upright—a kind of verbal ectoskeleton. Still, at first glance, few would call this toddler or her relationship with her mother disturbed. She is sensitive and articulate and can separate without obvious anxiety. She can grow up to be almost any one of our patients—any one of us.

Nonetheless, this child, like all children who are not comfortable in their own bodies, is not comfortable with her mother's body. She cannot relax into herself and take her mother's body for granted because her mother's body does not convey direct affective messages. The mother's mind–body dissociation makes it difficult for the child to connect to her. The mother is not fully present, and it is difficult for the child to read why. As an infant, this child needed her mother's body, not only for soothing and containment, but to poke and probe, to possess ruthlessly, to explore fearlessly. She now also needs her mother's body to be as resilient as a jungle gym. She needs an energetic, active body that can swoop her up, run after her, and release her when need be. This child's indirectness of gaze and body angulation suggests that she does not have free physical access either to her mother's body or to her emotional core. Because her mother's body does not accurately and safely communicate what she feels, the child is not safe to live in her own body. She must partially abandon it to search for and manage her mother. She is preoccupied with her mother's emotional state at the expense of what Winnicott (1949) calls "going on being" (p. 245). I mean to distinguish this preoccupation from the more usual need and wish a child possesses to reach the mother's inner emotional core (Loewald, 1970; Aron, 1991). It is distinguished by the extent to which this search is due to long-standing frustration and a feeling that it is necessary for social survival. It is a search that robs the child of personal liveliness.

This depressed mother, unable to process her own troubled feelings, cannot receive, contain, and detoxify Deedee's bad feelings (Slade, Coates, and Diamond, 1996). She does not dare to engage in mutual gaze with her daughter. She does not want to be explored and discovered. Disconnected from her own insides, she keeps her child emotionally mystified. Unless Deedee finds some way to challenge her mother's defenses successfully, she will be constricted in her ability to explore people and the world at large assertively.[8]

AGGRESSION, MIND–BODY HARMONY, AND THE MOTHER–CHILD RELATIONSHIP

Central to Deedee's psychosomatic breach and to her constriction in her relationship with her mother is the unavailability of aggression for constructive use. Anger, frustration, and sadness are locked into the bodies of both mother and child, and they are forced to do an unimaginative and careful dance. Deedee, a too good child, has had to forfeit her aggressive strivings and, consequently, her vitality, to accommodate to her rather fragile, disconnected mother. Her mother, handicapped by her own rigid yet tenuous mind–body connection, cannot make a safe space inside herself where she can hold her daughter. Deedee is not free to demand or to carve out that space. She is not free to spontaneously expand and contract what Raphel-Leff (1994) would call her "personal dominion," her ability to project herself intrusively into her mother's mind and body beyond body boundaries.

To discover and connect to others, we need to be free to use aggression in our conscious and unconscious imaginations and in our bodily interactions. Because the psychoanalytic relationship is a predominantly verbal process, it is especially difficult for patient and analyst to use aggression to enliven their interactions. It is difficult to keep the destructive and constructive aspects of aggression in a growth-promoting balance.

Analysts differ about whether and how they recognize a role for constructive and interpersonally adaptive aggression. There are also important differences in how the relationship between destructive and constructive aggression is understood. With respect to these important issues, I find Winnicott and his followers, and Bowlby and his successors, most comfortable theoretically and most helpful clinically.

Winnicott (1950), in a radical departure from Freud's (1915) "Death Instinct," and from Klein's (1932) idea that destructive aggression is rooted in an innate destructive envy of the breast, posited a constructive role for aggression. He saw innate aggression as something like a life force, synonymous with activity and movement, that becomes loving or hating, or both, through interaction with the caretaker. He located the developmental vicissitudes of aggression in the spaces between mother and child, and between the inside and outside of the body and the self. He saw the hammering out of boundaries between self and other as an inevitably aggressive process and one that is both interpersonal and intrapsychic. Aggression, Winnicott (1950) said, contributes to the development of the self, and an early recognition of me and not me.[9] He thought it a major task of both caretaker and analyst to survive aggression without diminishing the vitality of that life force. Winnicott (1969) warned against retaliating when aggression takes a destructive bent and exploitation when aggressive strivings are pleasurably erotic. He described how a child or a patient well-enough held could use aggression in the service of creativity and of whole and empathic relationships.

Attachment theorists (Bowlby, 1973; Ainsworth et al., 1978) and their intersubjective psychoanalytic successors (Stern, 1985; Beebe and Lachmann, 1988; Knoblach, 1997) also see a constructive role for aggression. They see an innate proclivity in the infant to find a homeostatic or mutually life-affirming relationship with the caretaking environment. This proclivity is evident in attachment-seeking and maintaining behaviors, such as smiling, reaching, grasping, gazing, crying. While these behaviors are clearly adapted for interpersonal survival, they can also be seen as aggressive in the conventional and potentially destructive sense. The infant or child protests angrily with crying, screaming, and clinging, and, later, with verbal bossiness or tantrums when the caretaker is emotionally or physically unavailable. Attachment theory allows for the possibility that the aggressive protest or even attack will get the mother to modify her responses to adapt better to the child's needs. We analysts must understand this adaptive and hopeful intention in aggression and use it to vitalize our interactions with our patients.

We need to understand the extent to which destructive aggression is constructive aggression turned to bitter, disembodied despair. This despair shows itself in the Kleinian imagery of dangerous or deadened body parts. While this persecutory imagery suggests a mental preoccupation with the body, it usually belies an abandonment of the experiencing and interpersonally related body. These patients deny and attack their needs for touch, closeness, and gaze. They have left their actual bodies and flown into a world of overideation and paranoia concerning the availability of the other. Winnicott's (1969) normal greedy attack has soured, becoming a destructive, deadening attack on the bodies of self and other.

Repeated failed attempts to connect with one's caretaker can result in rage, frustration, and despair (Bowlby, 1973). Such despair becomes a dead space between mother and child and between mind and body, a space where defensive pathological thought processes proliferate. André Green (1993) explores this phenomenon and describes the child's attempt to repair the psychic hole left by precocious body–psyche dissociation with compulsive sadomasochistic thought and fantasy. Eigen (1986) has provided a wealth of examples of the kind of "crazy" bodily imagery that can fill this dead space in psychosis. He says that in psychosis "what seems to be a spoiling process can be an attempt to put mind and body together in whatever ways are possible under the circumstances" (p. 293).

Psychotic thinking is only one of many consequences of rage and despair about not having comfortable access to the mother's body. In our work we more often see patients who have responded to their mother's psychosomatic disunity and unavailability with an avoidance of being fully alive. This fear is expressed through many symptoms, perhaps most commonly in psychosomatic, obsessional, or depressive illness. In all of these conditions there is a fear and avoidance of either loving or hating from an embodied place. The internal world is cut off from people, and the mind is cut off from affect and body.

In obsessional thought we try to control the past or the future with our minds by running away from the experience of the moment and from the body. Shabad and Selinger (1995) have described this flight from rootedness in the body and the spontaneous moment to an identification with vigilant mental activity as a counterphobic defense against disappointment by the environment.

In depression, the arms and hands, which would ordinarily reach out to touch and cling in hope, or gouge and penetrate in frustration, withdraw from the needed one and hang in limp despair. The mind of the depressed person is mostly involved in an attack on one's own body and on one's own body-based attachment needs. Lawrence Epstein (1984, 1987) has noted that a depressed patient will protect the analyst from negative feelings by turning them against the self and the body. Spotnitz (1976) calls this move, which he believes is originally learned to protect the parent, "the narcissistic defense." Both analysts believe that patients who are trapped in this cocoon of self-hatred must be helped to direct aggression toward the analyst in order to gain access to the interpersonal world.

Bringing aggression, either loving or hating, into the relationship and bringing it into the experiencing body are major tasks of psycho-analytic treatment. Here analyst and patient must rely on their attempts to stay informed by and grounded in bodily imagery and bodily experience.[10]

The following treatment vignette illustrates pockets of this kind of limp depression and dissociation, as well as primitive and paranoid thinking in a relatively sturdy, nonpsychotic person. It also is an example of clinical experience in which both patient and analyst use bodily experience and imagery to bridge"dissociative gaps" (Bromberg, 1996b).

SAMMY AND THE PIGS:
ATTACHMENT, THE BODY, AND RUTHLESS ATTACK

Sammy, the third of four children and his mother's favorite, came to treatment at age five expressing a profound discomfort with himself and, in particular, with his body. He felt that he was no good and should be left to live in the park, or to die, because his boy's body was not as good as a girl's body,[11] and his brain would not be good enough for the first grade and he was not good at riding a bike. His self-hatred reached this pitch several months after his mother gave birth to a baby sister. The delivery followed many months during which the mother was physically and emotionally unavailable owing to severe back pain.

Sammy's mother had suffered the back pain in denial and in dissociated, frantic activity. She was terrified of surrendering to her need for reduced mobility.[12] While she was pregnant and suffering the severe back pain, she did not lift and hold Sammy. Even before her injury, she was conflicted about being too available to Sammy, worried that her "soft spot" for him would spoil him. She felt guilty about her urge to cuddle and play with him and to let him grow up in his own time. Both she and Sammy's father had been brought up with "stiff-upper-lip" attitudes toward dependency needs. They had a glimmer of insight into the negative effects of this attitude on their children but needed help building on and using that insight. For the most part, they viewed frequent and prolonged separations from primary care-takers as character-building experiences that stoked ambition and pointed little boys toward the right gender orientation. They filled their children's lives with an unpredictable succession of relatively unempathic caretakers whose job was to deliver the children to end-less lessons and structured activities.

Sammy's older brother and sister went along with the program but suffered a variety of psychosomatic symptoms and received con-siderable admiration for their stoicism. Not so Sammy—he was the squeaky wheel. Long before the flamboyant symptoms that made him the only family member in history to be privileged with therapy, he had a reputation for being "spoiled." He demanded more attention than his siblings did, found fault with surrogate caretakers, and dug into his mother's emotional interior with such tearful questions as, "Why do you spend your life at meetings?" "Why can't we just hang out?" "Why don't your feet ever touch the ground?" His healthy ca-pacity to maintain attention-seeking and protest behaviors in the face of his parents' uneven availability had been given a boost by his solid memory of tastes of his mother's "soft spot" for him. But the memory was threatened with destruction in the face of recent deprivations. By the time he came to treatment, an "internal saboteur" (Fairbairn, 1952) had begun to persecute him for his attachment needs and all the bodily urges and experiences to which they are so intimately con-nected. That is why he wanted to banish himself and his needs to starve in the park.

Sammy had begun to accept the idea that he was bad and spoiled so as to protect his and his parents' belief in their goodness (Fairbairn, 1952; Spotnitz, 1976, Epstein, 1987). He was skillful at playing the part of a brat by anyone's standards. Thus the critical goal of his treat-ment was to help him and, if possible, his family to understand the difference between what Emmanuel Ghent (1992) has called "needi-ness and genuine need."

There were two avenues through which Sammy's attachment needs had been allowed expression and had stayed alive in his fam-ily. The whole family took pleasure in sharing and exploring food in quantity, quality, and creative variety. They also enjoyed the presence of animals in their home, dozens of animals, and gave full rein to and joined with the animals' urges for physical affection and raucous, aggressive play. Both avenues were invaluable for the treatment. They gave Sammy and me a relatively safe place to be connected to our bodies and to fuel up with life force. They offered a healthy perspective on, and a needed contrast to, the crippling consequences of frustrated attachment needs. In parent consultations and when the parents joined Sammy in conjoint sessions, playful talk about pets and restaurants relaxed them and their harsh superegos. It helped them to enjoy their delightful little boy and to allow him to have a relationship with me.

Throughout Sammy's three years in treatment, he let me know that he had little use for verbal interventions intended to enlighten him about his own disowned thoughts or feelings or even to demonstrate empathy for the obvious. Often, when I began to talk in any way that went beyond what was essential for the movement of our play, Sammy would say, "Just play. Just be." Eventually he would quiet me by rolling his eyes and saying impatiently, "You're doing it again." What he wanted from sessions was unselfconscious play, joint art projects, and, more important, just to be with me. He often wanted me to read to him. During the reading he sat very close to me and allowed our hands to touch as we turned pages and lingered over pictures of animals. Our art projects involved drawing and sculpting animals, usually animals in cages or behind fences. The animals loved being contained so that they and their zookeepers could easily "find one another." Often we would spend as much as 20 minutes imagining what it would be like to feel a polar bear's nose and how that would be for the polar bear. At those times, I was allowed no probing questions and no agenda other than appreciating the nature of things.

While I knew that in these activities we were doing exactly what Sammy needed to do, there were times when my work ethic, my analytic superego, and my own difficulty just being would make me concerned that I was functioning as nothing more than a high-priced nanny. Then I would feel impelled to say something "analytic," which would almost always disrupt the kind of connection that Sammy was looking for. The movement of the treatment relationship played back and forth between opposite poles of mind–body integration and mind–body dissociation. On one end of the continuum were experiences of simple embodied togetherness, in which our appreciation of our breathing in each other's company was the main event. At the other end were the enactments of struggle with our attachment-based problems of dissociation.[13][14] In these enactments, the healthy, demanding child tried to cure the mother/analyst of her difficulties with her own mind–body integration and with body and emotional intimacy. The less healthy child tried to accommodate to and cover for the mother's/analyst's difficulties by playing spoiled.

During these enactments I was often awkward and self-conscious of my own body, uncertain where to place myself in space in relation to him. When the demanding oedipal child was recognizably mixed with the "greedy spoiled" child, I found it difficult to be comfortable in my own body and to hear his real needs. I lacked trust in my intuition about where and how to be and when and when not to initiate talk or play. My interaction with him was derailed by the fear of spoiling, seduction, and pleasure. Like his mother, I had developed a soft spot for him and had trouble believing it was right just to enjoy this wonderful child. My voice would become false and high-pitched owing to the shallow breathing that accompanies disembodiment. If Sammy found me disconnected on a day when he was feeling hopeful and with plenty of emotional reserves, he would actively and often angrily try to help me connect, with "Where are you?" or "Oh, man, she's a goner today." As he became increasingly angry, he would sarcastically imitate my interventions and show me how ridiculous words could be.

If I could recognize and respond to his sarcasm as a legitimate attempt to get me back in connection with myself and with him, then we might accomplish a bit of important talk. The talk would often be about his problems connecting to both of his parents. On his more depressed and less resourceful days, he would react to my uptight behavior with diffuse discontent with the world and would pick on himself for his chubbiness, his untied laces, his school performance. On those days, I could not rely on his perseverance to get us back to our bodies in a healthy way. I had to work harder to find my way back to a belief in intuition, play, and embodiment. Here is a vignette from such a day.

Sammy, at this time in the second grade, came into a session on a rainy March day in bad shape. His parents had been away on a cruise for a week and were staying another week. He had a dreadful cold and was depressed and silent. He could not greet or look at me. He slumped into a chair and turned away to avoid my gaze. For a month preceding the trip, his mother had been spending three or four days a week away from the family to decorate the country house, and the father was busy at work. During that month, Sammy was under considerable stress but had held together well enough to carry on. The

most recent separation, however, was too much. He had run out of
emotional reserves and his immune system was compromised. He
was being cared for by grandparents who thought him spoiled and
wanted to use their time alone with him to shape him up. They gave
him little understanding about missing his parents. They told him
that, when his mother made her nightly telephone call to the children, he was not to show her he was sad and not to tell her he had a
cold. "If you don't sound cheerful," they said. "your mummy will never
get a rest and heal her back." "They must be right," Sammy said.

He was frightened and agitated by my attempts to show empathy or in any way open this up as a difficult situation. "It's hopeless. .
.I don't want to talk and I don't feel like doing anything else." Usually
Sammy loved his grandparents but had a realistic and often witty,
angry perspective on how insensitive they could be, a perspective
his considerably softer parents had shared a bit with him. Today,
however, he was a hostage in the enemy's camp. Another week would
be a very long time. The enemy, of course, was not literally the grandparents. The enemy was the internal saboteur that had crushed the
attachment needs over the generations.

We sat at a small table, his head down on his arms, he wanting to
stop his tears on his own for a long time. If my breathing or posture
suggested that I might be preparing to say something, he stiffened
and warded off my words. Sammy always knew when my mind was
circling over things to say, and he was rarely comfortable with my
thinking too hard, especially at a time like this. I took his instruction,
resisted my urge to talk, tried to get comfortable in my own body, and
hoped that good intuition would follow. I took some deep, relaxing
breaths and let my mind wander. Eventually I gathered up a cluster of
small farm animals out of a basket and fiddled around with them a
bit, just to take the pressure off him. After a time I saw that I had laid
out a farmyard with a mother sow and her babies in the center and
had encircled them with a fence. By and by, he watched me and picked
up the sow with six piglets attached to her teats. Then he picked up a
loose piglet, approached the sow timidly, and then retreated from
her three or four times. He weakly and limply tried once or twice to
line up the piglet on the mother's underbelly. When there was no place
for the piglet, he slumped back in his chair.

"Oh," I said, "he can't get to her." "Of course not, stupid," he replied. "Yes, of course not," I said, encouraged by the anger rising in
his voice. I went on, "It's like when your mother's back was so bad for
so long and then after that she was with Courtney more than you,
and nursing her." Sammy looked frightened, angry, and confused.

"Human beings don't nurse." "They don't?" I asked, looking at this well-informed zoologist with considerable incredulity. "No, no," he said angrily. "Mammals nurse and they have warm blood, and humans. . .they aren't mammals." Then, looking very confused and frightened, he dropped the piglet. "In fact," he said, "I think if you tried to nurse from a human mother, you'd just get her blood."

"How scary," I said, struck by this unprecedented break in his thinking. At this point, I too was frightened of falling into some dark hole, unable to help either of us before sending him back to the trenches. My survival response was spontaneous and aggressive. "Well, this piglet is scared, too, so I'll help him." I picked up the piglet and began to root aggressively at the sow, saying, "Give me some milk." Sammy said, "She won't, or she can't." I became more aggressive, banging at the sow. "I'm mixed up. You *won't* give? Or you *can't* give? . . . you mother pig?! You better give me milk . . . because I *need* it!" There was a pause. "Hey, I think I got a little."

Sammy said, "Well, maybe a little, but not enough to get by today or tomorrow, and she's not going to give it either." He turned his head away from me and from the pigs and mumbled weakly, "So now what can you do?" "Well, I've got to do something!" I said angrily. "I'm telling this mother pig I'm mad," I said, "and if that piglet can't have milk, we farmers are going to have pork chops, bacon, and ham!" This felt risky so I looked at him to see if he was still with me. He turned toward me, and made eye contact, his color and muscle tone showing new signs of energy.[15] Heartened, I went ahead with the greedy attack. For the first course, I made pork chops with apple sauce and mashed potatoes on the side. Daring to come alive, Sammy made Moo Shoo Pork and scallions with pancakes with Hoison sauce. We decided to let the sauce run down our arms and leave it there all day.

Next we had barbecued ribs with collard greens and black-eyed peas, followed by *puerco en mole* with tortillas. After that we had a burping contest, which Sammy won by a long shot. Then Sammy ripped off his school tie and coat which had added to his strangulation. He began to laugh and wave his arms in excitement. "I don't know where I'll put it, but we'll have to do ham with pineapple and potato salad before we're through." "You'll find a place," I said, "and we're not finished yet. Not until we put every scrap of hoof, ear, and tail into a soup! You can take that home with you if we don't finish it." My feet felt safely on the ground now. My movements broadened, and so did his. "Yeah, yeah," he laughed, "let's go for it." He scooped up everything in sight, saying lovingly to a little ear that was almost left behind, "You don't want to be forgotten . . . into the soup you go."

When we had eaten our fill and poured the soup into a five gallon jar for the future, Sammy breathed a long, deep breath. He settled into his body and rested for a few moments. Then he got up, tapped me on the knee, and said, "Okay, now I'm going to sing." He sang without self-consciousness, his breath and his sound reflexively generating from the deep place a baby breathes. His congestion had cleared; his voice was clear, steady, and full of joyous emotion. He sang three songs without stopping. All of them were odes to spring. When he finished, he looked at me, unembarrassed by the moisture in my eyes. I said, "Beautiful." "Yeah," he said, "I can be good. I have courage." As he said this, he underscored his conviction by running his hands down his torso.

SAVORING THE CLINICAL MOMENT: FINDING WELL ENOUGH AND LEAVING WELL ENOUGH ALONE

After the feast, his songs and Sammy's discovery that there was good in his needs and in their expression, there was nothing more for either of us to say. At that point, my therapeutic task was simply to allow myself quietly to enjoy the process, a process I would later conceptualize as laying down healthy memories in the body.[16] During this process, the analyst is bound to find the work pleasurable and may need help in understanding the importance of accepting the experience of this pleasure. We have been conditioned to take pleasure in the intellectual aspects of our work more than in the experiential. When we have been fully used by our patients, there will be pleasure in our bodies and in the hum of the movement on the bridge between psyche and soma. To strengthen that bridge, we need to stay in the moment and avoid abstraction.

Child and adult therapists know that there are times when commentary on immediate experience can disrupt the healing power of play. There is an especially fluid, imagistic dialogue between psyche and soma in play, in the reporting of a healing dream, or in experiences in which both patient and analyst have become grounded in their bodies and are feeling related to one another's body. This fluidity makes reorganization, healing, and growth possible. During such moments, the analyst's verbal commentary can push the patient back into a dissociative retreat from affect and bodily experience, and the mutative experience is minimized or aborted. In some measure, the mutative experience depends on the patient's own innate striving for wholeness. The analyst must believe in the striving and quietly let the mutative moment happen, and he or she help the patient hold and savor it. The patient will have taken some creative leap to assure that this moment happens and is his. The historical psychoanalytic overvaluation of the word and the postmodern stress on deconstruction can discourage savoring the clinical moment in this way. These stances encourage not only getting in the word, but getting in the last word in a way that cannot bridge the dissociative gap between mind and body. Both run away from saturation in experience and allow us to speak only *about* the body rather than *from* the body. It is so easy for us practitioners of "the talking cure" to inadvertently reinforce, rather than heal, premature ego development (Shabad, Selinger, 1995; Bion, 1962).[17]

With Sammy, I came to trust that he would comment on the therapeutic process in his own way when he was ready. During this kind of treatment experience, in which we found ourselves on newly built bridges between psyche and soma, Sammy would underscore the importance of the clinical moment by giving me a knowing look and a nod. Like the tap on my knee, this told me, "Take notice of where we are now and how it feels!" Following such a gesture, he would slowly move back into the world of abstract and conventionally shared language. He most often did this by wandering around the room and then stopping to linger over my seashell collection. He would stroke the shells inside and out, staying close to the body while verbalizing thoughts about the wonders of God, Creation, and procreation. Then he might begin to play with the more objective facts of biology that he had read in books.

During such moments, I could feel an easy two-way flow of energy from his mind to his body to the transcendent, his own area of faith (Eigen, 1981a). His interest in animal life was far from a hollow cognitive pursuit but came from his "body-centered" sense of reality (Lichtenberg, 1989) and was a living, creative force.

During a session in our termination phase, Sammy offered a few comments about the role of bodily experience in his treatment. "You know that Mom will be asking me if it's time to stop coming here, like she always does at the end of every school year." "Yes," I said, "do you think it might be time?" "Well, I haven't had any of the big problems I came with in a very long time. I think I would like to stay until next Christmas, just for good measure, but it wouldn't be the worst if I stopped before. It's hard to explain all of therapy to Mom. She gets the part about talking about worries and feelings now. She gets the need for it now, and she's better with me herself. But there are parts of therapy that are still hard for her to understand the need for, and those are the parts that would be hard to explain to anyone who hadn't been in it." "Do you feel like explaining it to me?" I asked. "Yes," he said. "It's the importance of having someone who knows all the parts of you, someone you have gotten very used to." "Used to?" I asked. "Yes, I'm used to the way you sit and move and talk, and to your seashells and how it smells in here. I'm even used to your funny nose and the way your hands shake a little when you put together Lego blocks."

Sammy's being "used to me" means that he felt he had comfortable access to my body, both literally and in his mind. He could use intimacy with me or distance himself from me. He could think freely about my body, consciously and unconsciously, with no harm done to either of us. Once he was able to take for granted access to my body on the level of his attachment needs, he was also free not to think about my body and to live in his own. His comfort with my body, and his own in relation to it, kept our verbal work grounded and promoted integration of thought, feeling, and bodily experience. Sammy's need to be known by an analyst he had grown "used to" has the same body-grounded quality I hear in Iris's need for an analyst she can "take for granted." I think Sammy and Iris are emphasizing the bodily dimensions of Bromberg's (1991) notions of "direct relatedness" and knowing one another "inside out."

In our time together, Sammy was able to bring me out of my head and into connection with him, and I was been able to do the same for him. He experienced his need for closeness in both quiet, mutual self-containment and in the aggressive reaching out and grasping and gouging and biting that Winnicott called the ruthless attack. He knew that all of this was fine with me. These events between us constituted what is meant both by mutual regulation (Beebe and Lachmann, 1988) and by mutual recognition (Benjamin, 1988).

Beyond that, our feast and his songs were a spiritual communion, a celebration of Sammy's recovery of his entitlement to be fully alive. When he sang spontaneously, he freed his urges to turn breath into sound (McClelland, 1990) and to project himself beyond his "personal dominion" (Raphel-Leff, 1994). Having followed my hungry and aggressive plunge into the bounty of the outside world, he was enlivened enough to create his own recipes and to take them in with pleasure. Then, having come to terms moment with issues related to his needs or "appetite," Sammy was able to enjoy his own sense of unpressured, unified, and continuous identity that comes with simply breathing and being alive (Eigen, 1981b). I see Sammy's singing as a special case of breathing and being alive. Singing is an especially spiritually and interpersonally connected form of breathing and living.

Winnicott (1945) suggests that breathing personalizes and solidifies our sense of self while connecting us to the world in a fluid and mysterious way. He sees a child's interest in intangible natural phenomena, such as bubbles, rainbows, and clouds, as clues to a capacity for illusion. He says, "somewhere here too, is the interest in breath which never decides whether it comes from within or without, and which provides a basis for the conception of spirit, soul, anima" (p. 154). Eigen (1981b) has suggested that breathing offers the possibility of rebirth "over and over again." Sammy's odes to spring voiced his belief in his own capacity and his world's capacity for rebirth. His songs celebrated the liberation of his life force and a belief that he and his body seemed to fit into the nature of things.

The bodily connected experiences that Sammy gathered up in his treatment not only made him more comfortable with himself but also buttressed his actual relationship to his mother. They gave him the courage to find new ways to connect to her, ways that wouldn't so often get him branded as spoiled. They also gave him the courage to know that failure to connect to her was not necessarily his fault and certainly not the fault of his needs. The treatment helped him reclaim dissociated, early healthy in-body experiences with his mother. It also gave him the experience of finding ways to have new, good body experiences in the presence of another. These were the memories he would take away from his treatment and, I trust, will be able to use.

CONCLUSION

Patients are healed in many ways, only a few of which have been described. They are healed through identifications with their analysts as collaborators (Freud, 1893–1895) and the investigation of human experience with a gentler superego (Strachey, 1934). They are also healed through their identification with their analysts' endeavor to be fully present (Schachtel, 1997),[18] fully alive and conscious of the shifts of the weight of experience as it moves over the mind–body continuum. This consciousness and grounding will make the thoughts of both patient and analyst—once spoken—voices rather than hollow words. The analyst's self-awareness on this body level, whether verbally disclosed or not, will make the analyst more usable for the patient. During moments that the analyst inhabits her own skin, she is more easily read by the patient. At such moments, the patient gets enough clear and useful information about the analyst that he is not stuck with reading the analyst's subjectivity at the expense of his own vitality.[19]

Bromberg (1996b) has written extensively about the importance of getting the patient to stand in the spaces of different pieces of his experience of self. He has emphasized that, in bridging self-states, language can never be a substitute for experience (Bromberg, 1991). I would expand on his ideas and say that working in the dissociative gap requires more than verbally based descriptions of the landscape on either side and of the terrors in the dark canyon below. It must include awareness of what it actually feels like in the body for both analyst and patient as they slip and fall and catch themselves and each other as they work in that gap. As Ferenczi (1912) said, "Conviction is felt in the body."

It is the analyst's unexamined mind–body disconnection that mystifies and ties the hands of the patient. This disconnection will be a tangible and critical feature of the enactment of disturbed relational patterns and therefore a major focus for the process of working through. The patient will be better able to tell the analyst how he needs to use her if the analyst is more interested in listening to her patient and to herself from an embodied place than in rushing to tell the patient what she thinks she knows. The patient will also be better able to mobilize the aggression needed to redirect the analyst when she is not there in the needed way. He will experience the enlivening sense of agency that comes with getting the analyst to "adapt to his needs" (Epstein, 1982). Working from this kind of grounded stance, rather than proceeding primarily from the mind, makes patient and analyst vulnerable to confusion and anxiety, and it requires a special kind of faith.

Sammy taught me something about the kind of faith this stance requires. Though his parents were agnostic, Sammy privately believed in God and made it clear to me that it was important for me to know and honor his belief. He was weary of having to be strong and smart, weary of carrying the weight of the premature ego development that had been his family's legacy. He drew some of his courage to use me fully in the treatment from his belief that there must be a way to be in balance with all of nature and to be a smaller part of a bigger whole. To help Sammy use this faith to become more whole, I had to match it and meet him there at a time when he was in need. I did not and could not have planned or conceptualized this ahead of time. We found our way through trial and error, using bodily experience and bodily imagery to guide us in the negotiation of boundaries and to keep us enlivened by immersion in the forms, textures, smells, and tastes of living things. We learned to tap into this life force through subtle shifts of attention and through the occasional daring leap. We learned how to use this force to inject new life into the psychosomatically frozen tableau of enactment, transforming it into vital and healing play. We could do these things together only after I learned really to listen to Sammy when he said, both angrily and lovingly, "Stop thinking and talking so much. Pay attention to how the moment feels. Why don't you put your feet on the ground?"

NOTES

[1]Khan (1977) described "cumulative trauma" as the "silent breeches in the mother's functioning as protective shield" that constitute the significant points of stress and strain in the evolving mother–child relationship over time. It is a concept that lends itself well to explaining the mind–body manifestations of that developing relationship. Throughout this chapter, I use the term dissociation descriptively, rather than diagnostically.

[2]The gains and losses of Freud's evolution of technique from hypnotic suggestion to free association (Aron, 1996b) have been discussed recently by a number of relational psychoanalysts in ways that touch on the problem of marginalization of the body. Bromberg (1996a) notes that this turn of events delayed our understanding of dissociation, which is, of course, a body-based experience. Benjamin (1996b) has said that free association and collaborative investigation have given psychoanalysts and patients the job of working backward from the word to the body.

[3]The neglect of lived bodily experience in psychoanalytic theory and clinical practice was the subject of presentations by Shapiro (1992) and Anderson, Balamuth, and Looker (1994). Shapiro (1996) has also elaborated on the suppression of bodily experience in Western culture since the enlightenment. Achterberg and Lawlis (1980), behavioral medicine practitioners and researchers who have contributed invaluably to mind–body medicine for over 50 years, note that, since the explosive development of the physical sciences in the 20th century the body has been viewed as a machine, separate from body and spirit.

[4]Clinicians involved in holistic medicine and in all the body therapies appreciate that "imagery is the golden cord between psyche and soma" (Achterberg, et al., 1980). Their knowledge of the use of imagery in healing has potential as a valuable resource for psychoanalysts.

[5]Winnicott's clinical genius and his unique ability to speak to analysts of all theoretical persuasions, as well as to the general public, was, I believe, greatly enhanced by his "hands-on" experience with parents and children in his pediatric practice. Usually, the psychoanalyst is deprived of this kind of experience.

⁶This was the Therapeutic Nursery at Jacobi Hospital directed by Dr. Leon Yorburg from 1970 through 1978. I am grateful to Dr. Yorburg (1974, personal communication) for making me aware that there are a great many things about human beings, and particularly about the mother–child relationship, that cannot be understood from behind a two-way observation glass. He believes that the clinician has a much better intuitive grasp of what is going on between mother and child when both clinician and patient have some freedom of movement and freedom to imagine and to engage in touch.

⁷These clinical observations of "Deedee" are abstracted from research findings previously reported by Looker and Wessman (1983).

⁸I have observed in my clinical practice that learning problems are often rooted in a child's frightened and stifled longing for the mother's body and for emotional contact. I find that, when aggression related to the child's connection to the mother's body becomes safely owned, learning problems often improve.

⁹It seems to me that the inherently difficult task of sorting out what is one's own and what is one's parents' gives an importance to the inside of the mother's body to the child that is probably even greater than the mystery of her procreative powers.

¹⁰Language, however, especially written language, will always be found wanting in conveying this sort of body-based experience. I am greatly indebted to my work with body therapists Marcia Lesser and Meeta l'Huillier for giving me experiences of enhanced awareness of the body–mind relationship. These experiences underpin and, I hope, texturize and enliven my use of words when I tell of my work with Sammy.

¹¹This was not a core gender identity problem as described by Coates (1992), but part of a shorter-lived reactive depression in a more solid core.

¹²Fran Anderson has called to my attention that frenetic activity in the chronic pain sufferer is referred to as "ergomania" in the pain literature (Blumer & Heilbronn, 1989).

¹³As Aron (1996a) has pointed out, enactments are not really discrete events. I prefer to call them "enactment leitmotifs" (Looker, 1996).

¹⁴Elsewhere (Looker, 1996), I have described the clinical importance of enactment in mind–body terms: saying that "during enactment the mutually constructed verbal narrative has gotten under the skins and into the bodies of both patient and analyst so that it feels 'real.'. . . Most often what is registered in the body during enactment is the discomfort of a break between psyche and soma that accompanies disturbed relational patterns."

¹⁵In a preconscious flash I considered whether my aggression was related to a manic defense that might not be helpful to him at the moment. I knew it was very important to monitor the impact of my move.

¹⁶The idea that neurological pathways that shape our behaviors and states can be repatterned, long important to other mental health professionals, is entering the psychoanalytic domain. One of the most recent and dramatic examples of this is Schore's (1994) work, which suggests that right-brain communication of pleasurable affect between parent and child builds neu-

rological structure. This kind of structural change, now visible by means of a PET scan, has long been the intuitive assumption of many psychoanalysts, child development experts, and body therapists.

[17]Shabad and Selinger (1996) warn us that psychoanalysis, characterized by rational dissection of the unconscious and a preference for observation over participation, can easily be practiced as a counterphobic leap into premature ego functioning. Bion (1962) also cautions us to understand the difference between just talking about psychoanalysis and actually doing it while we work with our patients. I know that this difference for me is whether or not my interactions with the patient are accompanied by bodily experience.

[18]Zeborah Schachtel (1997, personal communication) sees "being fully present" as the essential challenge of psychoanalytic work. My ongoing participation in a study group on the body with Drs. Schachtel, Ron Balamuth, and Fran Anderson has been invaluable to me in my attempts to persevere in this challenge.

[19]I agree with Joyce Slochower (1996) that there are times when the analyst's shared subjectivity is an impingement on the patient. I find that my intuition about the usefulness and limitations of mutuality and self-disclosure are impaired when I am not well settled in my body.

REFERENCES

Achterberg, J. & Lawlis, G. F. (1980), *Bridges of the Bodymind.* Champaign, IL: Institute for Personality & Ability Testing.

Ainsworth, M. D. S., Blehar, M., Waters, E. & Wall, S. (1978). *Patterns of Attachment.* Hillsdale, NJ: Lawrence Erlbaum Associates.

Anderson, F., Balamuth, R. & Looker, T. (1994), "Working Close to the Body in Psychoanalysis." Panel at New York University's Postdoctoral Program in Psychotherapy and Psychoanalysis.

Aron, L. (1991), The patient's experience of the analyst's subjectivity. *Psychoanal. Dial.*, 1:29-51.

——— (1996a), *A Meeting of Minds.* Hillsdale, NJ: The Analytic Press.

——— (1996b), From hypnotic suggestion to free association: Freud as a psychotherapist, circa 1892-1893. *Comtemp. Psychoanal.*, 32:99–114.

Beebe, B., & Lachmann, F. (1988), Mother–infant mutual influence and precursors of psychic structure. In: *Frontiers in Self Psychology: Progress in Self Psychology, Vol. 3*, ed. A. Goldberg. Hillsdale, NJ: The Analytic Press, pp. 3–25.

Benjamin, J. (1988), *The Bonds of Love.* New York: Pantheon.

——— (1995), Between body and speech: The primal leap. Keynote address, New York University Postdoctoral Program Conference, May 4.

Bion, W. R. (1962), *Learning from Experience.* New York: Basic Books.

Blumer, D. & Heilbronn, M. (1989), The treatment of chronic pain as a variant of depression. In: *Handbook of Chronic Pain Management*, ed. C. D. Tollison. Baltimore, MD: Williams & Wilkins, pp. 197–209.

Bowlby, J. (1969), *Attachment and Loss, Vol. I.* New York: Basic Books.
———— (1973), *Attachment and Loss, Vol. II.* New York: Basic Books.
Bromberg, P. M. (1991), On knowing one's patient inside out: The aesthetics of unconscious communion. *Psychoanal. Dial.*, 1:399–422.
———— (1996a), Hysteria, dissociation, and cure: Emmy von N. revisited. *Psychoanal. Dial.*, 5:55–71.
———— (1996b), Standing in the spaces: The multiplicity of self and the psychoanalytic relationship. *Contemp. Psychoanal.*, 32:509–535.
Bucci, W. (1985), Dual coding: A cognitive model for psychoanalytic research. *J. Amer. Psychoanal. Assn.*, 33:571–608.
Cassirer, E. (1944), *An Essay on Man.* New Haven, CT: Yale University Press.
Coates, S. (1992), The etiology of boyhood general identity disorder: An integrative model. In: *Interface of Psychoanalysis and Psychology*, ed., J. W. Baron, M. N. Eagle & D. L. Wolitsky. Washington, DC: American Psychological Association, pp. 245–265.
Davies, J. M. & Frawley, M. G. (1994), *Treating the Adult Survivor of Childhood Sexual Abuse.* New York: Basic Books.
Eigen, M. (1981a), The area of faith in Winnicott, Lacan and Bion. *Internat. J. Psycho-Anal.*, 62:413–433.
———— (1981b), Reflections on eating and breathing as models of mental functions. *Amer. J. Psychoanal.*, 41:177–180.
———— (1986), *The Psychotic Core.* Northvale, NJ: Aronson.
Epstein, L. (1982), Adapting to the patient's therapeutic need in the psychoanalytic situation. *Contemp. Psychoanal.*, 18: 190–217.
———— (1984), An interpersonal-object relations perspective on working with destructive aggression. *Contemp. Psychoanal.*, 20:651–662.
———— (1987), The problem of bad-analyst feeling. *Modern Psychoanal.*, 7:35–45.
Epstein, S. (1994), Integration of the cognitive and the psychodynamic unconscious. *Amer. Psycholog.*, 8:709–724.
Fairbairn, W. R. D. (1952), *Psychoanalytic Studies of the Personality.* London: Tavistock.
Ferenczi, S. (1912), Transitory symptom-constructions during the analysis. *First Contributions to Psycho-Analysis*, ed. M. Balint (trans. E. Mosbacher). London: Karnac Books, 1980, pp. 193–212.
Fosshage, J. (1997), The organizing functions of dream mentation. *Contemp. Psychoanal.*, 33(3):429–458.
Freud, S. (1893–1895), Studies on Hysteria. In: *Standard Edition*, 2:255–305. London: Hogarth Press, 1953.
———— (1915). Instincts and their vicissitudes. *Standard Edition*, 14:117–114. London: Hogarth Press, 1957.
Ghent, E. (1992), Paradox and process. *Psychoanal. Dial.*, 2:135–159.
Green, André (1993), The dead mother. In: *On Private Madness.* Madison, CT: International Universities Press, pp. 142–173.
Khan, M. (1974), *The Privacy of the Self.* New York: International Universities Press.

Klein, M. (1932), *The Psychoanalysis of Children*. London: Hogarth Press.

Knoblach, S. (1997), Beyond the word in psychoanalysis: The unspoken dialogue. *Psychoanal. Dial.*, 7:491–516.

Lichtenberg, J. D. (1989), *Psychoanalysis and Motivation*. Hillsdale, NJ: The Analytic Press.

Loewald, H. W. (1970), Psychoanalytic theory and the psychoanalytic process. In: *Papers on Psychoanalysis*. New Haven, CT: Yale University Press, 1980, pp. 277–301.

Looker, T. B. (1996), Impinging anxiety and bodily experience: A treatment enactment. Panel on Analytic Space for Bodily Experience. Meeting of Division on Psychoanalysis (39) American Psychological Association, New York.

———— & Wessman, A. E. (1983), Maternal mood and mother-child attachment behavior. Paper presented at the Second World Congress on Infant Psychiatry, March 31, Cannes, France.

McClelland, J. (1990), Freeing your natural voice. *Nature and Health*, fall: pp. 21–22.

Noy, P. (1969), A revision of the psychoanalytic theory of primary process. *Internat. J. Psychoanal.*, 50:155–178.

Putnam, F. W. (1989), *Diagnosis and Treatment of Multiple Personality Disorder*. New York: Guilford Press.

Raphel-Leff, J. (1994), Imaginative bodies of childbearing: Visions and revisions. In: *The Imaginative Body*, ed. A. Erskine & D. Judd. Northvale, NJ: Aronson, pp. 13–42.

Schachtel, E. (1957), *Metamorphosis*. New York: Basic Books.

Schore, A. (1994), *Affect Regulation and the Origin of Self*. Mahwah, NJ: Lawrence Erlbaum Associates.

Shabad, P. & Selinger, S. S. (1995), Bracing for disappointment and the counterphobic leap into the future. In: *The Mind Object Precocity and Pathology of Self-sufficiency*, ed. E. G. Corrigan & P. Gordon. Northvale, NJ: Aronson, pp. 209–227.

Shapiro, S. A. (1992), The discrediting of Ferenczi and the taboo on touch. Presented at meeting of Division on Psychoanalysis (39), American Psychological Association, April, Philadelphia.

———— (1996), The embodied analyst in the Victorian consulting room. *Gender & Psychoanal.*, 1:297–322.

Slade, A., Coates, S. W. & Diamond, D. (1996), New developments in attachment theory and research: Relevance for psychoanalytic theory and practice. Panel at meeting of Division of Psychoanalysis (39), American Psychological Association, New York.

Slochower, J. (1996), Holding and the fate of the analyst's subjectivity. *Psychoanal. Dial.*, 6:323–353.

Spence, D. (1996), In search of signs of healing: The quest for clinical evidence. *Contemp. Psychoanal.*, 32:287–305.

Spotnitz, H. (1976), *Psychotherapy of Preoedipal Conditions*. Northvale, NJ: Aronson.

Stern, D. N. (1985). *The Interpersonal World of the Infant*. New York: Basic Books.

Strachey, J. (1934), The nature of therapeutic action of psychoanalysis. *Internat. J. Psycho-Anal.*, 15:127–139.

van der Kolk, B. A. (1994), The body keeps the score: Memory and the evolving psychobiology of posttraumatic stress. *Harvard Dev. Psychiat.*, 1:253–265.

Winnicott, D. W. (1945), Primitive emotional development. In: *Through Pediatrics to Psychoanalysis*. New York: Basic Books, 1975, pp.

———(1947), Hate in the countertransference. In: *Through Pediatrics to Psychoanalysis*. New York: Basic Books, 1958, pp. 194–203.

——— (1949), Mind and its relation to the psyche-soma. In: *Through Pediatrics to Psychoanalysis*. New York: Basic Books, 1958, pp. 243–254.

——— (1950-1955), Aggression in relation to emotional development. In: *Through Pediatrics to Psychoanalysis*. New York: Basic Books, 1958, pp. 204–218.

——— (1969), The use of an object and relating through identifications. In: *Playing and Reality*. New York: Basic Books, 1971, pp. 86–94.

11

RE-MEMBERING THE BODY

A Psychoanalytic Study
Of Presence and Absence
Of the Lived Body

Ron Balamuth

The Uses of Not

Thirty spokes
meet the hub.
Where the wheel isn't
is where it is useful.

Hollowed out,
clay makes a pot.
Where the pot's not
is where it's useful.

cut doors and windows
to make a room.
Where the room isn't,
there's room for you.

So the profit in what is
is in the use of what isn't.

[Le Guin, 1992]

PRESENCE AND ABSENCE OF THE LIVED BODY

As that quote suggests, this chapter is riddled with a paradox. It is the paradox of absence. Specifically, how can an absence—in this case the absence of affect and its relation to the body, which has been described by such authors as Krystal (1988) and McDougall (1989)—be known, experienced and integrated in the analytic situation? The analytic case that I present here suggests that the lived body—the body as it is subjectively experienced—can become a touchstone for the recognition of the presence of an important absence in oneself. The immediacy of suddenly sensing one's own breathing, movement, and voice can be the vehicle that brings one centrally into the present, the here-and-now. Paradoxically, such moments straddle the boundary between presence and absence. For while one does achieve a broader, more encompassing perception of one's internal and external situation in these moments, they also reveal that one has thus far been absent, disconnected, and unaware of important aspects of self. When such moments occur in the presence of a patient whom one is analyzing, they provide richly unique information and opportunities for the analytic process.

Where Is the Body?

Jim is a tall, handsome, yet somewhat awkward person, with a deep, low voice and a seductive, shy smile. He plops himself heavily on the couch before he sits up, and he often takes a few moments to start.

On this early-morning session, five years into this analysis, Jim sets himself up with his coffee, carefully tears a little opening in the cover, takes a sip, and looks at me across the room. I am reminded of my dream of a couple of nights ago, which I suspect had to do with Jim. In it I am straining to remember what transpired at the last session with one of my patients. As much as I can recall, it was a young patient, but I am not sure even about that. In fact, I feel as if I hardly know him, and I begin to doubt that I have even met him. At the same time I feel that I should know him quite well. I can hear his parents in a voice-over, as I stare at my empty office, giving a description of a missing person, with details about his overall appearance, height, build. I desperately pull at strings and force myself to recapture some foggy glimpses of him as an eight-year-old boy, sitting on my couch with his feet dangling and not quite reaching the floor.

The feeling of anxiety about a lack, an absence, something not quite known yet lost, will recur at different times during this session.

I am aware of our little coffee ritual on these early morning sessions. I feel that it connects us through taste, temperature, and a measured gesture.

Somehow, the facts known to me about him—that he has young children, is a visual artist in his 30s—are all stored in a different file and seem quite irrelevant in bridging the distance between us. Recent sessions began just as this session has, and have proceeded in a rather predictable sequence, without either of us noticing or commenting about it. Jim starts this session by announcing that he has a lot to tell me. Professional work has been slow or practically nonexistent, and he is digging himself deeper into a financial hole day by day. He describes how insensitive his suppliers, his agents, and his family are to his predicament.

Narratives of desire, frustration, and longing have been part of our work since the beginning.[1] Were he to be asked about his analyst's contribution to this retelling of his life, he might describe it as an attempt to reflect, interpret, and ultimately to persuade him that he is compulsively reenacting scenes of abandonment by his father in adolescence.

He is silent now. He cautiously raises his eyes to check me as I remain quiet. Suddenly, the utter futility of trying to speak as the editor of his narrative silences me. I feel a sinking feeling in my stomach, a mounting discomfort. I am reminded of the lost boy of my dream. There is, unexpectedly, a pregnant silence between us, and yet, in a way that has become both new and familiar, I am suddenly surprised to find my body, my breathing. It is as if that lens through which this perception is visible has become less fogged up and cluttered by my ideas.

I now notice that I have been breathing all along, albeit in a shallow and tense fashion; that my back and my chest have been tense; that my face has an expression on it that I cannot readily interpret. Suddenly, and abruptly, another possibility of being emerges. One does not have to occupy the cramped, wordy, and irrelevant interpretive/symbolizing space. From this breathing-pulsating-moving place somewhere in myself I begin to see Jim now, almost as if for the first time. And with this shift in myself I find that I feel an all-encompassing sadness, as if my self-experience is filtered through an achromatic filter. This feels both familiar and new; it is a recognition, a refinding of something that was known.

The frequent concomitant to refinding one's lived body is a sense of familiarity and newness. It evokes the feeling of joy that comes with connecting with a part of oneself that had not been touched for a long time and a feeling sadness, as well, at the recognition of one's habitual fragmented state.

What is being discovered at such a moment is a certain truth about a mutual way of relating that was not accessible before. The feeling of loss echoed in my dream of the missing patient resonates with the sense of the absence of my aliveness (Ogden, 1995). I can find it in my experience of sadness and grayness, which is evoked in me as an inner metaphor of our state of nonrelatedness, and alienation. In a stance reminiscent of times when I felt compelled to absorb and contain experiences that were toxic for me, I feel as if my body is rebelling and will not let itself be coerced by the familiar pressure my mind is exerting on me, pushing me to resume a "knowledgeable" analytic posture that does not feel right for now. I associate this rebellious sensation with one I have felt when refusing to sit in a chair I suspect will be bad for my back or refusing to eat food that I know disagrees with me. Ogden (1994a) has described having an analogous, if milder, experience in relation to a disconnected patient. He writes:

> I could have taken up any one of these images as symbol of the themes that we had previously discussed, including the very detachment that seemed to permeate all that the patient was talking about as well as the disconnection I felt both from him and from myself. However, I decided not to intervene because it felt to me that if I were to try to offer an interpretation at this point I would only be repeating myself and saying something for the sake of reassuring myself that I had something to say [p. 6].

As the experience of near-repulsion and an organic protest in reaction to what I notice in myself subside somewhat, I return to listen to Jim, who, after a pause, resumes speaking. My interpretive voice is now absent. The bodies, his and mine, are now present to my awareness, with their weight and volume. The process of becoming aware takes place in this moment of paradoxical presence to our profound absence.

My listening to Jim seems to comes from a different place now. And yet it does not appear that I have done anything. Neither an interpretation nor a comment has been made, and still the change is unmistakable. The moment had the taste of Symington's (1983) enigmatically described yet evocative "inner act of freedom":

> I might just as well have spoken my thoughts out loud because she felt my inner act so that even an inner judgment

has some perceptible external correlate. I do not think that the mental, emotional and sensational spheres ever exist in isolation. The most inward mental act reverberates through the sensational and perceptual spheres [p. 287].

It is important to note that Symington does not see interpretations as useless; rather, he views them as by- or end-products, or as indicators that the critical inner process has already occurred. Interpretation remains essential as it brings to consciousness, and gives expression to, the shift that occurred moments before, when the analyst's inner act of freedom is perceived by the patient.

As Jim and I are constructing a new moment in our intersubjective field—by not taking our habitual postures—a new possibility emerges. Now, as he expresses longing to be with his child and describing how much he wishes that he could permanently live with him, his voice becomes more sonorous, his posture more erect, and he seems to be more alive. He speaks about his experience with authority and passion, as if the color has returned to him, whereas before he had seemed like a faded, second-hand version of himself. He says he wishes he could stay for a double session and that it feels significant for him to just speak about his feelings. He ends the session by describing how his young son has left him a huge mural "masterpiece" painted on his wall. He felt so connected to him as he gazed at it the day after his son left.

THE RE-MEMBERING OF BODY AND FEELINGS

As analysts, we are accustomed to noticing the emergence of our own feelings, fantasies, and thoughts in relation to a patient's material. We are less likely to consider the appearance of bodily sensations—tensions, contractions and pains, sudden changes in breathing and posture—as analytic data. Ogden (1994a), however, makes the following radical suggestion: "no thought, feeling, or sensation can be considered to be the same as it was or will be outside of the context of the specific (and continually shifting) intersubjectivity created by analysand and analyst" (p. 8). If one follows the implication of this position, the analyst's capacity to understand, perceive, and symbolize in the presence of the patient is embedded in the intersubjective field. My own focus here is on one dimension of the phenomenon by which the patient affects the analyst's state of mind in a manner that can facilitate understanding or limit it.

According to Bion (1962), projected, split-off fragments cannot be thought about or reflected upon. They must be encompassed in thought elements. (In other words, the thinker thinks only when he thinks about thinking.) The patient unconsciously creates in the analyst the required inner state in which the patient's projection can be encompassed and thus begin to become symbolized. This process made itself felt in my work with Jim. Many sessions were spent in rigid and repetitively collusive interactions. Only when the necessary shift in consciousness or self-state took place in the analyst, could the enactment be perceived, symbolized, and communicated.

I think of the process with Jim an almost physical re-membering of body, memory and, feeling, which have been dismembered by trauma. The vehicle for such re-membering was created in the analysis through the presence of bodily sensations. The body, with immediate here-and-now presence, has become the container in which such a broad integration of feeling and thought can take place.

Jim's body surfaced quite abruptly when he announced one day, about three years into the treatment, that he was going for a prostate biopsy. Rather flatly he discussed a swollen prostate nodule and his guilt and anxiety about how it may affect his sexual potency. A nagging pressure and discomfort in my groin in response to his matter-of-fact discussion of the biopsy stayed with me during our sessions until two weeks later, when he casually announced that he had received good news from the urologist. In fact, only then, when I allowed my body to relax, did I become aware of the tensions I had been carrying all along. I realized then that through his bland, matter-of-fact presentation, Jim had forced me to contain and carry much of what he could not let himself experience *in his own body.* Together, Jim and I had concretized the mind–body split, as I became the tense and anxious body while, taking refuge in his mind,he maintained his distance.

Discussing his experiences of undergoing the biopsy, Jim went into some detail about how invaded he had felt during the examination. He appeared vulnerable and upset as he spoke about how worried he had been regarding his potency after discovering blood in his body fluids. I felt the knots returning to my stomach. He described a panhandler, a veteran whom he saw on exiting the hospital, who sold flags and knickknacks and whose body was entirely mangled, almost unrecognizable. The panhandler had a sign that said, "I am a living proof to the strength of the spirit." Sobbing for the first time in our sessions, Jim said, "I am that guy." The deep, almost convulsive crying and the powerful image of a shattered, mutilated body spoke to the unbearable struggle between Jim's need to express his deep anxiety and pain and his need to ward these off. It seemed he was beginning to glimpse just how profoundly splintered from his body he had been.

Once he became more present and connected through our collaborative re-presenting and naming of his body, other traumatic memories, frozen and stored in the body, could emerge. He resonated with an earlier medical emergency, which further illustrated how disconnected he had felt from his body. A couple of years back, he had some mild stomach pains, which he attributed to having eaten some questionable Chinese food. He finally decided to go to the emergency room, though, and was immediately rushed to the operating room with acute appendicitis. He was operated on successfully, but shortly afterward developed a severe sepsis and was put on megadoses of antibiotics. "I was knocking at death's door. The doctors did not know what to do with me, and it was left to my body to either pull through or die." Jim described how his family flew in from out of town, preparing for the possibility of losing him.

The pain in my lower abdomen, the contortion of tension in my shoulder, all suggested that I was trying hard not to feel something. I had the peculiar sense that, for some unknown reason, Jim's body had chosen to survive and that this miracle might not recur. The panic that Jim's life could again be in jeopardy had to do with his bland, almost muted presentation, which made it seem as though he were saying that he did not understand what everyone was getting so worked up about.

My associations took me to my own recent visit to Israel, shortly after the Gulf War. I had asked one of my friends there how they coped with the repeated missile alarms and sirens and was amazed by his flatly stating that they simply ignored the sirens and after a while did not even go to the shelters. In contrast to his affectless response, his young son soon chimed in, saying that the only one who was still reacting to the loud sound of the sirens was the family dog, who, when he heard it, frantically ran to hide under the bed, refusing to come out. With this jarring image in mind, I said to Jim that he seemed to respond to his bodily emergency signals like a person who has been hearing a fire alarm go off for so long that he has grown habituated to living with it and no longer perceived it. Jim began sobbing uncontrollably and continued for a very long time before he could stop. He was still sobbing, his face wet with tears and contorted with pain when we had to end the session.

After Jim left, I stared for a long time at the tear-drenched tissues

scattered all over my office. The pain in my lower abdomen, the contortion of tension in my right shoulder, both suggested that his body
and my body had been touched and had come to life. The abruptness
and the urgency with which his body made itself known in the room,
its vulnerabilities, transformed our previously disconnected ways
of working together.

Jim's father, who died when Jim was 15 years old, became more
present in our sessions shortly after the biopsy. His father had left
him his cowboy boots, and, although they have become too tight for
him, he still likes the way he looks in them and occasionally wears
them. He brought some happy pictures of himself as a young baby
with his father. The pictures depict the years up to age four, at which
time his father mysteriously disappeared from the pictures and from
his life as a living presence. He could not remember where his father
had been and why he was not present between that time and the time
of his death 11 years later. Jim associated his father's disappearance
at the time with the birth of his sister. This, however, felt like a very
incomplete explanation for such a long stretch of absence, and I began to wonder what else might have taken place then. As we explored
this question, it became easy for us to lose touch again in our zeal to
uncover the facts. Jim seemed lost and unable to find a place in his
life. He could not find work and was feeling increasingly hopeless about
his financial situation and his marriage. In this bleak state of mind he
was angry and felt misunderstood and unappreciated. We needed
another opportunity to experience and become aware of the distance
between us.

Shortly thereafter, Jim shared his concern about a recent diagnosis of hypertension. He had spent many sessions discussing his intense workout in the gym, which was an attempt to lower his blood
pressure. Describing his grueling routine workout at the gym, he recalled his father's sudden death of a heart attack at a gym in the
midst of a basketball game. "His friends revived him when he first
collapsed," Jim said. "Then they called the ambulance and waited
for the paramedics. On that day there was a big train accident and all
the ambulances were on call, so they never made it in time. Had they
come in time they might have saved him."

In connection with his extremely demanding exercise schedule,
Jim said that he was satisfied and proud to strengthen his heart and
that he was confident that he would be able to avert a heart attack.
Since he was neither drinking nor smoking as his father had, his risk
was very low. I was reminded of my own magical/compulsive efforts
in struggling with similar fears during my adolescence. My father died

unexpectedly during my adolescent years. My own years spent in swimming training in an unrelenting effort to build up strength were coming back to me. The compelling wish for a magical cure to the fear of a fatal coronary that killed my father was very much with me as I listened to Jim. I was only peripherally aware of the strong oedipal aspects of my situation, which involved intense weekly swim competitions and, ultimately, the victory of outliving my father. Recalling the thrill and terror of pushing my body past its limits, I found myself closer to Jim's inchoate fears. I commented that he seemed to be intent on averting, but was also thrilled to come as close as possible to having, a heart attack in the gym just as his father had. In this way he would neither win nor lose in his battle with his father but would simply come as close to him as he could. Jim was profoundly struck by this interpretation. He felt that it addressed his wish to know everything about his father as directly as possible as a way of "getting into him."

This elaboration of Jim's father's death and its significance to his identification with him is strikingly reminiscent of what Herzog (1982) and Lewis (1991) have termed "father hunger." The fatherless boys they studied had crystalized their fathers' absence and the circumstances surrounding it as their main way of having a relationship with their fathers. Thus, every memory of the father was mediated through this insatiable hunger for the paternal object. The circumstances of the father's disappearance had become an inseparable aspect of the object itself. "The story of the abandonment constitutes each boy's main experience with his father and thus, forms the basis of his internalized object relationships with him" (Lewis, 1991, p. 274).

Jim's father hunger intensified and ultimately drove him away from his family. He was, unconsciously, building bridges to his father by persistently re-creating crucial moments in his father's life as he had witnessed it.

After his father's death, Jim did not give up on being fathered. He was taken under the wing of a powerful, highly educated man, a psychiatrist who was an adjunct art history teacher in Jim's high school and lived a few blocks away from his family. This man took personal interest in Jim. Jim recalled spending time doing homework and being tutored by Dr. K. Memories of the ebullient and charismatic Dr. K ebbed and flowed during the treatment, emerging in crucial moments of confluence when loneliness and need for a father came to the fore most powerfully. Jim recalled the time he had touched his first girlfriend in the school yard. Dr.K's thundering, if facetious, voice booming, "Take your hands off this girl!" still resonated with him now.

Wistfully, he described that he could not take his hands off the girl, and Dr. K continued mockingly to reprimand him. It is as though that voice came to represent the sound of the affirmation of Jim's manhood, for here was a towering father both reprimanding and recognizing the man that had taken the place of the boy.

After graduation from high school, Jim was invited by Dr. K to spend a year of study abroad in Italy. He reminisced about his wonderful time there; he had his first sexual encounters and felt he was coming into his own away from his family. Curiously, he did not recall having spent any of his time abroad with Dr. K, but he attributed this to their living in different parts of town. For Jim, Dr. K carried an aura of a generous, powerful, yet absent and even mysterious man.

For many years, Jim believed that after he returned from Italy, he and Dr. K lost touch. Browsing through some old letters recently, though, he was startled to discover check receipts indicating that, while in Italy, he had financially supported his benevolent father figure. A fuller story now emerged. A few years after Jim's return from abroad, he received a call from Dr. K inviting him for a visit in a hotel. Jim arrived at the dilapidated downtown hotel only to find Dr. K and another man, his lover, drinking themselves to death on hard liquor. Dr. K demanded money and a regular supply of alcohol, and Jim, capitulating, began regularly to deliver money and liquor to his old-time benefactor. When he eventually decided to stop this supplying, the two lost touch. Shortly afterward he came across Dr. K's newspaper obituary.

Jim was left with a gnawing, unanswerable question about his relationships to father figures: Is there something inherently self-destructive in anyone who ever tries to father him? It is likely that Jim's interest in art was sparked through his mentorship with Dr. K and that his long-standing work-blocks, unsuccessful attempts to find an artistic mentor, and professional isolation are related to the traumatic losses of both fathers. With uncanny, tragic resonance, the experience with Dr. K reactivated and repeated the earlier loss of Jim's father.

As the treatment continued, Jim's persistent search for the lost connection with himself, his body, and his father was so overwhelming that it ultimately led to his leaving his family. Now, the empty space the father had left—in which neither his father nor his body existed—was periodically filled with sexual escapades that paradoxically brought him closer to his father and at the same time made him realize how diminished and powerless he felt in comparison with him. He became particularly attracted to a woman with whom he felt free enough to share his sexual fantasies and to listen to hers. She was seductive, enticing, and unavailable. He pursued her almost addictively, feeling humiliated and hurt yet unable to stay away. An aspect of this tenacious pursuit became somewhat clearer when he spoke about how she showed her love for him: "She told me that she always has fantasies of bondage and pain with anonymous men's bodies only. They are always faceless. I am the only man with whom she puts a face on that body." The promise of becoming that one body—held by her gaze and her desire—was intoxicating. He was determinedly, if unconsciously, seeking the opportunity to heal his inner splits and was willing to endure much pain in repeated humiliations and rejections in order to achieve it.

Jim's struggle with the separation from his children was one of the saddest and most moving parts of his analysis. As I witnessed his unraveling of his family's fabric, I had to remind myself that in the process he was recreating the negative space, the void that his father's absence had opened in his life. I was given the task of containing the intense tension between his search for an authentic way of living and the tragic reenactment of his abandonment. Jim described a scene that evoked for me an image of Harlow's monkeys, which were desperately grasping their mothers—his young son clasping his leg and not letting him out of his sight day and night. The boy could let himself fall asleep only when he was firmly clutching Jim's body. Comforted by this embrace, Jim was also deeply troubled by it. It seemed to echo his past longing, of which only a faint echo was now audible. Meanwhile, I was trying to contain my own sadness and the powerlessness I felt in my struggle to prevent another traumatic abandonment, one I knew I neither could nor should try to prevent. As I spoke to Jim, I felt as though I were almost physically hurling my words across to try to hitch him just as he was about to let his son fall away into a void he unconsciously knew so well. At no other time in my work with him did the image of mountaineers—attached to each other with ropes and totally dependent on each other for survival—come so readily to me. Hoping, I imagined that, somehow, our work would trickle down to Jim's connection with his son. My own father's infrequent and precious hugs became my anchors on the slippery slope we were scaling.[2]

As Jim's desperate search for his father in his own son's frantic grasp gradually became more conscious, he became intensely sad and remorseful, able to recognize his son's terror. While still intensely ambivalent about how vulnerable he could let himself become, he now reconsidered his plans to move out of the city, and decided instead to move to a nearby apartment and remain connected.

Against this shifting context of longing and abandonment, Jim recalled a long-forgotten memory of a whole day spent in his father's car, waiting—for what probably felt like forever—for his father to return from a visit to a girlfriend. And yet, almost in the same breath, he said that he had never felt closer to his father as when there were women around. Memories of father's male friends, who were rich, famous, and powerful and sometimes brought his father home after he had too much to drink, soon followed. These memories conjured a locker-room atmosphere of camaraderie, with sweaty, odorous male bodies joined in competitive and sexual pursuits.

Jim identified with the exciting father of sexual escapades. In his internal world he had identified with his father on visits to clubs and glittery hangouts. I found myself carrying the feelings of the abandoned child who waits for his father all day. Those parts of him that felt cheated out of father's love were safely deposited in me. As we embodied these splits in the transference, it was almost impossible to recognize that these were parts of a whole. Once again, I felt that we had lost contact. Jim was speaking the language of desire, of sex, of feeling hypersexual and wishing to be admired. I spoke to him in the language of longing for a lost father. My words seemed to define the empty space left by his father's absence, but they could not fill it. During this phase of our work, he could not resonate with the longing and sadness I was attributing to him. One day, we passed each other on the street, literally as strangers, for, as he saw me walking toward him from a distance, he looked away. He had no recollection of this encounter when I later brought it to his attention. I felt that he was retreating into a familiar cocoon.

Jim appeared to become more deeply aware of, and empathic with, his son's acute distress over his leaving the family. In the context of his impending departure, the memory of that fateful day when Jim's mother found a pack of condoms in his father's golf bag suddenly emerged. This event was the last straw that led to his father's banishment from the family. It crystalized Jim's mode of identification with his father as a phallic, exciting, yet abandoning object. Father's condoms evoked the venturesome, potent phallus, which had driven him away from his son and family.

Jim's identification with his father as a superpotent object became apparent in his discussion of his own use of condoms. Somewhat embarrassed but proud, he confessed that his penis was too large to fit in any generic condom and therefore he was using them inconsistently. With some self-consciousness he reported that previous lovers had always admired his penis' unusual size. He was visibly uncomfortable in discussing this topic and upon inquiry said that he was concerned that I might feel diminished by, and envious of his huge penis. This he said with a smile, while looking straight at me. An unusual silence ensued. We took stock of the fact that, for the first time, we had made contact as phallic rivals, quite literally sizing each other up.

Jim's unblinking assertion of his phallic superiority caught me by surprise. I was pleased at his openly and personally taking me on as a worthy opponent. I somewhat enviously imagined myself asserting my prowess to my father, my teachers, and my analysts. I appreciated Jim's spontaneous phallic gesture and was mostly pleased in the coy pleasure he took in doing so. He seemed to be present in body and feelings in a way that I had not witnessed before. We had made the transition from a parallel to a more mutual play, which allowed for the inclusion of competitiveness and rivalry. These enlivening moments allowed us to share a new level of intimacy.

Jim's associations moved to his son, who was age-appropriately curious about, and admiring of, Jim's genitals. He pursued Jim into the bathroom, wished to urinate next to him, and was eager to reach and touch his father's penis. As we discussed Jim's phallic admiration of his father I suggested that, from the perspective of a young child, a father's penis is likely to appear gigantic. Quite upset, Jim responded by recalling an incident when he was told by his stepmother that his father was rather modestly built. Anxiously amused, he said, "All these women were pursuing my father, for a reason," adding, "since his penis was small, I guess he made up for it by owning a stretch Mercedes-Benz, and huge motorbikes." Apparently caught in this contradiction, Jim began to smile astutely and soon broke into a loud laughter.

In the space that was defined by his father, his son, and his analyst, Jim could find his masculine voice in a distinctly male body. The body, previously fragmented and splintered, was coming to life with new feelings. While his body and feelings were more present now, it was striking to discover how much of what he had known about his and his father's bodies came from hearsay, rumor, and conjecture rather than "full-bodied" conviction born of exploration and self-awareness. I was reminded of the Egyptian myth of Isis and Osiris. I felt as though, as analyst, I had been given Isis's task of collecting Osiris's severed body fragments from across many times and places. This process—of gathering perceptions and memories—was akin to feeding, in which the memories reconstitute not only the missing body that was long forgotten and stored in pieces, but also the original healthy appetite for such an integration.

And, with the restoration of Jim's "father hunger"[3] (Herzog, 1982), his voracious, assertive attempts to take apart and creatively destroy his father and to take him in gradually began to emerge. He described how he had persistently beseeched his father, shortly before father's death, to sit for him for a portrait. His father kept brushing him off impatiently until, Jim said, "I insisted, and I finally sat him down and took the picture. My father was restless, smoking his cigar, and he would not give me any eye contact. He refused to look into my camera." Jim brought in the photograph and as we looked at it he said, "I may appear tame and passive, but I stood behind the lens like a cheetah and I was ready to leap at him, to tear him up and to get inside of him and find out who he is."

Jim's 40th birthday was quickly approaching, and he experienced its imminent arrival as a turning point. He discussed at length a plan to visit his father's grave, to which he had not been since his father's funeral 25 years earlier. There was a frenzy of activity surrounding his trip. He was leaving his home, wife, and children and was planning to go from the graveside straight to his new apartment. The fateful and tragic aspects of these events were not lost on us; he was discussing his visit to the cemetery as a pilgrimage. He described his heart-wrenching struggle to peel his son off him as they embraced upon his departure.

Jim packed pictures of his children, "since my dad had never seen them," and brought his father's old cowboy boots, which he had outgrown. He intended to leave them in the cemetery by the tombstone. He also brought a pack of tissues, a camera, and a book. He was ready to take pictures of himself and to write down his feelings: "I knew that I would feel a lot and would not remember much of it later, so I wanted to have the pictures and the words so that the memory can stay."

Jim did not return from his trip a transformed man. We still had much work ahead of us. His body, his feelings and his mind were still at odds with each other. These absences, and lack of "I- ness," however, had begun to trouble him enough to mobilize him to look after his body. He began a specialized diet and a systematic workout plan designed to lower his blood pressure, and he was pursuing alternatives to medication to manage his hypertension. I think he had come to anticipate more of the abruptness and the intensity by which his body made itself known. He began to remember enough to catch himself at those moments when presence dissolves into absence. Those absences have become clues to the possibility of his becoming more of who he is.

Jim recently became involved in an intimate relationship, which for the first time seems quite satisfying. He was able to stay connected to his children and has become intensely connected to his girlfriend's children as well. In one of our final sessions, finding himself in the role of a surrogate father to these children, he wondered about how readily he would channel his "father longing" to these new children, who were quick to adopt him and call him daddy. He could easily recognize their father hunger, and, struggling between his need for a father and his need to father, he is resisting the pull to father them, fearing that it might undermine his loyalty to his own children. When Jim and I met to discuss this chapter after he had read it, he remarked that his girlfriend, who has suffered the loss of her father, asked poignantly, "Does anyone ever resolve this father hunger?"

I have changed too. My work with Jim, and with other people who struggle with similar issues, has taught me to trust a much more open-ended form of analytic listening. One can conceive of it as the silent counterpart of free association, with the lived body as its base. It reveals that at some unexpected point the process of disappearance has the potential of becoming more conscious, and a new opportunity for integration can present itself. Each time, a deeper trace is left, which renders the disconnection of body, mind, and feelings less pervasive and compelling. These moments of cohesion and integration are now held and sustained by patient and analyst both.

THE DIALECTICS OF EMBODIMENT AND PSCYHOANALYTIC CLINICAL THEORY

What is the place of bodily experience in analytic work? How does a lived bodily experience—the analyst's and patient's—inform the work? How does the lived body figure in the clinical situation just described with Jim?

This chapter is an inquiry into the part played by the lived body, its mass, its breathing in one analysis. It is taken in the spirit of an expedition into a region of the analytic landscape from which findings cannot easily be retrieved, stored, and transported into the laboratory of the symbolized form where they may be preserved. The discoveries exist, at least initially, in the moment of experiencing and recognition. This region is defined by the indefinite space that Winnicott (1949) depicted as "potential space" and Ogden (1994a) referred to as the "analytic third." It involves an inner state akin to Freud's (1912) "evenly suspended attention" and Bion's (1962a) "reverie," requiring subtle attentiveness and perception, which is often lost through premature comments or interpretation. For example, in the initial case illustration, as the analyst becomes aware of how blocked his own interpretive stance has made him, and "lets go" of it, he becomes much more open to listening to the patient. Only then can absence become an "analytic object," revealed in the lack of connection that is discovered in the session.

In this light, the premonitory absent-patient dream I described earlier may be seen as generating an experience similar to the one Ogden (1995) highlights in connection with patients' missed sessions. Ogden suggests that the analyst should write process notes even for those sessions patients do not attend.

> I operate under the assumption that the patient's physical absence creates a specific form of psychological effect in the analyst and in the analysis, and that the analytic process continues despite the analysand's physical absence. In this way, the specific meanings of the patient's presence in his absence are transformed into analytic objects to be fully experienced, lived with, symbolized, understood and made part of the analytic discourse [pp. 701–702].

The dream, remembered in the presence of my absent patient, becomes such an analytic object that is saturated with meanings regarding our situation.

Of the many clinical facts that become accessible in such moments when one's awareness turns toward oneself, I have chosen to elaborate the direct somatic experience of embodiment. As the clinical material suggests, the path to this form of awareness in the analytic situation is nonlinear and quite unpredictable. Paradoxically, however, this perception and awareness cultivate a kind of gradual trust in the possibility of more moments of such confluence of knower and known, moments that connect and bridge bodies and minds.

Viewed from the perspective of current relational psychoanalytic theory, embodiment can be thought of in relation to those psychoanalytic events that are often described as enactments. Enactments—a patterning of psychoanalytic interactions that are repetitive of past events in the analysand's life and are largely unconscious—have been described by Poland (1992), Mclaughlin (1991), and Jacobs (1991). These writers usually present from a vantage point from which enactments are already recognized or at least suspected to be what they are. The authors do not fully elaborate on the central question of how an enactment becomes recognized. What impels analyst and patient to attend to such a repetition, saturated with personal meanings, and make it stand out as figure when it had previously been ignored as irrelevant background?

I propose that the type of immediate, lived body experience described in my work with Jim is a frequent concomitant of the first recognition of an enactment. Authors such as Jacobs (1991) and Poland (1992) often describe having vivid bodily sensations—such as tensions, discomfort, or simply a dawning consciousness of the presence of their bodies—at the moments when they become aware of a rigid, collusive, and repetitive interaction with a patient (see Hirsch, 1996, for a fuller discussion of these authors). While none explicitly focuses on the lived body as a focal point, all have alluded to it. Ogden (1994b) provides a clinical/developmental frame from which to consider the same type of phenomena under his "autistic-contiguous" mode of experience, a protosymbolic, sensation-dominated mode, or psychological organization, more primitive than the positions delineated by Klein:

> Such conception represents an elaboration and extension of Bick, Meltzer, and Tustin. . . . It is associated with a mode of generating experience that is of a sensation-dominated sort and is characterized by protosymbolic impression of sensory experience that together help constitute an experience of a bounded surface. Rhythmicity and experiences of sensory contiguity (especially at the skin surface) contribute to an elemental sense of continuity of being over time [p. 36].

It is the immediacy of the experience that includes the enlivened body, in the here-and-now, that permits analyst and patient more fully to recognize an aspect of their interaction as an enactment. The patterns of tension and bodily sensations that are evoked in the analyst in response to a patient's associations, are, in turn, evoking personal associations in the analyst, which, as part of the process, have become "analytic objects." Thus, my associations to my own swim training days, or to the sound of air raid sirens, while personally meaningful, could not be considered in isolation from the transference and countertransference interaction.

Ogden (1994a) often refers to this mode, in which bodily sensations are experienced as significant clues to unconscious and split-off parts projected into him by the patient. He has, for example, written, "I could feel a cool breeze wash across my face and enter my lungs relieving the suffocating stillness of an over-heated, unventilated room" (p. 7). This mode of experience guides Ogden when he interprets to the patient: "I then said that I had the sense that he sometimes felt so hopelessly stifled in the hours with me that he must have felt like being suffocated in something that appears to be air, but is actually a vacuum" (p. 7). And later in the same description, "the physical sensations of breathing freely and suffocating were increasingly important carriers of meaning" (p. 10).

How is this type of self-transforming knowledge created in the analytic encounter? It appears that a change in the way of knowing oneself in relationship to one's patient has to take place in order for the analyst to begin to realize, and to be able to articulate, his participation in the transference–countertransference enactment with the patient (Davies and Frawley, 1994; Ogden, 1994a; Bromberg, 1996). Once recognized, repetitious rigidification and falsification of the authenticity of the analytic encounter—which is the stance that characterizes enactments—clues the analyst to how far he and his patient have drifted from a real encounter. The potential for something new to be discovered is found, paradoxically, in those moments when one becomes open and is willing to surrender to a receptivity (Ghent, 1990), a perception that can include both participation and observation. It is an inner act of attention (Symington, 1983) that reveals what has thus far been obscure, vague, or barely visible. I suggest that the expansion of the field must include the body. As I became aware of my rigid routinized interactions with Jim, the presence of my body— tense and unfree to breath and to be—was the first clue to how strapped we both had become.

This subtle shift in listening, in the deployment of the analyst's attention, can, for example, be thought of as analogous to one's noticing that one is tensing a muscle unnecessarily. The awareness that one is holding one's pen too tightly as one is writing can, by itself, lead one to release some of this tension without any sacrifice in efficiency.

I find my questions resonating with ideas put forth by Bion (1970), Ogden (1994a,b), Symington (1983), and Bromberg (1996), who ask: what permits the analyst to listen in a new way? What frees his or her attention to truly "free associate" to the patient's material? (Bollas, 1997).

I would like to emphasize that the analyst needs to be able to "free associate" to his own body, to take his body as an object.[4] In that mode of experience, (captured by Ogden's [1994a] formulation of the autistic-contiguous mode), the subjectively experienced body—as an organic breathing energetic field with contours, texture and myriad of movements and stirrings,—stands in dialectic tension to the splintered and split "schizoid paranoid" and to the symbolized and more integrated "depressive" bodies. The body has a specific and essential part to play in our understanding of the process of discovering unarticulated and inchoate meanings. Ogden has written of such body-centered reveries as signs not of narcissistic self-involvement or inattentiveness, but rather of the presence of psychological activity through which the unarticulated, often unfelt, experience of the analysand takes protosymbolic form in the "intersubjectivity of the analytic pair" (p. 12). This mode of experience may even have its own access to memory, as the clinical material suggests.[5]

Jim's relationships with his body demonstrate well how the body can become objectified, looked on from a distance, as if from the perspective of an outsider. In such an instance it is the mind that imagines and feels the body to be separately localized, as if it were situated externally and can be verbalized at a distance.[6]

At every juncture in Jim's treatment, when bodily sensations appeared, the accompanying feeling was of longing, sadness, and often specific memories of loss and trauma followed. How can we understand this confluence of sensations, loss, and trauma?

To situate this discussion in a developmental context, I suggest that it is Winnicott's (1949) contribution that provides the important link between early trauma and the loss of authentic and direct sense of self grounded in the body. Further, Winnicott's ideas provide us with a basis for understanding the way in which a patient who has left his body as a result of early trauma of poor caretaking has "a tendency for identification with the environment aspect of all relationships that involve dependence, and difficulty in identification with the dependent individual" (p. 247). Jim's relationships with his son can be characterized by his inability to see his son's dependence and anxiety about his father's—Jim's—leaving. Similarly, in the transference, Jim could identify himself with his father's adventurous and risk-taking self, but he could not also allow into awareness identification with the dependent son who badly needed a father.

Following Winnicott, Gordon and Corrigan (1995) aptly describe the role of the "mind-object." The mind is seen as the usurper, a compensation. It is a function that has evolved from the failure of good-enough caretaking. The mind-object represents the infants attempt at self-care, an attempt by the mind to maintain the self in the absence of adequate mothering. Thus, according to Phillips's (1995) reading of Winnicott, "Where there is a mind object at work there is a loss, or a violation, that cannot be acknowledged" (p. 230). As the severance of mind functioning from a grounded bodily experience begins to reverse in the course of an analysis and the body reemerges as the place that the patient had once inhabited—a place from which he was seduced or coerced to leave—the feelings of loss and longing also begin to resurface.

Winnicott's and Gordon and Corrigan's formulations shed some light on the link between Jim's absence of bodily and affective experience and trauma, caused by a failure in early caretaking. Whenever the body became more present in Jim's treatment, it was immediately associated with memories of abandonment, longing, and environmental failures. These seem to be the fault lines in caretaking through which Jim has taken refuge from his body.

Patients' striking instances of somatic cut-offness—Jim's distant relationship to his appendix emergency is one—can be understood as the body's attempts to bring the mind back to the body. As Winnicott (1949) has described:

> In these terms we can see that one of the aims of *psychosomatic illness* is to draw the psyche from the mind to the original intimate association *with the soma*. . . . One has to also be able to see *the positive value of the somatic* disturbance in its work of counteracting a "seduction" of the psyche into the mind [p. 254].

The mind-object acts as a perpetual signpost of emotional and somatic emergency, which can alert the analyst, and call for his attention. The mind-object's goal is to abolish both the need and the object. As soon as the mind object is exposed in its brittleness and its futility, it reveals the generative, destructive, but also life-sustaining voracity that underlies it. Thus, in Jim's struggle to find his father, his "father hunger" emerged and brought him into fuller contact with his feelings and his body.

As the study of lived experience, psychoanalysis can develop greater tolerance of the imprecision and ambiguities that are inherent in it. Convictions and absolute certainties, when they crop up, can serve as reminders that one has left the lived body and is again in the presence of a mind-object.

Phillips (1995) has commented on Descartes' lifelong search for certainty in a way that also highlights the tension between states of conviction and the mind-body split.[7] Phillips states that, in our search for an element of objectivity and reliability in our knowledge, we are often inevitably pulled away from the body, which is seen as a source of error and distortion: "It is not exactly, Descartes implies, that we need to get away from the body, but that once we go in search of trustworthy foundations, of states of conviction, the body is the first casualty" (p. 230).

Do we need to give up entirely the possibility of convictions? I do not think so. I feel that there may be a place for conviction and even authority in analytic experience and that these do not need to be kept in the mind and isolated from actual lived experience. That analytic knowledge which is felt, lived, and experienced contains the, paradoxically, temporally ephemeral, and yet full-bodied conviction at the moment when it is held by the two subjectivities of patient and analyst. This knowledge, initially unstable and precarious, can evolve and become recognized and discursive. I consider Jim's pilgrimage to his father's grave, 25 years after the funeral, to have been taken with such a sense of conviction. Unsaid, but clear to both Jim and me, was that we had come to a watershed in his life in and out of analysis. His visiting his father's *body* and "picturing" himself next to it, his son's grasping *body*, and the emergence of our phallic *bodies* in the room all carry this visceral recognition that something lost had been retrieved.

The unique opportunity in which the dialectic of presence–absence can be transformed unfolds at the very moment when this dialectic is held in the consciousness of the analyst and gradually also of the patient. The role of the analyst in these moments can be described, using Bromberg (1996), as "standing in the spaces" between presence and absence. The analyst himself struggles to become a container, to hold in his awareness a link between what the patient may experience as discreet and unbridgeable self-states.

"The Uses of Not," quoted at the beginning of this chapter, is a honed attempt to bridge the abyss between what is and what is not and transcends it. Like a Zen Koan, but with a more subtle punch, it can reveal something that lies hidden. In psychoanalysis we often look far and wide for subtle and hidden meanings. We often miss an experiential center in ourselves from which to perceive the intersubjective field in which we are immersed. The experience of the body as a container and a source of our immediate experience of aliveness (Ogden, 1995) provides an essential orientation to our total situation with our patients.

But the body itself, like the spokes, the clay, and the windows and doors in the Tao Te Ching, is not what is useful. It is in the discovery of the possible relationships among the mind, feelings, and the body that its usefulness can emerge, and its absence become known.

NOTES

[1]Since this chapter is focused primarily on the lived body experience, other important clinical and theoretical aspects of the treatment were intentionally omitted. Thus, much of the clinical work addressing early object relationships, issues of self-regulation and sexuality, and more specific work in the transference were largely left out, with the goal of staying as close as possible to the bodily based clinical material.

[2]Much exploratory and interpretive work took place at this juncture in the treatment, primarily attempting to differentiate the traumatic past from the present situation in his current family.

[3]Father hunger is a tenacious affective state of longing experienced by all of the more than 70 children of divorce studied by Herzog (1982). Interestingly, even in early development that is unmarked by divorce, the father's greater distance allows the child to form cognitive representations of him earlier than of the mother, who is always present (Brooks-Gunn and Lewis, 1979). Abelin (1971) wrote of father as a "non-Mother" object that encourages "elated exploration" and "bridges to the outside."

[4]This is intended in a sense similar to Bollas's (1987) notion of taking the "self as object."

[5]This idea has been explored by various writers on trauma and is specifically related to Bessel van der Kolk's (1994) work on the different storage and recall systems for traumatic events.

[6]Similarly, the analyst can experience himself as operating from within, embedded in the intersubjective field (Ogden, 1994a). Altenatively, he can experience himself "objectively," at a distance from himself and his patient. These vastly different modes of experiencing oneself in relation to one's patient were recently discussed very thoroughly by John Steiner (1996).

[7]Drew Leder's (1990) study, which raises interesting questions about the phenomenology of embodiment, provides an inspiring discussion of this topic. Leder compellingly suggests that the absence of the body from awareness is no accident but is an inherent quality of the lived body. Thus, the often-mentioned split and distance from corporeal existence in Western culture is not accidental and is not the primary factor in the mind–body split.

The body's tendency to disappear from sight, or from experience, is seized on by the Cartesian project of our culture. Therefore, Leder contends, Descartes's doctrine of an immaterial mind trapped inside an alien body rests on a phenomenon of bodily absence that experientially supports such a dualistic understanding.

The body and its states of needs and satisfactions, its desires and appetites, its multifarious energies, its perpetual inner movements, defy any attempt to pin it down in definition and in words. Only a mind split-off and imagined to be held constant in time can generate the experience of conviction and certainty, which, starting with Descartes, has been influencing Western thought. Leder's work suggests that the work of correcting Descartes's epistemology is not intellectual work. Rather, the reversal of the split has to begin by its recognition, and the analytic setting presents a unique opportunity for this type of project.

REFERENCES

Abelin, E. (1971), The role of the father in the separation-individuation process. In: *Separation Individuation,* ed. J. B. McDevitt & C. F. Settlage. New York: International Universities Press.
Bion, W. R. (1962a), *Learning from Experience.* New York: Basic Books.
——— (1970), Attention and interpretation. In: *Seven Servants.* New York: Aronson, 1977.
Bollas, C. (1987), *The Shadow of the Object.* New York: Columbia University Press.
——— (1997), The Goals of Psychoanalytic Treatment. Presented as the Edmund Weil Memorial lecture of the Institute for Psychoanalytic Training and Research, New York City, May 16.
Bromberg, P. M. (1996), Standing in the spaces: The mulitiplicity of self and the psychoanalytic relationship. *Contemp. Psychoanal.,* 32:509–535.
Brooks-Gunn, J. & Lewis, M. (1979), "Why mama and papa?" The development of social labels. *Child Devel.,* 50:1203–1206.
Davies, J. M. & Frawley, M. G. (1994), *Treating the Adult Survivor of Childhood Sexual Abuse.* New York: Basic Books.
Freud, S. (1912), Recommendations to physicians practising psycho-analysis. *Standard Edition,* 12:109—120. London: Hogarth Press, 1958.
Ghent, E. (1990), Masochism, submission, surrender. *Contemp. Psychoanal.,* 26:106–136.
Gordon, P. E. & Corrigan, E. G., ed. (1995), *The Mind Object.* Northvale, NJ: Aronson.
Herzog, J. M. (1982), On father hunger: The father's role in the modulation of aggressive drive and fantasy. In: *Father and Child,* ed. S. H. Cath, A. R. Gurwitt, & J. M. Ross. Hillsldale, NJ: The Analytic Press, 1994, pp. 163–174.
Hirsch, I. (1996), Observing-participation, mutual enactment, and the new classical models. *Contemp. Psychoanal.,* 32:359–383.
Jacobs, T. (1991), *The Use of the Self.* Madison, CT: International Universities Press.
Krystal, H. (1988), *Integration and Self-Healing.* Hillsdale, NJ: The Analytic Press.
Le Guin, U.K., trans. (1997). *Lao Tzu: Tao Te Ching, A Book About the Way and the Power of the Way.* Boston: Shambala.

Leder, D. (1990), *The Absent Body*. Chicago: University of Chicago Press.

Lewis, O. (1991), Parental absence. *Contemp. Psychoanal.*, 27:265–287.

McDougall, J. (1989). *Theaters of the Body*. New York: Norton.

McLaughlin, J. (1991), Clinical and theoretical aspects of enactment. *J. Amer. Psychoanal. Assn.*, 39:595–616.

Ogden, T. (1994a), The analytic third: Working with intersubjective clinical facts. *Internat. J. Psycho-Anal.*, 75:3–20.

———— (1994b), *Subjects of Analysis*. Northvale, NJ: Aronson.

———— (1995), Analysing forms of aliveness and deadness of the transference-countertransference. *Internat. J. Psycho-Anal.*, 76:695–709.

Phillips, A. (1995), The story of the mind. In: *The Mind Object*, ed. P. E. Gordon & E. G. Corrigan. Northvale, NJ: Aronson, pp. 229–240.

Poland, W. (1992), Transference: An original creation. *Psychoanal. Quart.*, 61:185–205.

Steiner, J. (1996), Problems of psychoanalytic technique: Patient-centered and analyst-centered interpretations. In: *The Kleinians of London*, ed. R. Schafer. Madison, CT: International Universities Press, pp. 372–382.

Symington, N. (1983), The analyst's act of freedom as agent of therapeutic change. *Internat. Rev. Psychoanal.*, 10:283–291.

van der Kolk, B. A. (1994), The body keeps the score: Memory and the evolving psychobiology of posttraumatic stress. *Harvard Rev. Psychiat.*, 1:253–265.

Winnicott, D. W. (1949), Mind and its relation to the psyche-soma. In: *Through Paediatrics to Psychoanalysis*. New York: Basic Books, 1958, pp. 194–203.

12

PSYCHIC ELABORATION
OF MUSCULOSKELETAL
BACK PAIN

Ellen's Story

Frances Sommer Anderson

Musculoskeletal back pain brings the body into the consulting room in an unavoidable, compelling way. Consider Mr. H, age 59, who was a vigorous, physically active executive until six weeks ago, when he developed acute musculoskeletal back pain due to Tension Myositis Syndrome (TMS).[1] Our initial session was on the phone because he is immobilized by severe pain. When I enter my waiting room to meet

I deeply appreciate Ellen's participation in our psychoanalytic quest and her consent to share it in this format. I am grateful to the following colleagues and teachers for their help in the creative process. The intellectual stimulation and emotional support of my Body Study Group—Ron Balamuth, Tamsin Looker, and Zeborah Schachtel—made it possible for me to find my voice expressed in the manuscript. Tamsin Looker and Eric Sherman tirelessly read and meticulously edited multiple drafts of this chapter. Lewis Aron, Philip Bromberg, Virginia Goldner, Stephen Mitchell, and John Sarno helped me clarify my thinking at crucial junctures. Adrienne Harris, Joyce McDougall, and Lawrence Friedman persistently encouraged me along the way. My colleagues Lucia Kellar, Neal May, Virginia Kelley, Pasqual Pantone, Elaine Martin, and Barbara Gold were always available to help me through the rough spots.

him for our second session, he is lying on the floor with his wife at his side. He needs her assistance to enter my office. Once we are inside, Mrs. H and I use all my pillows to support him in a semireclining position on my analytic couch so that he and I can face each other during the session. He asks that his wife remain with him during the consultation. Fully aware that Mr. H is in great physical discomfort, I nonetheless press forward with the psychoanalytic inquiry that I began in the phone session. [2]

When a patient's bodily functioning enters the treatment in such a striking way, I am confronted immediately with decisions about how to vary the frame, for example, phone sessions, providing physical assistance to the patient, allowing a companion to remain in the session. While these decisions can be difficult, even more challenging questions arise that reflect the dichotomous thinking that characterizes our psychoanalytic training: Can I treat someone in acute pain? Shouldn't Mr. H be in a medical office? If I undertake a psychoanalytic inquiry about the emotional circumstances in which Mr. H's pain began and is sustained, isn't Mr. H likely to think that I don't believe that his pain is "real," that I think it is all "in his head"? Mightn't Mr. H infer that I believe that he is somehow "to blame" for his pain? Where does an analyst turn for authorization to undertake a psychoanalytic exploration?

PSYCHOANALYSIS AND PAIN

Physical pain, including musculoskeletal back pain, is a major public health problem that affects over 50 million Americans, accounts for over 80% of all physician visits, and costs over $70 billion annually in health care costs and lost productivity (Gatchel and Turk, 1996, p. xi). A recent article in *The New York Times* (1997), describes the burgeoning of retail businesses that target back pain sufferers. Anyone who has experienced Mr. H's kind of pain can attest to the intensity of the experience and to the anxiety and fear that accompany it. When this pain leads to decreased mobility, every aspect of one's daily routine can be severely disrupted, which leads to greater anxiety and fear. At this juncture, the body needs care, and we have been taught to consult a physician, not a psychoanalyst, for a diagnosis and treatment plan.

On consulting a physician, the patient encounters the dichotomous thinking inherent in the traditional biomedical model of illness and pain, which dates back to the ancient Greeks and was codified by

Descartes in the 17th century (Turk, 1996). In this model, pain originates from a "specific disease state represented by disordered biology, the diagnosis of which is confirmed by data from objective tests
of physical damage and impairment" (pp. 3–4). Accordingly, to treat
pain, we must identify a diseased organ or organ system and provide
treatments to correct organic dysfunction or pathology. The patient
soon discovers that there are many specialists (e.g., neurologists,
orthopedic surgeons, physiatrists, osteopathic doctors, and chiro-
practors) with seemingly contradictory diagnoses (e.g., TMS, herni-
ated disc, spinal stenosis, spondylolisthesis) and treatment plans (e.g.,
bedrest, healthy back exercises, physical therapy, electrical stimulation, back and neck braces, pain medication, antiinflammatory agents,
muscle relaxants, trigger point injections, and various surgical pro-
cedures). To complicate matters further, medical doctors are not
trained to ask about the psychological context in which the pain
began.

   If the back pain sufferer is in psychoanalytic treatment, the danger is that the analyst as well may begin to feel that only physicians
have a contribution to make to the patient's recovery. While there is
a large research and clinical literature on physical pain, much of it
behavioral and cognitive-behavioral,[3] there are comparatively few
references to it in the psychoanalytic literature. Szasz (1957) reported
"the surprising lack of psychoanalytic contributions to the problem
of pain" (p. 53). He commented on the "widespread tendency to differentiate between 'physical' and 'mental' pain" and observed that
the "physical" had been "excluded from the domain of psychoanalysis altogether and is assigned to physiology and organic medicine"
(p. 53).

   More recently, Anzieu (1989) and Mikail, Henderson, and Tasca
(1994) noted the relative lack of attention given to pain by psychoanalysts. Mikail, Henderson, and Tasca cite the observations of Szasz
(1957), Pilowsky (1986), and Melzack (1973) to support their conclusion that Freud abandoned consideration of somatic experience as
his interest moved from neurology and medicine to psychoanalysis, thereby reinforcing the dualism underlying our psychoanalytic
heritage.

   Psychoanalysts who have explored the complex concept of pain
usually begin by citing Freud's contribution, notwithstanding the inherent dualism (e.g., Szasz, 1957, pp. xviii–xix; Engel, 1959, p. 917).
Grzesiak (1992), a relational psychoanalyst and pain researcher/cli-
nician, reviews Freud's central references to physical pain, first when
he was developing his concept of the protective barrier (Freud, 1895,

pp. 281–397), in subsequent elaborations of it (Freud, 1926, pp. 169–172), and in his discussions of Elisabeth von R.'s pain (Breuer and Freud, 1893–1895, p. 174) and Dora's pain (Freud, 1905, pp. 3–122).

Engel (1959), an internist with psychoanalytic training, elaborated on the developmental process underlying an individual's "concept" of pain and "pain memories." He held that pain can serve as a warning and as a mechanism of defense and identified the ways in which pain acquires special meanings.[4] In describing "pain-prone personalities," Engel identified features of early life experience that contemporary analysts would think of as potentially traumatic[5] and concluded that pain is a "psychic phenomenon." In 1980, McDougall stated that *"pain is basically a psychological phenomenon"* (p. 423). Her current position is that

> pain is basically a psychosomatic phenomenon, but it is always possible that the psyche refuses to allow a mental representation of the physical pain, in which case the patient is not consciously aware of his/her physical suffering. As we know, such a split between body and mind may have serious consequences of either a somatic or a psychological order [personal communication, December 2, 1997].

Grzesiak (1992) holds that contemporary psychosomatic diagnosticians often ignore an important observation that Freud made in his discussion of Dora's pain: "intractable physical symptoms can be divorced from their original biological origins" (pp. 2–3). Elaborating Engel's concept of "pain-proneness," Grzesiak[6] has developed the concept of the "matrix of vulnerability" to chronic pain. He defines the matrix as the "hidden, usually unconscious, foundation for pain proneness that is a consequence of psychosocial and developmental experiences that involve illness, pain, aggression, guilt, and suffering" (pp. 23–24). Here he includes the effects of early childhood trauma that have been encapsulated or dissociated until a physical or psychic trauma or illness in the present provides an avenue for "expression of these long-hidden conflicts in chronic suffering" (p. 2).

THE PLACE OF AFFECT IN THE PSYCHOANALYTIC TREATMENT OF MUSCULOSKELETAL BACK PAIN

As noted, until recently psychoanalytic treatment of musculoskeletal back pain was marginalized largely because of the dichotomization inherent in our medical and psychoanalytic heritage. In addition, "pain patients" have been considered refractory to such a treatment approach, that is, not capable of introspection and insight. Coen and Sarno (1989), laying a foundation for a psychoanalytically informed treatment approach to TMS pain, identified a relationship between the inability to tolerate one's affective life and the development of TMS.

In subsequent elaborations, Sarno (1991, 1998) holds that TMS is initiated by unconscious emotional processes and that TMS represents defenses against powerful, frightening, unacceptable, unconscious feelings, particularly anger and rage. Essentially, he sees TMS as a psychological distraction or avoidance process. Sarno advances the position that self-induced pressures stemming from perfectionism and "goodism" are the primary reasons for the repressed anger and rage. He also cites the etiological significance of childhood experience, along with the hassles and stresses of everyday life, as contributors to TMS (personal communication, March 31, 1997). In other contexts (Anderson, 1994, 1996), I have discussed case material that identifies the significant role of affective functioning in the onset and maintenance of TMS.

Contemporary psychoanalytic theorists[7] cite the place of affects as central in their models of health and illness, for example, Taylor (1987, 1992, 1993; Taylor, Bagby, and Parker, 1997).[8] Schore (1994, 1997)[9] and Beebe and Lachmann (1988, 1994), investigating the significance of affective life in early development, are documenting the nature and impact of the affective interchanges between the infant and its caretaker on the origins of self- and object representations. Lachmann and Beebe (1996), discussing applications to adult treatment of their three organizational principles of interactive regulation, state that "intense affect" is a "sufficiently unique dimension" of interactive regulation to "justify its inclusion as a third principle" of interactive organization (p. 6).

In another area of psychoanalytic theorizing, Spezzano (1993) has provided a comprehensive review of the place of affect in psychoanalytic theory. He concludes that psychoanalysis is essentially a theory of affect. Citing the work of Tomkins (1962, 1963), he presents a detailed argument that "interest-excitement" is the affect that organizes behavior. Stating that "character is the container and regulator of a person's affects" (p. 183), Spezzano goes on to make a case that therapy/analysis "must provide a means of containing and regulating the patient's affects" (p. 184). His work has been cited by Schore (1997) and by Taylor et al. (1997) as support for their affect regulation models.

In the following presentation of my psychoanalytic work with Ellen, who was referred with a diagnosis of TMS back pain, I advance the position that a relational, intersubjective approach that is attuned to the affective functioning[10] of the analyst *and* the analysand can be used successfully to treat musculoskeletal back pain and other physical symptoms. My psychoanalytic data provide additional support for the inclusion of the analyst's bodily experience in the psychoanalytic process, a dimension identified previously by Balamuth, Anderson, and Looker (1994), Schore (1994, 1997), Shapiro (1996), and Anderson et al. (1996). I am also placing my work in the context of contemporary psychoanalytic models of psychobiological functioning that identify affect regulation as a fundamental construct. Object relatedness is also a major consideration in somatization, as Blaustein (1995; Blaustein and Tuber, 1998)[11] documents in her investigation of affectivity and object relatedness in somatization. My position in this presentation, however, is that the affective dimension of the patient's *and* the analyst's experience has not been given enough attention in our attempts to coconstruct meaning. This is true even though the fundamental role of affect in trauma (Krystal, 1988) and in psychosomatic illness (Krystal, 1988; McDougall, 1985, 1989, 1995) has been established. I have articulated my point of view (Anderson, 1994, 1996) in other contexts, in accord with Schore (1994, 1997), Aron (1996), and Maroda (1995).

ELLEN'S STORY

Ellen, now 46, was referred by her physician, who told her that the musculoskeletal back pain she had been experiencing for nine years was due to Tension Myositis Syndrome. During those nine years, Ellen had consulted numerous traditional and nontraditional health practitioners, always stopping short of surgery. None of the treatments had relieved her back pain. Her life had become quite constrained by the limits on physical activity that were prescribed by her physicians. In fact, she had developed a fear of physical activity because she had come to believe that it would make her pain worse. In the interval between the TMS diagnosis and our initial consultation (about eight weeks), Ellen experienced a gradual and significant reduction in her pain level (she estimated a 35% reduction), and she began to resume physical activity. After the first three months of our psychoanalytic work, she reported another pain reduction of about 40% and she continued to increase her physical activities. The residual pain resolved by the end of the first year of treatment. Ellen and I have identified a pattern of pain eruption during times of great emotional stress. The analytic process can resolve the symptom within a few sessions, or sooner.

In the following discussion of my analytic project with Ellen, I, using dreams and other clinical material, demonstrate the process of psychic elaboration of Tension Myositis Syndrome across a period of several years of analytic work and within a single session . I hope to enrich the psychoanalytic literature 1) by showing how dissociated affect contributed to Ellen's physical symptoms, 2) by illustrating how my affective functioning in the relational matrix, often at a somatic level, constituted a key element in the process of psychic elaboration of her musculoskeletal pain and other somatic symptoms, and 3) by underscoring the challenge that analyst and analysand face when their attempts to psychically elaborate physical symptoms result in serious, sometimes life-threatening, illness. My discussion of the full psychodynamics of the case is necessarily incomplete because of the limited scope of the chapter.

I acknowledge, at the outset, Ellen's collaboration with me in the analytic process—through the journals that she has kept during our work, through her active pursuit of knowledge of the psyche–soma relationship outside our sessions, and through her permission for me to use material from our analytic endeavor in this chapter. I have included Ellen's voice from our analytic process whenever possible. In addition, I have integrated her editorial comments on my penultimate manuscript[12] into the text.

Dissociated Affect: The Boxer Dog

The Tension Myositis diagnosis made sense to Ellen, so our analytic work began—eight years ago. At that time, Ellen had been divorced from her husband, Ted, for nine years. Her parents are living, and she has one sibling, a brother, Joe, who is three years older. She lives alone and has had a married lover, Mark, for nine years.

The analytic process started for me as I listened to Ellen's voice on her answering machine when I returned her initial call. Her way of speaking had an impact immediately. Her voice was flat; her pace was slow, deliberate, and measured. As we spoke in the initial interview, I noticed that she paused frequently and swallowed audibly. After a few sessions, I realized that her speech pattern was heightening my awareness of her lack of emotional response to what I was often experiencing as highly affectively charged material. I noticed that I would feel tense at these times because I was feeling stirrings of anger or outrage or disappointment that I, the analyst, could not express as Ellen described various interpersonal situations that had turned out badly for her.

Early in the treatment I began to feel mildly distressed that Ellen was not experiencing affects that could be protective for her (Krystal, 1988, pp. 3–20). For example, I noticed that she spoke in great detail about her relationship with her ex-husband, Ted, but with almost no affective response as she talked about the way their marriage had failed and about the many ways she continued to be involved in his life, even after he had remarried and had two children. I remember being especially surprised to hear that she had used her considerable talent as a landscape architect to specify the plantings for the grounds of Ted's new family's home, only a few houses away from her own. Given how painful she said that their breakup had been, I wondered silently how she could continue to be involved in his new marriage in such an intimate way, especially since her own intimate life with a partner continued to be frustrating and largely unfulfilling. How could she tolerate these interactions? Weren't they at least somewhat painful? Ellen also described work and other personal situations in which she appeared not to be sensing that her own interests could be endangered by the agendas of colleagues and friends. Meanwhile, quite early, I was already able to anticipate that she was going to get "hurt" when she entered interpersonal situations without seeming to use knowledge of past experience that could help her protect herself.

I was familiar with this apparent "absent affect,"[13] having encountered it frequently during the last 18 years treating people who have TMS pain. In analytic work with a patient referred with a diagnosis of Tension Myositis Syndrome, reaching the affect is usually a fundamental part of the analytic process. With Ellen, I guessed that a big challenge lay ahead because her "absent affect" was so striking *and* because my somatic response to her was so strong: while I waited eagerly, yet apprehensively, to hear what was to happen next, I would often feel a visceral sense of dread and notice an increase in my heart rate. At the same time, I would often be holding my breath, which I have learned is my unconscious somatic response when I do not want to experience fully my emotional reactions.

A dream that Ellen brought after five months of treatment illustrates further this aspect of her psychological functioning, my response to it, and the implications for our elaboration of her musculoskeletal pain. We had been identifying the emotional circumstances in which her back pain had started and persisted. Briefly, Ellen's back pain had begun about six months after her divorce from Ted was final—after a separation of about a year and a half. She had described that separation as a period of unrelenting activity that analysts call the "manic defense." In her words, "I was a human doing, not a human being." We had come to understand that this activity was, unconsciously, a way to avoid dealing with her emotional reactions to the marital separation and the pending loss of the marriage.

I had also learned that, through her marriage to Ted after college at age 22, she had gained a place of respect in her family for the first time. She had remarked several times that she felt that her mother was "in love" with Ted and that he had found in her mother the kind of maternal care and attention that was not available to him from his own mother. Ellen had also reported that the only support her family gave her was for her to take the "wife/mommy track," despite her obvious considerable talent in two professional areas. In our initial session, in fact, she had stated that her family had always "championed" (her word) her brother, Joe. She felt that they had never championed her.

While Ellen was married to Ted, she worked full-time to support him through his postgraduate professional training and went to school at night for a master's degree in one area of interest. Ted was actively discouraging and disparaging of her efforts to get this degree; her parents were ambivalent. When Ted completed his degree, she could not overcome his active discouragement of her pursuing additional career goals, and she settled for work in a variety of situations in which she always felt frustrated and unfulfilled. When she separated from Ted, at his request and to her family's dismay, she felt, in her words, "like throwing myself on the railroad tracks" because of the shame and the enormous threat to her self-image. Ted's stated reason for wanting a divorce was that Ellen was too "controlling" of him in her need for "neatness" and "cleanliness" in their household. As the divorce was approaching, and prior to the onset of her back pain, Ellen had been preparing to enter a training program to get a long-cherished professional credential. She had to relinquish this goal after the onset of the debilitating back pain and a subsequent fracture to her left arm when she was hit by a motorcyclist. Forced to find a new career path, she entered a profession that is still chosen predominantly by men.

Ellen told the following dream at the beginning of a session. She introduced it by saying that she'd had a "nightmare":

> I was out in the countryside somewhere, riding bikes
> with Ted. It started out pleasant. We had a boxer dog
> with us. My family got one, a male, when I was six
> months old and we had it 'til I was seven. The second
> boxer was when I was in fourth grade and we had it
> 'til I was a junior in high school–a female.
>
> Both became overprotective, and we had to get
> rid of them. Ted and I were in Minnesota for three
> years, and then we came to Princeton and after one
> year we bought a house. The neighbors had two
> boxers. The fawn one lived with us in the evenings.
> Shortly before we broke up, one morning we found
> him dead on our porch—rat poison. The dog in the
> dream was nice looking—running along with us. The
> first part was euphoric. Somewhere in the middle, the
> dog was not keeping up. I knew it was sick. It keeled
> over dead, rolled over on its back; its chest cavity
> was open and deteriorated.

As I listened, the tension mounted for me, but Ellen seemed very calm. She had told me that this was a nightmare. I was wondering, "What's going to happen?" The way she was interweaving the history of the boxers was heightening the tension by delaying the nightmare ending. I also noticed that there was no detectable change in her affect as she related this "nightmare." There was just Ellen, telling me the story in calm, measured tones.

When she finished telling this dream, she continued by giving more useful factual associations in her now familiar detached, objective manner. Meanwhile, the image of the damaged, dead boxer persisted for me as I cringed inside and wanted to clutch my chest protectively. I was wondering what had happened to the boxer, what could this signify? What had happened in the marriage that I hadn't heard about? Why was euphoria followed by—by what?—by physical trauma to the boxer dog and what I experienced as a blank space where I had expected to hear an affective response. Bromberg (1994, 1995) would call this a "dissociative gap." Meanwhile, I silently filled in the gap—I was horrified. Nothing in our discussions to date, nothing in the "facts" she had provided, had given me any indication that her experience in the marriage had been this traumatic.

As I listened to her associations to the dream, I waited for her to show some feeling for the boxer, clearly an important attachment figure given her story, but she showed none. Also, I still wasn't clear about what had made it a nightmare for her. Finally, I wondered aloud what her reaction was to what had happened to the boxer. She looked stunned, she was speechless, she couldn't find a reaction to report.

This was an early pivotal moment in the treatment, one to which we have referred often. One of my roles as analyst was taking shape—I was to register affective responses when Ellen showed none, or none that I deemed appropriate, that is. Through my silent, but visceral, affective response to hearing about the physical trauma to the boxer, I was entering a lengthy enactment with Ellen: I would silently experience pain and rage for the boxer and Ellen as she represented herself again and again as a sick and damaged boxer in her dreams and as she described herself over and over as the victim of aggression in interpersonal relationships. Early in the treatment, she would report this information to me with apparently little reaction while I was left holding all the violent images and their associated affects and trying to find a way to elaborate them, to make sense of such violent, physically destructive aggression.

I think of what happened in this session as an example of extreme dissociation of "cognitive awareness" from "affective experiencing." Specifically, in this dream, Ellen had "cognitive awareness" that something was wrong with the boxer. The dream ended as she was "observing" what was wrong, but she showed no affective response to that knowledge. That is, there was no "experiencing I," but rather an "affective paralysis" noted by Laub and Auerhahn (1993, p. 288). I agree with their position that integration of traumatic experience requires the development of an "experiencing I," or an "ownership," of the experience. One of my early roles as Ellen's analyst was to be the "experiencing I," to register and bear the painful and violent affect that she had been unable to tolerate and symbolize.[14] Fully elaborating the "emotional context" has been particularly important with Ellen, especially at the beginning of the analysis, because she is skilled at presenting details and rich associations, but often without their associated affects.

When Ellen told this dream, and I heard what had happened to the boxer and I noted her lack of affective response, I immediately speculated that there was a significant relationship between her persistent back pain and what had happened to the boxer. I conjectured that she was symbolizing in the damaged, dead boxer dog some kind of traumatic experience that she had not integrated and that I had not yet learned about. I hypothesized that the blank space that I experienced in Ellen's telling of the dream referred to her failure to integrate an affective response to what had happened with Ted. In line with this hypothesis, I wondered if her inability to integrate what had happened in the marriage and her inability to mourn the loss of Ted had led to back pain, that is, I wondered if the back pain had come to serve as a defense against painful affect.

It was not until a year and a half later that Ellen began to fill in that dissociative gap when she began to disclose, very slowly, traumatic experiences with Ted that she "knew" about but had not affectively integrated. In a session near the 11th anniversary of her divorce, she mentioned, fleetingly, that he had been physically violent toward her. Disclosing this fact, without any details, was retraumatizing: Not only did she have to relive the experience in reporting it, but she also felt tremendous shame and humiliation that the violence had occurred. Perhaps worse, she felt that she was betraying Ted.[15]

Months later, I learned that Ted had once hit her in the chest in a violent outburst: we had finally made a link between the decayed chest of the dream boxer and a violent physical and affective experience that had happened in the marriage. Still later, she revealed that she was, in her words, "living in danger the whole time." To keep him from "flying off the handle," she felt as if she were "stretching a rubber band as far as possible." "Just to sleep with somebody with that kind of violence is unreal," she said. When I asked how she was able to do it, she replied, "I kept myself in a bloody straitjacket."

In June, 1994, the O. J. Simpson story triggered an apparent reliving of the violence with Ted when Ellen developed a sudden, intense relationship with a man she had met in a singles bar. He quickly became emotionally violent and controlling, and there was reason to believe that he could be physically violent as well. Ellen developed a serious abdominal infection of unknown etiology, her second such condition during the analysis. This infection required hospitalization and prevented her from having intercourse with this man. In our analysis of this repetition and my overprotective reactions during it, we elaborated further the violence that she had experienced with her ex-husband. Ellen stated, "When Ted took my life in his hands, I had no reaction. The mindset I had was that it didn't matter. When he hit me, I thought I dreamed it." The power of dissociation as a survival mechanism can hardly be more evocatively described. These vivid images helped us make even more sense of her chronic muscle tension and its relationship to the underlying fear and rage that she could not experience (see Coen and Sarno, 1989; Sarno, 1991, 1998).

Living in a situation where there is chronic emotional tension of the kind Ellen experienced with Ted has long-term physical effects

(McDougall, 1985, 1989, 1995; Krystal, 1988; van der Kolk, 1994, 1996a). In psychobiological terms, van der Kolk (1994) states that "the body keeps the score," that is, the "psychological effects of trauma are stored in somatic memory and expressed as changes in the biological stress response" (p. 253). In my analytic and psychotherapeutic work with people who live with chronic emotional stress, I have seen that it can lead to upper and lower back pain, headache, temporal mandibular joint pain, and other somatic symptoms. This has been documented by Sarno (1974, 1976, 1977, 1981, 1984, 1991) and elaborated by Coen and Sarno (1989) in the psychoanalytic literature. In the pain literature, Turk (1996) reviews research showing that psychological factors can have a direct effect on physiological parameters associated with the prediction or exacerbation of the perception of pain. For example, thoughts can lead to sympathetic nervous system arousal and increased muscle tension. If the activation is chronic, as is often the case in posttraumatic stress disorder, this increases skeletal muscle tone and can set the stage for hyperactive muscle contraction and possibly for persistence of contraction following conscious muscle activation. Flor, Turk, and Birbaumer (1985) have shown that discussing stressful events can lead to an increase in EMG activity localized to the site of back pain. Sarno (personal communication, 1997) would say that this EMG activity and the associated physical pain that is experienced at this site is due to mild ischemia of involved muscle tissue.

Chronic emotional stress can also have a compromising impact on the immune system (Maier, Watkins, and Fleshner, 1994). In our analytic work, Ellen's back pain essentially resolved after a few months in treatment. However, she began to manifest an extreme susceptibility to a wide range of unusual, difficult-to-diagnose eye, mouth, throat, thumb, and pelvic infections. Two of the pelvic infections required hospitalization. These infections always followed sessions in which she discussed material that was highly affectively charged, but the time constraints on the session had prevented her from fully processing or symbolizing (Bromberg, 1996) the powerful associated affects (van der Kolk, 1994; 1996a). Turk (1996) cites the work of O'Leary et al. (1988), who have documented the effects of thoughts on biochemistry (on suppresser T-cells). McFarlane and van der Kolk (1996, p. 571) cite recent unpublished data by van der Kolk et al.(1996) on the effects of trauma on the immune system. McFarlane and van der Kolk (1996) and May (1996) refer to research (Pennebaker and Susman, 1988; Speigel, 1993) suggesting that verbalization of emotional distress can have significant positive effects on the immune system.

The latter data can be taken as support for an analytic undertaking like the one in which Ellen and I have been engaged. The immediate frightening physical consequences of experiencing affects associated with traumatic material in sessions has, however, underscored for me the importance of working very slowly and carefully to help Ellen learn to tolerate and symbolize strong affect that is activated during the integration process. Ellen strongly agreed that I needed to underscore caution in this discussion of psychic elaboration of physical symptoms. Analysts have always been advised to proceed carefully when analyzing somatic symptoms (e.g., Krystal, 1988; McDougall, 1985, 1989). The stress on the analyst, also, can be considerable when the process of psychic elaboration results in the patient's becoming physically ill. While I have not become physically ill in reaction to the analytic work with Ellen, I have been actively engaged in sometimes painful deliberation about this aspect of our work by reading and consulting with colleagues as I try to tolerate experiencing the ambiguities associated with our work. I have been made acutely aware that the impact of the analytic process is paradoxical in that our very attempts to treat the condition underlying symptoms can also prove painful and, sometimes, perilous.

Integration of Traumatic Affect: The Rabbits

To illustrate further our psychic elaboration of Ellen's physical symptoms, I offer a dream that she brought about one year after the preceding dream. She told it at the end of a session in which the theme had been "keeping secrets." She introduced the dream by talking about a movie—*The Prince of Tides*—she had seen the night that she had the dream. Her remarks focused on the "enduring relationship" that the central male character had with the female psychiatrist/analyst. She had cried for hours after seeing the movie. She also noted that she had had an intense conflictual phone interaction with her brother the day before the session. Then she said, "My back started to hurt when I started to tell you the dream."

> I was in Switzerland, skiing,[16] which I don't do now. I learned to ski with Ted the first year we were married. We were skiing, trying to get on one lift to go to a scenic run. We missed it, got on another one. We were skiing through mountains, we paused. I looked over and I could see a tiny white rabbit. A rabbit sitting

inside the carcass of a twin bunny. It was dead. The first rabbit was eating the carcass of the rabbit it was sitting in. It pushed the dead rabbit off the cliff. A bloody scene. The live rabbit was sitting on the edge of the cliff wriggling its nose. A harmless, cute rabbit that had done this deed. Ted and I were watching. Three or four ugly men came up and confronted us. It's giving me a chill to tell you. The dream shifted. I was with my family—mother, father, brother, my family of origin. We were watching a home movie documentary about the white rabbit eating the carcass. When it ended, I was sitting on the floor. I had a leather-embossed story book with the words, "My Story" on the cover. I had a Windex bottle in the shape of a little girl. I was spraying it clean, only the cover.

There, my back doesn't hurt so much.

First, I want to note Ellen's progress in integrating traumatic experience. Specifically, in this dream, Ellen moves from being merely an onlooker at a scene of disturbing physical violence to portraying herself as the subject of the violence: She takes the scene of trauma to the rabbit's body into her family home where it becomes "Her Story." But, as in many previous boxer dreams, she is still telling "Her Story" with animals as the characters representing the trauma.

Although Ellen reports no affective reaction within the dream, this time she tells me that her back started to hurt when she started to tell me the dream. This time she knows there is a connection between her body's reaction and the content and telling of the dream. She has learned to read her body's signals, an important first step on the road to eliminating the physical symptoms. Further, she gets a "chill" while telling the dream—this time I was not alone in feeling a visceral response to the horror of the dream image. Then, Ellen says she feels better after telling me the dream—another linking of psyche and soma.

In the five and a half years of analytic work since this dream, Ellen and I have continued to elaborate one of her "secrets"—the theme of violence in her family, the violence she depicts in the many damaged boxer dream images and in the image of the horror and destruction of the rabbit that becomes "Her Story." To date, the clinical material has pointed us to Ellen's powerful, conflictual attachment to her brother, Joe, three years older.

Ellen seems to have received highly contradictory messages from her parents about her status in the family compared with Joe's, reflected, for example, in many dreams about "unequal playing fields." Her increasing awareness of this discrepancy has been an extremely painful theme running throughout our work. She recalls, from an early age, family stories about her mother's first pregnancy, which ended in the miscarriage of a male child. Further, she has been told that both parents were hoping that she would be a boy; they had even chosen a name for him in their eager anticipation of his birth.

She has always felt that Joe is the favored sibling, whom she also adored, whose cowboy outfits she wore when he outgrew them, and whose toys she preferred to hers. One source of confusion was that her parents did not make an appropriate age and "sexual" differentiation between her and Joe—in many ways they treated them as "twin boys." On the other hand, she felt that her mother had treated Joe preferentially, exemplified in a letter that Ellen had written to Joe when she was in first grade. It read: "I love you but you be bad to me. Mom gets me and lets you free." When Ellen read my penultimate manuscript, she told me that my including this letter was the most painful disclosure for her, but she felt strongly that I must include it because it was such a critical piece of information about "Her Story."

Goldner (1991), working to develop a "critical relational theory of gender," has made the following observations, which shed light on Ellen's pervasive dream images of bodily violence:

> Since complying with contradictory gender injunctions and reifications is tied to sustaining the child's primary object relations, the child must accommodate to these impossible terms by performing acts of internal "violence" on the self. In so doing, the relational complexity of the internal world fragments, and ambivalence devolves into splitting and false self operations [p. 268].

It was not until much later in the treatment that we began to appreciate just how painful the relationship with Joe had been. I have learned about scenes of emotional and physical conflict with Joe that Ellen has depicted in the following way: "My parents would let stuff go on til I screamed in pain and would get hurt. I knew I was going to get picked on; I just never knew when. My whole life with my brother was that way. They were right there letting it happen, so the violation was more intense." She would rail out to her parents, "How can you let him do this?" but they would not intervene.

In writing this chapter, I became aware that I did not understand clearly what the "stuff" was that went on with Joe. When Ellen and I discussed my lack of knowledge in this area, she identified two kinds of "stuff" that went on: sibling competition with regard to physical strength, that is, "You can't bend my finger back"; and verbal combat, that is, Joe would tease her by calling her a "stupid" girl and refer to her as "my idiot sister" when she took too long in the family's only bathroom.

When Ellen gave me these examples, I could see that she was starting to be overwhelmed with emotional pain—her eyes filled with tears and her neck and face reddened—and I remembered that sessions like this would often be followed by a severe somatic reaction, usually an infection. Here I was reminded of Laub and Auerhahn's (1993) description of the dilemma we all face in dealing with trauma. They state, "We all hover at different distances between knowing and not knowing about trauma, caught between the compulsion to complete the process of knowing and the inability or fear of doing so" (p. 288). Further, they point out, "To protect ourselves from affect we must, at times, avoid knowledge" (p. 288). Our interaction in this session acutely exemplifies this dilemma. As the session progressed, Ellen acknowledged that she was feeling overwhelmed and said that she thought we should go more slowly. I agreed. In the discussion that followed, she asked me if I thought that I had been afraid to know more about some areas of her experience. I answered that I thought that was likely, given the number of instances when I had failed to "pursue the particulars" about her early conflictual encounters with Joe, for example.

Because the information that Ellen and I have thus far does not adequately account for the degree of violence and bodily damage in her dream images and in her physical illnesses, I have to wonder what else there is for us to learn. Nevertheless, Ellen's gradual ownership of the traumatic experience with Joe that we do "know" about has increased her awareness of how she leaves herself open to boundary violations in the present. She has begun to realize, with great shame and fear, that she has repeated these scenarios with Joe in her relationship with Ted, with her married lover, and in other personal and professional relationships.

Subsequent elaborations of the rabbits dream and other clinical material have referred to sexual betrayal in power relationships. When these themes came up initially in sessions, Ellen treated references to sexual abuse as largely symbolic rather than actual. Nevertheless, she is slowly and cautiously starting to let me know more about Ellen the "seductress"—about how she has been attracted to powerful men, often her bosses, and how she has taken risks and used her sexuality to try to secure the relational tie. After reading my manuscript, Ellen elaborated further: "I appear to be an attractive, intelligent woman who has it all. The men put me on a pedestal—my father never did. I'm in a power position sexually and use it. The men get thwarted because there's no way I'll go to bed with them. Then they're angry." They then disrespect her and treat her badly in business negotiations, in ways that are painfully similar to what has happened to her in her family. She said, "In my family, male equals power. I'm after power. Women can level the playing field by countering male power in using their femininity." This strategy "backfires" when she does not follow through sexually. In her words, "I have never had a job situation where my superior didn't abuse the power situation." More recently, she has been using the awareness that she has gained in the analysis to anticipate and negotiate these power dynamics to protect herself better. We agree that much analytic work remains to be done in this area.

In the last three years of our work, we have been involved in intense enactments of the violent situations that she experienced in her family of origin. We have been analyzing all the positions that she and I have been taking in these enactments, along the lines delineated by Davies and Frawley (1994) and by Frawley-O'Dea (1997).[17] We have linked my experiences of hurt and impotent rage when listening to her stories of being treated badly to those times when Joe would torment her and her parents would not respond to her cry for help. Ellen has been in the position of the uninvolved parent and the abuser when she reports abuse with no reaction. I have been the silent, neglected, suffering Ellen, who believed that the only way to survive was to endure and to try not to feel overwhelmed in response to what was happening.

Another version of this enactment developed in a session where I, in the position of the neglected and abused child, could no longer silently tolerate hearing about another painful situation she had set up for herself. Finally, in an angry tone of protest, much like Ellen's cry to her parents, "How can you let him do this?" I told her how painful it was to listen. Ellen said, "This will sound bizarre. I have this slight amount of comfort that I've transferred my pain to you at the same time I'm not taking care of myself. I think, okay, if Fran's got it, we'll nail it." She then reported that she had been increasingly aware that I would become upset when she hadn't taken care of herself. I replied, "I'm the one who feels the pain and says 'This hurts.' " She replied, "I make you do this, I want you to say it; then I'll know it's really true. I want you to feel every step of this, be with me when I feel this. I'm afraid to feel this without you in the room."

In our analytic process, we have learned that, for Ellen, experiencing anger/rage can be emotionally overwhelming and somatically dangerous. In a session in which she tried to recall whether she had ever felt angry at her brother, she said, "My mind just went." She "saw red" and almost blacked out, stating that anger at Joe "looms as a convulsion." These responses are suggestive of dissociated rather than repressed rage because the affect is so overwhelming (Bromberg, personal communication, 1997). Bromberg (1996) suggests that this kind of "traumatic affect flooding" occurs when an individual is unable to "hear in a single context the voices of other self-states holding alternative realities that have been previously incompatible" (p. 530).

Ellen's fear of interpersonal confrontation was also vividly illustrated to us in a dream in which she was riding with her family in the family car. She was angry about what was happening in the car and decided to get out and walk. When she got out, she asked her mother to get her suitcase from the car trunk. When her mother handed her the suitcase, Ellen threw it at her. When Ellen told this dream in the session, she almost "blacked out" when she started to experience the rage that she felt toward her mother. We learned that she was fearful that she would destroy her mother and was ashamed that she experienced such destructive impulses toward her mother. These "aggressive" and "destructive" versions of her "self" were impossible to integrate. She stated, "This is why I get back pain and get sick, because I don't use this realm. I'm afraid to use [healthy] boxer emotions, afraid to make the connection." At these junctures, Ellen has frequently reported that she "can't think and feel at the same time."[18]

When Ellen refers to "healthy boxer emotions" in this context, she is referring to the optimal use of anger and aggression in interpersonal relationships. Mitchell's (1993) relational perspective on aggression and its impact on the definition of self is helpful in understanding her experience. Mitchell defines aggression as a "biological response to the subjective experience of endangerment and being treated cruelly" (p. 163) or "a psychological experience embedded in and accompanied by a physiological surge" (p. 165). He states that unintegrated intense anger can "shatter and diffuse other concerns and intentions, generating mental disorganization" (p. 165). Thus, one's sense of self is "transformed by altered physiology" (p. 166), and this sense of self can be difficult to contain alongside other versions of self.

In our analytic dyad, Ellen is increasingly able to tolerate her anger at me when I confront her if I sense that she is not taking care of herself in interpersonal situations. After five years of analytic work, she said, "You're less of an authority figure now. This is a revolution. Previously I was looking for mirroring; now I'm looking for arguing." She is still frightened, however, of losing closeness with me, afraid of destroying a positive connection with me if she experiences and expresses anger at me, as she did with her mother in the preceding dream. While exploring her experience of feeling angry at me, she has said,

> You're the first person for the longest period who supported me. If I showed anger at you . . . we'd be equal combatants on the playing field. Instead, I become a stone. The only time I can remember summoning anger at you, I got a little terse tone. I squeezed shut the floodgate, contracted the gluteus maximus. I don't let my anger out and screw up my back instead. I can't reverse it all at once.

We continue to identify and analyze Ellen's anger and aggression toward me. This is always an aspect of the psychoanalytic process, but it is particularly important for a severely somatizing person like Ellen for whom dissociated rage and aggression have been directed toward the body.

Commenting on the role of the analyst in such a situation, Bromberg (1996) holds that, in order for the patient to move from "dissociation to intrapsychic conflict," the patient and analyst must engage in the "messy" parts of the analytic relationship. In the preceding observations, Ellen was forecasting the stormy weather that lay ahead in our analytic undertaking. This and numerous other examples of how Ellen feels overwhelmed when she experiences anger and rage underscore the necessity of moving slowly and carefully as she integrates self-states that have violent associated affects. This integration is essential if Ellen is to use those affects to take better care of herself. Here the importance of being able to recognize, tolerate, and "reexperience" (Novey, 1961, cited by Krystal, 1988, p. 17), affect is critical in order that Ellen's affects can serve a protective function.

THE ANALYST'S AFFECTIVE PARTICIPATION
AS A MUTATIVE FACTOR

When Ellen says that she wants me to "feel every step of this," to be with her in the room when she feels it, I believe that she is directing us to a mutative aspect of the analytic process. Schuman (1991), exploring the relevance of an Eastern philosophical paradigm for our Western psychoanalytic treatment approach, stresses the importance of the therapist's capacity to "be" with the patient, to "attend to the present moment" (p. 619). She cites Guntrip's emphasis on the patient's need for the analyst to be in a "stable" state in order for the patient to "feel real and find his own proper self" (p. 619). Schachtel (1996) has stressed the importance of the analyst's being "fully present" in the analytic process. Schore (1994) advocates a state of "vitalizing attunement" (p. 449) to the patient, which requires that the analyst's affect state resonate with changes in the patient's internal states. The analyst's awareness of countertransferential visceral-somatic responses is essential.

In our analytic dyad, Ellen's first requirement was for me to tolerate hearing about situations that evoked painful, frightening, violent affect, the first step in helping her to tolerate experiencing it. If our pace was too quick, she became ill, much as the boxers in her dreams had. In describing our roles in the early phase of the analysis, Ellen said, "I'll tell you in monotone, with no inflection in my voice. I can pass it through you. Once I pass it through you, the jig is up. I have to feel it." Thus, the boxers also represented feelings that she needed to experience. I, in the role of the boxer, have had to suffer a great deal as we symbolize such violent, bodily destructive dream images as the boxer who vomited a half-decayed capon and had a bowel movement of two whole, half-decayed turkey carcasses containing three half-decayed rats; the boxer who was knocked senseless in a violent fight with another dog; and the boxer who was injured by a stake in her back and went into convulsions and died because of the pain.

To elaborate further on the importance of my affective response to Ellen, I am including, on her recommendation, a boxer dream from an early phase of our work which has always been in the background but never adequately analyzed. The dream occurred shortly after Ellen's hospitalization (the first during the analysis) for a life-threatening pelvic infection, initially thought to be toxic shock syndrome but later said to be "of unknown etiology." This infection occurred about three weeks after her mother's hysterectomy for uterine cancer.

In the week prior to the onset of the acute infection, we had a session in which Ellen *experienced* the realization intensely, for the first time, that the very bedrock of her identity had been to bear emotional pain for others, in particular her mother, her ex-husband, and her married lover, Mark. She almost fainted on the couch just before she articulated her situation in this way: "I abandoned my body and soul and jumped into theirs." While she was in the hospital, we arranged for a phone session on a weekend day and she called me at my home office. In that session, she revealed that she had felt suicidal after she left the session in which she had had the painful insight about a primary source of her self- esteem. Soon after the phone session, she had a dream in which she came to visit me in my home in New York City (she lives outside the city). She opened the door to my home and let my four boxers run out into the street.

After reading my disclosures about the pain I have experienced during the analysis, Ellen said that she finally understood the dream about my boxers. She conjectured that, early on, she must have been aware that I was reacting to "Her Story" and that she must have unconsciously needed me to feel for her so that she could begin to tolerate feeling for herself. Certainly my concern for her was apparent during the somatic aftermath of the traumatic session.

The importance of my showing affect became clearer to both of us when we discussed Ellen's reaction to reading my description of her voice as "flat." At first she was surprised and hurt. On further reflection, she realized that this aspect of her speech pattern has probably been interpreted by friends and others as an indication that she is very "laid back" and able to tolerate a great deal of upset. She also appreciated, for the first time, that neither of her parents showed a range of emotional reactions. Only her brother, Joe, recognizably expresses affects, particularly anger, as did her ex-husband, Ted. She speculated that her parents' constricted range of affect expression had impaired the development of her own affective functioning, and left her unprepared to recognize and tolerate affect, particularly anger.

From a relational perspective, what I believe has been mutative in the work with Ellen is my role in the analytic process as participant, both onlooker *and* experiencer—that is, as integrator of painful affects. In this context, the boxers can be thought of as symbolizing a "protective shield" (Laub and Auerhahn, 1993) or a "good object" (Kirshner, 1994) that protects against traumatic experience. Laub and Auerhahn propose that the essential experience of trauma is a disruption of the link between the "self" and the "empathic other," usually thought of as the mother. On an intrapsychic level, this means that the maternal introject, or mothering function, is deficient or "damaged" in some way. In a similar vein, Kirshner (1994) attempting to find the common ground in theories of trauma (e.g., Ferenczi, Freud, Klein, Winnicott, and Lacan), holds that the essence of trauma is the constant threat of destruction or loss of the "good object." He defines the good object as a "function of symbolic representation of the human world of cultural meanings and value" (p. 235). He suggests that psychoanalysis of trauma involves maintaining or restoring the symbolic function of the good object.

Ellen's descriptions of the ways in which she has needed me to participate in our analytic encounter are in line with Aron's (1996) elaborations about the subjectivity that the analyst reveals in all interpretations (pp. 118–121). Aron identifies three dimensions of interpretations and other interventions that make them mutative: the affect/experiential, the cognitive/insight, and the relationship/interaction dimensions. Stating that he believes that the dimension of the analyst's affective responsiveness has been neglected, Aron suggests that "patients need to feel that they are having an emotional impact on their analysts" and that they know this "only if the objects, the targets of their emotional expression—separate subjects—*respond* in some way that demonstrates that they have been *affected*, moved, changed" (p. 120). Aron cites Maroda's (1995) description of this aspect of the intersubjective analytic process as "completing the cycle of affective communication" (p. 120).

In essence, my ongoing ability to recognize, differentiate, tolerate, and symbolize painful, violent affect in the analytic process with Ellen constitutes the repair of a damaged protective shield, or maternal introject, or "good object." Ellen has needed me to function as a protective shield or good object by tolerating and symbolizing emotional pain without being irreparably damaged or destroyed by it, as her internal boxer, or "good object," has been. This work is still in progress. On a cautionary note, remember that in telling the first dream in session, Ellen volunteered that, in her family, the boxers were sent away when they became overprotective. While she was married to Ted, the boxer she had been strongly attached to died of poisoning. I have wondered about the implications of this for my fate in the analytic process. In particular, I puzzle about the multiple meanings of the interruptions in the treatment because of Ellen's dire financial circumstances. In editing my manuscript, Ellen acknowledged for the first time that she had sent me away many times when I became too protective.

SUMMARY

Ellen came for treatment because of bodily pain that was persistent and disabling. From my analytic perspective, this kind of bodily experience presents a compelling challenge and sometimes frightening dangers. In the preceding discussion, I have shown that Ellen was extremely dissociated from the affective significance of a great deal of her life experience. I illustrated our discovery in the analytic process that this dissociation resulted in somatic symptoms—musculoskeletal pain and a variety of infections of varying degrees of severity.

In this undertaking, I also elucidated how somatic symptoms appear and can be resolved in the treatment process. In the first few months of the analysis, Ellen's musculoskeletal pain essentially resolved, and she resumed most of the physical activities that she had previously avoided on the instruction of her physicians. I documented that she occasionally experiences a return of the back pain when greatly stressed; that is, her back pain returned as she prepared to tell me the "rabbit" dream, and the pain remitted as she finished telling me the dream. I also reported that in the psychic elaboration of the symbol of the boxer dog, twin rabbits, and other dream images, new and frightening symptoms, usually infections, appeared. I view this as an example of symptom substitution in that Ellen's inability to tolerate and symbolize traumatic affects continues to result in a traumatic somatic reaction. I consider this an indication that the treatment process is extremely powerful *and* that it must continue, even more carefully and cautiously.

CONCLUSIONS

The psychoanalytic quest that Ellen and I have undertaken documents the impact of affective life on physical health. The rapid resolution of Ellen's nine-year history of musculoskeletal back pain, and the symptom substitution, strikingly demonstrates the power and utility of a relational, intersubjective psychoanalytic approach to the treatment of somatic symptoms. Ellen's recovery was accomplished without a "laying on of hands" or any other "medical" intervention. The dramatic effect of psychoanalytic listening, interpretation, and what I call the "experiencing cure," is clearly revealed in the psychoanalytic process with Ellen. This kind of power can be "empowering" to analyst and analysand *and* it can be frightening. I have presented similar material to psychoanalytic audiences and found that some analysts are skeptical about the proposed connections between affective functioning and back pain. Others have been frightened by the severity of the physical symptoms that patients may develop in the course of the analytic process. Reflecting on these reactions, I suggest that they reflect our ambivalence as analysts about the power of the unconscious and our emotional life to affect our health. Further, these concerns may be another indication of the degree to which we are still affected by the dichotomization of mind and body in our psychoanalytic legacy.

While I have focused on somatic symptoms in this chapter, I believe that my findings can be of use to all analysts in that they underscore the importance of affective attunement and affective engagement in a psychoanalytic endeavor. I have found that an intersubjective, relational perspective on psychoanalytic treatment offers options for engaging a wider range of people with musculoskeletal pain than I believe has been possible using a more classical approach (see also Ehrenberg, 1992; Mitchell, 1993; Bromberg, 1996; Aron, 1996). Listening for the often subtle, elusive dissociations embedded in the flow of the patient's and analyst's associations has been particularly helpful to me in working with Ellen, whose elaborate dreams and rich associations can easily obscure her lack of affective connection to her material. An awareness of mutuality in the psychoanalytic process encourages me to attend to all of my experience in the intersubjective field. For instance, as I reflected on who I am for Ellen in my participation in the process (attuned parent, critical parent, sadistic torturer, dissociated onlooker, abandoned child), I was challenged to explore my internal object world as I learned more about hers and how she came so easily to dissociate cognitive awareness from affective experiencing.

In our analytic journey, Ellen and I have discovered the importance of the analyst's ability to tolerate painful and violent affect. I believe that this aspect of the treatment process has been overlooked, especially in the treatment of people with musculoskeletal back pain. The analyst is challenged to consider, "How much pain can I tolerate—and how much am I willing to tolerate—as my analytic partner learns, or seems not to learn, through his or her experience, what is painful and how much he or she can and should tolerate?" In my work with Ellen, she and I came to see that this was a fundamental issue as we discovered that we were involved in enactments of situations from her childhood. As she and I continue to analyze these enactments, I have learned that she feels that I still am not always able to "stay with her" as she describes more situations in which she is treated with disrespect and hostility. She recently said that all she wants from me is to tolerate being with her in the moment when she is struggling to make a decision about a course of action to take. We have identified that *I* am the one who dissociates at these moments, for example, by registering discomfort directly, through a change in the tone of my voice, and by interpreting her "sadomasochism" prematurely.

I believe that, in these moments, I am presented with a most difficult challenge—the challenge to "surrender" to Ellen's experience. Here I refer to Ghent's (1990) discussion of "masochism as a perversion of surrender" in which he distinguishes between "receptive" and "outreaching, penetrative" versions of surrender. Receptive surrender is characterized by a "longing to be recognized, deeply known, penetrated" (p. 125). In the outreaching, penetrative version, there is a "desire to deeply know, penetrate, discover the other." My position, like Maroda's (in press), is that the analyst, when confronted with an analysand's repetition of painful relational encounters, is challenged to "surrender" to the analysand's experience so that the analytic couple can discover the analysand's longing to be known, to be recognized, or, in Ellen's words, to be "championed."

Ellen recently reminded me of a dream in which she was rushing to get on a commuter train and saw that I was already on the train. The door closed as she rushed to enter. She readily interpreted the dream in terms of our analytic dyad: "You get on the train without me." I have been challenged to look inward to understand my resistance to "staying with her" as she discovers dissociated longing and anger/rage. Looker's (1996; Balamuth et al., 1994) attunement to the subtle ways in which the analyst dissociates at these junctures has deepened my understanding of this aspect of my work with Ellen. I have had to confront my family's history of dissociated grief and rage and the ways it has contributed to my own dissociative tendencies, as well as the ways in which it has enabled me to be attuned to the affective functioning of my patients.

Another challenge that the analyst confronts is how to use aggression in the analytic process, particularly when the patient is already in pain. In my work with people who present with Tension Myositis Syndrome pain, I have learned that engaging the analysand in psychic elaboration of physical pain means that we will inevitably encounter affect(s) that have been intolerable for him or her to experience. In fact, I have had many patients say, after they have begun to integrate dissociated affect, that they would rather have their back pain than go through such an intolerable experience. Indeed, some patients leave treatment because these affects are too difficult to bear.

This emotional experience can create resistance in the analyst that can manifest as a kind of "hovering countertransference" described by Looker (1996; Balamuth et al., 1994).

I have found myself hovering at various points throughout the analytic work with Ellen. For example, early in the treatment, after hearing the boxer dog dream, I realized that the degree of pain and destruction in the image of the damaged boxer had to be psychically elaborated in our analytic dyad. This dream image, together with the long duration of her back pain, suggested to me that the work ahead would be difficult and that we should proceed carefully. On the other hand, Ellen brought that boxer dream quite early in the treatment, and I took that as both an invitation and a sign of trust in our developing analytic bond. Thus, I proceeded cautiously, sometimes too cautiously, and carried that image with me to serve as a guide. When the rabbit dream appeared some time later and took the image of horror and destruction into her family home, I felt that the dream was confirmation that my cautious yet curious analytic attitude had been the necessary one. When she began to develop severe, sometimes life-threatening infections in reaction to the analytic process, my caution and awe of the power of our emotional life to affect our physical health were intensified. At these times I was concerned about the "injury" and "damage" that I was inflicting on her in my role as her analyst.

An additional consideration of the power dynamics in my analytic partnership with Ellen pertains to my decision to write about our work. Briefly, "Her Story" was compelling from the outset. As the treatment unfolded, I realized that aspects of the analysis related to dissociated affect and musculoskeletal back pain had not been addressed in the psychoanalytic literature that I had been reading. I decided that I wanted to contribute my experience. Then I immediately encountered my great concern about the impact on Ellen of my speaking and writing about the analysis: Was I a "cannibal rabbit" in desiring to use our work to tell "Her Story" to a psychoanalytic audience? I was concerned that I was "exploiting" her contribution for my own advancement. The image of "unlevel playing fields" was persistent, along with our many discussions about the ways in which her colleagues often found a way to take credit for her work. In addition to the usual concerns about the inevitable intrusion and gratification that come with writing about an analysand, I knew that I could not write about any aspect of the analytic process that I had not adequately worked on with Ellen without feeling that, indeed, I had exploited and betrayed her trust in our confidential bond. Thus, the process of writing about our analytic endeavor was infused with the very power dynamics that we were analyzing! My resolution of this dilemma was to ask Ellen's permission at the outset, to "level the playing field" by asking her to be an editor and to include her voice whenever possible. We continue to analyze the impact of this undertaking on our psychoanalytic process.

The exacting process of psychic elaboration with Ellen has often proved viscerally, affectively painful for me and sometimes perilous for her. In her words, "It'll make you crazy to feel 40 years of what was repressed in such a concentrated fashion. . . . I'm afraid I'll go mad [like one of the dream boxers] if I feel the pain." Nevertheless, Ellen's courage and determination have been inspiring. She states, "When I come to the session, I bring a bag of courage. Let's go." It seems to me that our analytic process has been, in large part, a kind of "championing" of Ellen by attempting to tolerate hearing about "Her Story" and to stay in the room with her as she is trying to tell us. By giving me permission to share our work in this chapter, Ellen said that she hopes that her experience in the analysis, presented in this way, will prove helpful to others. Our shared belief in the benefits of attempting to integrate traumatic affects in order to relieve physical symptoms has helped us endure and prevail.

NOTES

[1]TMS is a psychically-induced myoneuralgia, or muscle-nerve pain, that is mediated through the autonomic nervous system (Sarno, 1991, 1998). Sarno, a physician who specializes in physical rehabilitation medicine (physiatry), contends that the physical pain that accompanies TMS is due to mild oxygen deprivation in the involved tissue. Sarno differentiates TMS from "chronic pain," defined by other pain researchers and clinicians as "that which persists beyond the expected time of healing, with three months taken as the most convenient point of division between acute and chronic pain" (Mikail et al., 1994, p. 2). His earlier work (Sarno, 1974, 1976, 1977, 1981, 1984) lays the foundation for his current theoretical position and treatment approach.

[2]In Mr. H's case. I had been authorized by his referring physician to begin an analytic investigation. After making a diagnosis of TMS, Sarno begins the treatment process by educating his patient, in a series of lectures, about the interdependence of the physical and psychological variables in creating and sustaining their pain. Sarno reports that the majority of his patients do not need psychotherapy because they are able to achieve relief from the pain through the insight that he provides in his treatment program. In certain cases—5% to 10%—the patient's psychological functioning is more re-

sistant to the process of insight that his lectures provide. When a patient is referred for psychotherapy or psychoanalysis, the physical rehabilitation medicine "team" approach is used in which the therapist/analyst refers the patient back to Sarno if the symptom does not resolve, if it worsens, or if new symptoms appear. This arrangement assures that the analyst *and* analysand collaborate with the medical doctor about the analysand's body. This rehabilitation-medicine model encourages the patient to reclaim "ownership" of her or his body (McDougall, 1985, 1989, 1995; Krystal, 1988).

³It is beyond the scope of this chapter to provide a review of this literature. I refer the reader to Feinblatt, Anderson, and Gordon (1986), Grzesiak (1994), Mikail et al. (1994), Grzesiak, Ury, and Dworkin (1996), Turk (1996), and Gatchel and Turk (1996) for overviews of the field and for contemporary biopsychosocial models of pain.

⁴1) Pain warns of damage to or loss of the body, and thus becomes intimately connected with protection from injury and, consequently, with learning about the environment and its dangers and the body and its limitations. These experiences contribute to the development of "pain memories," which Engel described as "ideational complexes, conscious and unconscious, associated with past pain experiences, stimulation of which may later give rise to pain" (p. 901). These pain memories contribute to a "body pain image" consisting of parts of the body that have been sites of pain, one's own pain or the pain of others. 2) Pain is very involved in object relations from infancy because pain, or discomfort, leads to crying, which leads to comforting by a loved person, which leads to relief of the pain or discomfort. While pain itself is not pleasurable, its association with a "reunion" with a love object and relief of pain is clearly powerful and can lead to the experience we call "sweet suffering." 3) Pain and punishment are linked in early object relations. Punishment for being "bad" leads to pain, which can become a signal for guilt. Thus, pain can become a medium for expiation of guilt. 4) Pain is early associated with aggression and power when it is experienced as one of the outcomes of aggression toward the self by the other or by oneself. We can also control our own aggression by suffering pain such that the pleasure of aggression is retained but the self is the target. 5) Pain is easily associated with threatened, or fantasized, loss of a loved one. In this context, pain can expiate guilt if there is guilt for aggressive feelings toward the lost one.

⁵The features were 1) verbally or physically abusive parents, 2) harsh or punitive parents who overcompensated with rare displays of affection, 3) cold or emotionally distant parents who were warm only when the child was ill, 4) a parent with chronic illness or pain, and 5) parent–child interactions involving guilt, aggression, or pain.

⁶Grzesiak (1992, 1994; Grzesiak et al., 1996) believes that "pain-proneness" can lead to chronic pain syndrome. He defines chronic pain syndrome as "pain that continues for extended periods of time with or without objective physical findings to account for its existence and that is accompanied

by dysfunctions in virtually all areas of psychosocial activity" (Grzesiak, 1992, p. 1)

[7]LeDoux (1996), a neuroscientist, also reports a recent increase in neuroscience research on the "emotions" (P· 304).

[8]Taylor (1987, 1992) has attempted a synthesis of contemporary psychoanalytic theories with research in developmental psychology, developmental biology, and the biomedical sciences. In an application of his new psychosomatic model, Taylor (1993) states that "the psyche is conceptualised not merely as the origin of conflicts that might produce prolonged states of emotional arousal with pathogenic effects on the body, but also as one component within the hierarchical arrangement of reciprocally regulating subsystems" (p. 582). Elaborating a psychoanalytic approach to treatment, he states that the aim is to overcome "psychological deficits involving affect regulation and the maintenance of a stable sense of self" (p. 582).

In a recent comprehensive work, Taylor, Bagby, and Parker (1997) place affect regulation at the core of their extension of Taylor's earlier psychobiological model. They define affect regulation as a "process involving reciprocal interactions between the neurophysiological, motor-expressive, and cognitive-experiential domains of emotion response systems" (p. 14).

Taylor et al. (1997) argue that the major psychopathologies (e.g., somatoform disorders, anxiety and depressive disorders, substance use and eating disorders) and physical pathologies (e.g., coronary heart disease, essential hypertension, diabetes mellitus, rheumatoid arthritis, and inflammatory bowel diseases) are manifestations of disorders of affect regulation. The authors hold that the failure to regulate distressing emotions cognitively can lead to illness by exacerbating autonomic nervous system and neuroendocrine system activity, thereby creating conditions conducive to physical disease.

[9]Schore (1994) places patterns of affect regulation at the core of a sense of self, in that these patterns afford an integrated sense of self across state transitions. His central hypothesis is that the infant's early affective interactions with the social environment, especially the mother in her role as regulator of the environment, "directly and indelibly" (p. xxx) affect the development of postnatal maturation of brain structures that will underlie all future interpersonal emotional functioning. Further, in his discussion of a possible rapprochement between psychoanalysis and neurobiology, Schore contends that there is "evidence to argue that affect regulation, the regulation of patterns of energy dissipation by internal images, is a potent explanatory concept that clarifies and elucidates infant developmental, affect, and memorial phenomena" (p. 534). Self-regulation is the successful outcome of adequate early affective interchanges between the infant—a developing brain—and an adult who regulates the environment. Schore sees self-regulation as the result of the modulation of subcortical energetic processes by higher cortical activity and believes that this represents a "potential con-

tact point between psychoanalysis and neurobiology" (p. 534). Schore cites the work of Beebe and Lachmann (1988) as support for his conceptualization of the fundamental role of affects in the development of the self.

[10]In referring to "affective functioning." I use the information-processing analysis of affects described by Krystal (1988). In this view, an affect comprises 1) a cognitive component, that is, the meaning of, or "story behind," the affect; 2) an "expressive," or physiological, component; 3) hedonic elements, that is, consciousness of pleasure, gratification, or pain, and 4) activating aspects or affects that influence arousal and speed of response to an event.

[11]Blaustein (1995) provides an excellent review of the somatization literature in the presentation of her clinical research data. She found strong relationships between shifts in object relatedness and somatic processes compared with affectivity. She concludes that people who experience chronic somatic distress can benefit from psychoanalytic treatment that is attuned to the quality of relatedness in the therapeutic encounter in order to "rework and rebuild problematic self- and object-representations resulting from experiences of early and profound empathic failures" (p. 242).

[12]Pine's (1990) discussion of the considerations he used when planning to publish material from an analysis was helpful to me in this undertaking.

[13]Balamuth's (1996; Balamuth et al., 1996) illuminating discussion of the ways in which an awareness of "absence" brings the analyst's attention to subtle dissociative processes has heightened my own awareness of this aspect of the analytic endeavor.

[14]See Krystal (1988) for a discussion of the importance of affect recognition, affect naming, affect tolerance and affect differentiation in the desomatization process. McDougall (1985, 1989, 1995) holds that it is the role of the mother, as primary caretaker, to name all the affects. Accordingly, the analyst fills this role in the treatment process. Levenson's (1988) recommendation that the analyst "pursue the particular" is useful in helping analyst and analysand fully elaborate the emotional context in which a symptom appears.

[15]I refer the reader to the work of Goldner (1992; Goldner et al., 1990; Walker and Goldner, 1995) for a discussion of the "gender paradoxes in volatile attachments" between members of a couple in which the man is physically violent toward the woman.

[16]In a discussion of this dream many months later, Ellen told me that her skis were on backward, a detail that she had discovered in her journal.

[17]In their work with adult survivors of childhood sexual abuse, Davies and Frawley (1994) identified eight transference–countertransference relational positions, within four dyadic constellations, that require analysis. The dyadic constellations are 1) the uninvolved, nonabusing parent and the neglected child; 2) the sadistic abuser and the helpless, impotent enraged victim; 3) the idealized, omnipotent rescuer and the entitled child who demands to be rescued; and 4) the seducer and the seduced (p. 166). Frawley-O'Dea

(1997) added a fifth constellation, the chronic doubter and the unyielding believer (p. 12).

[18]In puzzling about the mechanisms underlying Ellen's statement, I have found LeDoux's (1989, 1996) work helpful in understanding why emotions sometimes interfere with thinking. LeDoux (1989) accumulated evidence that "emotion and cognition are mediated by separate but interacting systems of the brain" (p. 267). Detailed exploration of his work is beyond the scope of this chapter, but I refer the reader to LeDoux (1996) and van der Kolk (1996a, b; van der Kolk, van der Hart, and Marmar, 1996) for an explication of the neurobiological underpinnings of traumatic memory and the implications for the fate of affects and cognitions during traumatic experience and its recall.

REFERENCES

Anderson, F. S. (1994), Trauma, affect, and the body. Presented at annual research conference of the New York University Postdoctoral Program in Psychotherapy and Psychoanalysis, Tuxedo, NY.

—— (1996), Psychic elaboration of chronic physical pain and suffering in an analytic dyad. Presented at annual meeting, Division of Psychoanalysis (39), American Psychological Association, New York City.

—— Balamuth, R., Looker, T. & Schachtel, Z. (1996), Creating analytic space for bodily experience. *Psychol. Psychoanal.*, 16:39–40.

Anzieu, D. (1989), *The Skin Ego.* New Haven, CT: Yale University Press.

Aron, L. (1996), *A Meeting of Minds.* Hillsdale, NJ: The Analytic Press.

Balamuth, R. (1996), Presence and absence of lived body experience in psychoanalysis. Presented at annual meeting, Division of Psychoanalysis (39), American Psychological Association, New York City.

—— Anderson, F. S. & Looker, T. (1994), Working close to the body in psychoanalysis. Presented at annual research conference, New York University Postdoctoral Program in Psychotherapy and Psychoanalysis, Tuxedo, NY.

Beebe, B. & Lachmann, F. M. (1988), The contribution of mother-infant mutual influence to the origins of self- and object-representations. *Psychoanal. Psychol.*, 5:305–337.

—— (1994), Representation and internalization in infancy: Three principles of salience. *Psychoanal. Psychol.*, 11:127–165.

Blaustein, J. P. (1995), Knowing the unspeakable: Affectivity, object relatedness and the processes of somatization in individuals suffering with chronic somatic distress. Unpublished doctoral dissertation, The City University of New York.

—— & Tuber, S. B. (in press), Knowing the unspeakable: Somatization as an expression of disruptions in affective-relational functioning. *Bull. Menn. Clin.*

Breuer, J. & Freud, S. (1893–1895), *Studies on Hysteria. Standard Edition*, 2. London: Hogarth Press, 1955.

Bromberg, P. M. (1994), "Speak! that I may see you": Some reflections on dissociation, reality, and psychoanalytic listening. *Psychoanal. Dial.*, 4:517–547.

———— (1995), Psychoanalysis, dissociation, and personality organization. *Psychoanal. Dial.*, 5:511–528.

———— (1996), Standing in the spaces: The multiplicity of self and the psychoanalytic relationship. *Contemp. Psychoanal.*, 32:509–535.

Coen, S. J. & Sarno, J. E. (1989), Psychosomatic avoidance of conflict in back pain. *J. Amer. Acad. Pychoanal.*, 17:359–376.

Davies, J. M. & Frawley, M. G. (1994), *Treating the Adult Survivor of Childhood Sexual Abuse.* New York: Basic Books.

Ehrenberg, D. B. (1992), *The Intimate Edge.* New York: Norton.

Engel, G. L. (1959), "Psychogenic" pain and the pain-prone patient. *Amer. J. Med.*, 26:899–918.

Feinblatt, A., Anderson, F. S. & Gordon, W. (ed.) (1986), Psychological and vocational considerations. In: *Principles of Physical Medicine and Rehabilitation in the Musculoskeletal Diseases,* ed. J. C. Leek, M. E. Gershwin & W. M. Fowler, Jr. Orlando, FL: Grune & Stratton, pp. 217–234.

Flor, H., Turk, D. C. & Birbaumer, N. (1985), Assessment of stress-related psychophysiological responses in chronic pain patients. *J. Consult. & Clin. Psychol.*, 35:354–364.

Frawley-O'Dea, M. G. (1997), Who's doing what to whom? Supervision and sexual abuse. *Contemp. Psychoanal.*, 33:5–18.

Freud, S. (1895), Project for a scientific psychology. *Standard Edition*, 1:281–397. London: Hogarth Press, 1966.

———— (1905), Fragment of an analysis of a case of hysteria. *Standard Edition*, 7:3–122. London: Hogarth Press, 1953.

———— (1926), Inhibitions, symptoms and anxiety. *Standard Edition*, 20:75–175. London: Hogarth Press, 1959.

Gatchel, R. J. & Turk, D. C., ed. (1996), *Psychological Approaches to Pain Management.* New York: Guilford Press.

Ghent, E. (1990), Masochism, submission, surrender: Masochism as a perversion of surrender. *Contemp. Psychoanal.*, 26:108–136.

Goldner, V. (1991), Toward a critical relational theory of gender. *Psychoanal. Dial.*, 1:249–272.

———— (1992), Making room for both/and. *Networker*, March/April:54–61.

———— Penn, P., Sheinberg, M. & Walker, G. (1990), Love and violence: Gender paradoxes in volatile attachments. *Fam. Proc.*, 29:343–364.

Grzesiak, R. C. (1992), Unconscious processes and chronic pain: On the foundations of pain-proneness. Presented at annual meeting, American Psychological Association, Washington, DC.

———— (1994), The matrix of vulnerability. In: *Psychological Vulnerability to Chronic Pain,* ed. R. C. Grzesiak & D. S. Ciccone. New York: Springer, pp. 1–27.

———— Ury, G. M. & Dworkin, R. H. (1996), Psychodynamic psychotherapy with chronic pain patients. In: *Psychological Approaches to Pain Management,* ed. R. J. Gatchel & D. C. Turk. New York: Guilford Press, pp. 148–178.

Kirshner, L. A. (1994), Trauma, the good object, and the symbolic: A theoretical integration. *Internat. J. Psycho-Anal.,* 75:235–242.

Krystal, H. (1988), *Integration and Self-Healing.* Hillsdale, NJ: The Analytic Press.

Lachmann, F. M. & Beebe, B. A. (1996), Three principles of salience in the organization of the patient–analyst interaction. *Psychoanal. Psychol.,* 13:1–22.

Laub, D. & Auerhahn, N. (1993), Knowing and not knowing massive psychic trauma: Forms of traumatic memory. *Internat. J. Psycho-Anal.,* 74:287–302.

LeDoux, J. (1989), Cognitive-emotional interactions in the brain. *Cognition & Emotion.,* 3:267–289.

———— (1996), *The Emotional Brain.* New York: Simon & Schuster.

Levenson, E. A. (1988), The pursuit of the particular: On the psychoanalytic inquiry. *Contemp. Psychoanal.,* 24:1-16.

Looker, T. (1996), Impinging anxiety and bodily experience: A treatment enactment. Presented at annual meeting, Division of Psychoanalysis (39), American Psychological Association, New York City.

Maier, S. F., Watkins, L. R. & Fleshner, M. (1994), Psychoneuroimmunology: The interface between behavior, brain, and immunity. *Amer. Psychologist.,* 49:1004–1017.

Maroda, K. (1995), Show some emotion: Completing the cycle of affective communication. Presented at annual meeting, Division of Psychoanalysis (39), American Psychological Association, Santa Monica, CA.

———— (in press), *Surrender and Transformation.* Hillsdale, NJ: The Analytic Press.

May, N. (1996), Uses of the written word in psychoanalysis. Presented at annual meeting, Division of Psychoanalysis (39), American Psychological Association, New York City.

McDougall, J. (1980), *Plea for a Measure of Abnormality.* New York: International Universities Press.

———— (1985), *Theaters of the Mind.* New York: Basic Books.

———— (1989), *Theaters of the Body.* New York: Norton.

———— (1995), *The Many Faces of Eros.* New York: Norton.

McFarlane, A. C. & van der Kolk, B. A. (1996), Conclusions and future directions. In: *Traumatic Stress,* ed. B. A. van der Kolk, A. C. McFarlane & L. Weisaeth. New York: Guilford Press, pp. 559–575.

Melzack, R. (1973), *The Puzzle of Pain.* New York: Basic Books.

Mikail, S. F., Henderson, P. R. & Tasca, G. A. (1994), An interpersonally based model of chronic pain: An application of attachment theory. *Clin. Psych. Rev.,* 14:1–16.

Mitchell, S. A. (1993), *Hope and Dread in Psychoanalysis*. New York: Basic Books.

The New York Times (1997), Back remedies are on a roll. September 25, pp. F1, F8.

Novey, S. (1961), Further considerations on affect theory in psychoanalysis. *Internat. J. Psycho-Anal.*, 42:21–32.

O'Leary, A., Shoor, S., Lorig, K. & Holman, H. R. (1988), A cognitive-behavioral treatment for rheumatoid arthritis. *Health Psychol.*, 7:527–544.

Pennebaker, J. W., & Susman, J. R. (1988), Disclosure of traumas and psychosomatic processes. *Soc. Sci. & Med.*, 26:327–332.

Pilowsky, I. (1986), Psychodynamic aspects of the pain experience. In: *The Psychology of Pain*, ed. R. A. Sternbach. New York: Raven Press.

Pine, F. (1990), *Drive, Ego, Object and Self.* New York: Basic Books.

Sarno, J. E. (1974), Psychogenic backache: The missing dimension. *J. Fam. Prac.*, 1:8–12.

——— (1976), Chronic back pain and psychic conflict. *Scand. J. Rehabil. Med.*, 8:143–153.

——— (1977), Psychosomatic backache. *J. Fam. Prac.*, 5:353–357.

——— (1981), Etiology of neck and back pain: An autonomic myoneuralgia? *J. Nerv. Ment. Dis.*, 169:55–59.

——— (1984), *Mind Over Back Pain*. New York: Morrow.

——— (1991), *Healing Back Pain*. New York: Warner Books.

——— (1998), *The Mindbody Prescription*. New York: Warner Books.

Schachtel, Z. (1996), Discussant: Creating analytic space for bodily experience. Presented at annual meeting, Division of Psychoanalysis (39), American Psychological Association, New York City.

Schore, A. N. (1994), *Affect Regulation and the Origin of the Self*. Hillsdale, NJ: Lawrence Erlbaum Associates.

——— (1997), Interdisciplinary developmental research as a source of clinical models. In: *The Neurobiological and Developmental Basis for Psychotherapeutic Intervention*, ed., M. Moskowitz, C. Monk, C. Kaye & S .J. Ellman. Northvale, NJ: Aronson, pp. 1–71.

Schuman, M. (1991), The problem of self in psychoanalysis: Lessons from Eastern philosophy. *Psychoanal. Contemp. Thought*, 14:595–624.

Shapiro, S. A. (1996), The embodied analyst in the Victorian consulting room. *Gender & Psychonal.*, 1:297–322.

Spezzano, C. (1993), *Affect in Psychoanalysis*. Hillsdale, NJ: The Analytic Press.

Spiegel, D. (1993), Cancer and interactions between mind and body. *J. Natl. Cancer Inst.*, 85:1198–1205.

Szasz, T. S. (1957), *Pain and Pleasure*. New York: Basic Books, 1975.

Taylor, G. J. (1987), *Psychosomatic Medicine and Contemporary Psychoanalysis*. Madison, CT: International Universities Press.

——— (1992), Psychoanalysis and psychosomatics: A new synthesis. *J. Amer. Acad. Psychoanal.*, 20:251–275.

——— (1993), Clinical application of a dysregulation model of illness and disease: A case of spasmodic torticollis. *Internat. J. Psycho-Anal.*, 74:581–595.

—— Bagby, R. M., & Parker, J. D. A. (1997), *Disorders of Affect Regulation*. Cambridge: Cambridge University Press.

Tomkins, S. S. (1962), *Affect/Imagery/Consciousness, Vol. 1*. New York: Springer.
—— (1963), *Affect/Imagery/Consciousness, Vol. 2*. New York: Springer.

Turk, D. C. (1996), Biopsychosocial perspective on chronic pain. In: *Psychological Approaches to Pain Management*, ed. R. J. Gacthel & D. C. Turk. New York: Guilford Press, pp. 3–32.

van der Kolk, B. A. (1994), The body keeps the score: Memory and the evolving psychobiology of posttraumatic stress. *Harv. Rev. Psychiat.*, 1:253–265.

—— (1996a), The body keeps the score: Approaches to the psychobiology of posttraumatic stress disorder. In: *Traumatic Stress*, ed. B. A. van der Kolk, A. C. McFarlane & L. Weisaeth. New York: Guilford Press, pp. 214–241.

—— (1996b), Trauma and memory. In: *Traumatic Stress*, ed. B. A. van der Kolk, A. C. McFarlane & L. Weisaeth. New York: Guilford Press, pp. 279–302.

—— van der Hart, O. & Marmer, C. R. (1996), Dissociation and information processing in posttraumatic stress disorder. In: *Traumatic Stress,* ed. B. A. van der Kolk, A. C. McFarlane & L. Weisaeth. New York: Guilford Press, pp. 303–327.

—— Wilson, S., Burbridge, J. & Kradin, R. (1996), Immunological abnormalities in women with childhood histories of sexual abuse. Unpublished manuscript.

Walker, G. & Goldner, V. (1995), The wounded prince and the women who love him. In: *Gender, Power, and Relationships*, ed. C. Burck & B. Speed. New York: Routledge, pp. 24–25.

INDEX